INSTANT POT COOKBOOK

550 Simply Delicious Everyday Recipes for Your Instant Pot Pressure Cooker

MICHELLE DORRANCE

Copyright © 2017 by Michelle Dorrance

All rights reserved. No part of this publication may be reproduced, distributed, or transmitted in any form or by any means, including photocopying, recording, or other electronic or mechanical methods, without the prior written permission of the publisher, except in the case of brief quotations embodied in critical reviews and certain other non-commercial uses permitted by copyright law.

Limit of liability/Disclaimer of Warranty: The publisher and the author make no representations or warranties with respect to the accuracy or completeness of the contents of this work and specifically disclaim all warranties, including without limitation warranties of fitness for a particular purpose. No warranty may be created or extended by sales or promotional materials. The advice and strategies contained herein may not be suitable for every situation. This work is sold with the understanding that the author is not engaged in rendering medical, legal or other professional advice or services. If professional assistance is required, the services of a competent professional person should be sought. Neither the publisher nor the author shall be liable for damages arising herefrom. The fact that an individual, organization, or website is referred to in this work as a citation and/or potential source of further information does not mean that the author or the publisher endorses the information the individual, organization, or website may provide or recommendations they/it may make.

Trademarks: Instant Pot® and the Instant Pot® logo are registered trademarks of Double Insight, Inc. and are used throughout this book with permission.

Photography © 2017
Stockfood/Benjamin Cohen, Stockfood/Giada Harper, Despositphotos.com, Stockfood/Jeff Walker, Stocksy/Sarah Remington, Stocksy/Sarah Canu, Stockfood/Harald Wasserman, Shutterstock.com, Stockfood/Kimberly White, Shutterstock.com

Illustrations © Tim Johnson

Cover design by Angie Gerard

Cover hand lettering by Laura Foster

Manufactured in China

To all my Instant Pot Cookbook fans, this book is dedicated to you. Without your loyalty and support, this book would never have been possible.

To my favorite taste-testers – my husband, Todd, and my lovely girl Toma – thanks for trying all my cooking experiments (the good and the bad!) and for your love and throughout this amazing journey!

CONTENTS

ABOUT THIS BOOK 1

INSTANT POT BASICS 3

CHAPTER ONE
BREAKFAST 23

CHAPTER TWO
BEANS & GRAINS 71

CHAPTER THREE
VEGETABLES & SIDE DISHES 120

CHAPTER FOUR
SOUPS, STEWS & CHILIES 169

CHAPTER FIVE
BEEF, LAMB & PORK 219

CHAPTER SIX
POULTRY & CHICKEN 269

CHAPTER SEVEN
FISH & SEAFOOD 324

CHAPTER EIGHT
VEGETARIAN MAINS 376

CHAPTER NINE
INSTANT POT STOCKS & SAUCES 425

CHAPTER TEN
DESSERTS 473

COOKING TIME CHARTS 523

ADDITIONAL RESOURCES 526

ABOUT THE AUTHOR 527

RECIPE INDEX 529

About this Book

I want this book and the recipes in it to be accessible to everyone. You'll find basic recipes here for the newcomer, as well as slightly more challenging recipes for those who want to take their pressure cooking to the next level. I believe that every recipe in this book is something anyone can make.

In addition, I want to make sure that there are lots of options in this book for all kinds of cooks and so I included a vegetarian main dishes section, as well as included vegetarian recipes throughout the other sections of the book.

The recipes in this book were tested with various pressure cooker. Where you might see instructions for cooking batches of food, you can probably save time and cook more at once. In addition, you might also find that you can shave a few minutes off the cooking time.

Regardless of what sizes instant pot you are using, understand that much like cooking in an oven or on the stovetop, timing may vary a little based on a number of factors – the size of your food, the size of the cuts of foods, etc....

Use your better judgment when cooking to determine when foods are cooked to your liking.

Instant Pot Basics

Instant Pot® is the brand name of an electronic pressure cooker, just like Crock Pot® is a brand name of a slow cooker. There are several different brands of EPC but I have the instant pot® IP-DUO60 7-in-1 multifunctional Pressure Cooker.

The 7 functions of Instant Pot are: Pressure Cooker, Slow Cooker, Rice Cooker, Sauté/Browning, Yogurt Maker, Steamer & Warmer.

I used to have a stove-top pressure cooker. Oh my, what a difference! No need to babysit the pressure cooker any more. And it's not loud like my old pressure cooker. When I was a kid, my mom's pressure cooker once exploded (!) and there was turmeric-colored dal (lentil soup) all over the ceiling and walls!! I shudder just thinking about it. No need to worry about such scary things with the Instant Pot. It has lots of safety features including automatically regulating pressure.

The Instant Pot is a magical device powered by leprechauns (while it seems magical, I'm pretty sure it just runs on electricity) pressure cooker.

This thing has tons of different options – besides using it as a slow cooker, rice cooker, and yogurt maker, it can sauté and do a ton of other stuff. Using this one device to replace so many others has saved me a lot of space, but the best thing about the Instant Pot is that it saves this busy mama TIME.

Throughout this book, I'll explain which food combinations are best suited for your instant pot. I'll also give you basic formulas to use so you can whip up super-quick healthy recipes that don't compromise on flavor. At the same time, I've made sure that all the recipes are low in calories yet hearty enough to provide a full meal on their own or when paired with a side salad. Best of all, unlike many instant pot recipes calling for extensive prep, most of these recipes require less than 15 minutes to prepare the ingredients, with little to no precooking requirements.

Whether you're new to the Instant pot or just looking for new tips and tricks, you're going to love these recipes!

Happy Pressure Cooking!

Benefits of Pressure Cooking

Pressure cooking as a kitchen technique has been in use since the late 1600s. From the first-ever steam digester to the 3rd generation pressure cookers, the idea served miles to bring revolution in the cooking techniques. As of today, pressure cooking has achieved an even bigger milestone through instant pot electric pressure cookers. The technique was first introduced to reduce the cooking time significantly. But time conservation is not the only benefit pressure cooking offers, it also preserves all the nutrients and reduces any chance of food contamination. Experts believe that pressure cooking has not only brought ease to the kitchen, but it also provides healthy and nutritious food.

- **Healthy and Nutritious Meal**:

When food is cooked under high pressure, it takes less time. As prolonged and excessive boiling of ingredients in water can reduce the number of nutrients they carry, it is more appropriate to cook the meal in a shorter amount of time with less liquid. Food, when cooked at a faster rate in a closed vessel never loses its true color, aroma, and flavor. With every tick of the clock, food being cooked in an open vessel will lose its moisture, essential minerals, and nutrients through continuous evaporation of its steam. In contrast, the food in pressure cookers actually bathes in its own steam which leaves it more enriched.

- **Time and Energy Conservation:**

Life today is much busier than ever and spending several hours in the kitchen to cook yourself a decent meal is a luxury that few can afford. With the pressure cooking technique, we can save time due to its effective steam mechanism. With pressure cookers, the cooking time is reduced up to 70% compared to the time taken by open pots or vessels. Moreover, such cookers are also energy efficient. Pressure cooking saves us from using multiple pots and different burners to cook a single meal. It allows us to cook a single pot recipe in less time, which in turn reduces the energy consumption per meal.

- **Cleaner and cooler kitchen:**

With pressure cooking, all the heat and steam is contained inside the sealed container. Hence it does not emit excessive heat to the surroundings. As a result, the kitchen's temperature remains the same. Whereas when the meal is cooked in open pots, the heat flows with the steaming vapors and raises the kitchen temperature. Pressure cooking makes it convenient to stay in your kitchen even in hot summers. Another great benefit that comes with pressure cooking is that it keeps kitchen atmosphere, walls, and appliances clean. With open pot cooking the steam along with oil settles on nearby surfaces. Thus, the kitchen demands constant cleaning. Whereas when you pressure cook food, all the vapors and oil particles stay inside the vessel and does not settle on the kitchen walls and appliances.

What to Look for When Buying an Instant Pot Electric Pressure Cooker

Pressure cooking has never been easier than today, as Instant Pot electric pressure cookers have brought great ease and convenience to every home. The third generation one button electric miracle allows you to cook a meal with extremely simple steps. It has crammed all the cooking options into a single control panel. Just by selecting the appropriate mode for your recipe and setting the time limit, you can cook any meal using the instant pot. As the technology has taken over the market, Instant pot Electric pressure cookers are available everywhere, in many different sizes and designs. Each new model comes with additional features and smarter technology. Consider the following options when selecting an electric pressure cooker.

Available Sizes

Instant pot pressure cookers are mainly categorized according to their size and volume. Available in various models, each model has a different size and external features. Currently, there are three different sizes available in the market, which includes 5-quart, 6 quarts, and 8-quart pressure cookers. To recognize a pot for its size, look for its model number. IPDUO50 has a volume of 5 quarts, IP-DUO 60, IP ULTRA, IP LUX 60 V3, IP Smart Bluetooth and IP-DUO plus 60 has a volume of 6 quarts, and IP DUO80 has a volume of 8 quarts. With the increase in size and capacity, the price range of each pressure cooker also increases. However, each model provides the same basic standards functions for cooking. While looking for a particular model and size, one must also check its weight and dimensions. The weight of all the models varies from 12lbs. to 16lbs. approximately. To pick the right pot for you, first look for the desired size and related model then compare the weight, dimensions, and individual prices of each pot.

Sr. no	Model	Volume	Power Supply	Weight	Dimensions	Caliber of inner pot
1.	IPDUO50	5 QT	120V/60Hz	11.68lb	13x12.2x11.8 inch	5.5x9.45 inch
2.	IPDUO60	6QT	120V/60Hz	14.57lb	13x12.2x12.6 inch	6.3 x9.45 inch
3.	IPDUO80	8QT	120V/60Hz	15.21lb	14.8x13.3x14.2 inch	7.09x9.45 in

Model Specifications

It is important to recognize and inspect the specific features of an electric cooker before buying the product. As instant pot pressure cookers are available in a variety of designs, each model offers additional features for customer satisfaction. Thus having sound knowledge about a particular model of your need is necessary before making a final decision. Listed below are all the models of Instant Pot electric pressure cookers currently available in stores.

IP-DUO60

Its optimum size and affordable price have made IP DUO60 the most popular model among all the instant pot pressure cookers. It is a multifunctional electric appliance which offers 7 different functions in a single cooking unit. Whether you are looking for the pressure cooker, slow cooker, yogurt maker, warmer, steamer or a rice cooker now you can get all in one countertop kitchen appliance. This device offers 14 different cooking modes for all the recipes with an additional pressure adjusting option.

IP-DUO Plus60

It is a modified version of IP-DUO 60, available with certain additional features. Along with the standard modes, it also provides the egg, cake, and sterilizing options. The display unit has been modified into a blue LCD screen that shows icons for the selected cooking mode. The marking system is more defined, and fine gradation lines are engraved on the inner pot.

IP-DUO80

With greater volume and internal capacity, IP-DUO 80 provides you with all the standard features of IPDuo50 and IP-DUO 60. It has an 8-quart capacity, which gives you the option to cook larger meals. This cooker is a perfect option for people with larger families.

IP-ULTRA

IP ultra is the latest innovation in town. It is not simply a modified version of IPDUO60, but it has entirely different features like the adjustment dial. Using additional buttons, you can customize cooking time, pressure, and temperature settings. It also has options for cake, egg, and sterilize. The display screen also indicates the stages of its cooking process. Moreover, the device adjusts automatically according to the altitude.

IP Smart Bluetooth

IP Smart Bluetooth is also available in stores now. It has the same standard features and volume as IP DUO60. However, it has Bluetooth connectivity and allows users to connect the appliance to their Mobile phones or Tabular devices. Using the Instant pot application, you can control the modes, pressure, and timing of the pressure cooker.

Basic Structure of an Instant Pot Pressure Cooker

Although an instant pot is a countertop single unit appliance, it consists of several different components which are provided in the complete package. These components are assembled into the basic cooking unit for the efficient functioning of the product. Before making the purchase inspect all the components with their specifications.

1. Base unit:

It is the basic functional unit, which has a built-in electric system with special pressure sensors and temperature controller. The base unit is a cylindrical vessel that consists of a rigid outer body, with a control box and a control panel fixed outside. The open end of this unit has cooker handles, a lid stands, and lid open/close markings. The heating element is under the base of this unit.

2. Control box with Control panel:

A standard Instant pot IP DUO 60 has an attached control panel fixed inside its control box. This panel consists of a LED display; pressure, mode, and function indicators; function and operation keys. This panel allows you to select a specific mode of cooking through one-touch button system. With a function key, you can adjust time and the suitable pressure for cooking. The 7 in 1 multifunctional instant pot pressure cookers have the following programs to support the range of different recipes:

1. Soup	2. Rice	3. Meat stew	4. Multigrain
5. Bean chili	6. Porridge	7. Poultry	8. Steam
9. Slow Cook	10. Yogurt	11. Sauté.	

There are separate keys for each mode, including time and pressure adjustment, manual operations, and Keep warm function.

3. Stainless-steel Inner pot:

Each instant pot pressure cooker comes with a stainless-steel inner pot, which is also dishwasher safe. For easy cleaning, it is mirror polished from inside out. While its bottom consists of 3-ply material, so the heat is distributed evenly. Size of the inner pot varies for each model. It is marked with grading lines from inside.

4. Lid:

Lid maintains and controls the pressure inside the cooker effectively. On the underside of the lid, there is a sealing ring fixed inside the sealing ring rack. A sealing ring is important to maintain the pressure. Make sure the ring is intact. It prevents steam leakage from the sides. Its lid also has the anti-block shield, float valve, pressure release outlet and lid locking pin. On the outside, the lid has the lid handle, lid fin, lid position marks, venting position markings, float valve, and pressure release handle.

Anti-Block shield: This shield covers the venting system and allows unhindered flow of steam. It prevents clogging of the float valve and pressures releasing outlet.

Pressure Release handle: This handle covers the pressure release outlet and controls the mechanism through the rotation. To seal the cooker for pressure cooking, the bar of the handle is positioned to "sealing" point. And to release the steam, the bar positioned to the "venting" mark.

Float valve: The float valve also controls the internal pressure and adjusts accordingly. When the cooker is switched to the "cooking" mode, it has to be pressed down to seal the vessel. However, when we release the steam, the float valve pushes outward until all the steam is released.

5. Condensation collector:

The primary function of the condensation collector is to store all the steam and vapors produced inside the vessel during cooking. A condensation collector is affixed outside the cooker base and can be removed for cleaning. After each cooking session, condensation collector needs to be drained and cleaned.

6. Accessories:

The list of items does not end here; the product is available with a few other accessories to ease the cooking process. It comes with a durable silicon ring, a tempered glass lid, a silicon cover, a silicon mini mitt, a measuring cup, rice paddle, soup spoon, a stainless-steel steam rack, and a trivet.

The Step-by-Step Guide to Instant Pot Electric Pressure Cooker

Once you learn all about the basic functioning of the Instant Pot pressure cooker, your kitchen time will be greatly reduced and cooking will become nothing but a delightful experience. In order to avoid any mistakes while handling the appliance, it is important to know the standard functions of your electric cooker. To initiate the cooking operation for the first time, it is essential to assemble all the parts and accessories as needed.

1. Prepare the appliance:

Unbox the appliance and take out all the accessories and base unit. Check all the components carefully and place the device on a countertop near an electric supply. Before the initial use remember to follow the following steps:

a. Install Condensation Collector:

As the condensation collector is not attached to the base of the cooker, it has to be placed in a specified slot. Gently slide the condensation collector into this slot and fix it. For cleaning, reverse this movement to remove the collector from the base.

b. Install the Anti-Block Shield:

The anti-block shield prevents the vent from clogging. Hence it has to be installed and removed before and after cooking respectively. For installation, simply place it in the right position and press it down gently. To remove the shield for cleaning, push it to the side and then pull outwards.

c. Install the Sealing Ring:
A sealing ring is most important to maintain the internal pressure. In order to install it, push it inside the sealing ring rack under the lid and press it down section wise. To remove the ring, simply pull it outwards.

2. Lid handling:

Proper lid control is crucial for personal safety. The whole mechanism is a bit complex with all the valves involved. But with clear understanding, lid handling will not cause any nuisance while cooking.

a. Before opening the lid, ensure that the pressure cooking program is complete. If the program is not complete, then press the "Keep Warm or Cancel" key to end the ongoing program.

b. Do not open the lid right after the termination of the selected program. First, release the pressure built inside.

c. To release the pressure, the Instant Pot pressure cooker provides you with two different options:

- Quick release.
- Natural release.

For quick release, turn the pressure release handle to the "Venting Position." Let the steam out until the float valve goes back to the dropped position. Remember the quick release is not appropriate for food with large volume like soup or porridge etc. Use natural release of such recipes.

For natural release, let the cooker cool down for 15 or more minutes. The steam will escape naturally and the cooker will automatically switch to Keep Warm mode. When the float valve drops down, it indicates that all the steam has been released from the cooker.

d. Now you can open the lid through its lid handle. Hold the handle and turn it counterclockwise until it clicks to open position. Keep pressure release valve to the "Venting position" to avoid vacuum suction. Now simply lift the lid to open the cooker.

3. How to cook:

It's about time to learn all about the working mechanism of Instant Pot pressure cooker and ways to operate the appliance. Certain sets of steps are required for the preparation of any meal. Whether it's breakfast, lunch or dinner with instant pot cooker, you get it all in minimum cooking time.

a. Open the lid:

To open the lid hold the handle and rotate the lid to 30 degrees in counterclockwise direction. When the arrow mark on the cooker lid aligns with the marking of the base unit, remove the lid.

b. Inspect Components:

Before initiating any program, check all the components of the lid carefully. Inspect float valve, pressure release handle, sealing ring and anti-block shield. Ensure everything is completely fixed in the right position. Then plug in the device.

c. Put all the ingredients in the Pot:

Remove the inner pot from the base unit and add all the ingredients of the recipe into it. Use a measuring cup to add ingredients accordingly. Consider the inner markings on the side wall of the pot. Make sure that the volume of ingredients remains under the safety limit, which is about 23 full of the pot. Avoid adding ingredients which can produce foam or froth inside the vessel. If ingredients can expand while cooking, then keep the level to the half of this pot.

d. Place the inner pot inside the base:

After adding all the required ingredients in the pot, place it gently inside the base unit. Make sure that outer base of the inner pot is clean and dry. If not, use a soft cloth to wipe it out.

e. Close the lid properly:

After placing the inner pot, cover the base with the lid. When you place the lid back on, the "open" mark on the lid and cooker base aligns. Now twisting the lid 30 degrees clockwise will set it to the closing position and the close marks on the base and lid will align. Press down the float valve to ensure secure locking.

If the lid is not closed tightly, then the cooker will not function properly. The display screen will flash "LID" sign continuously. Ensure secure lid locking for every cooking mode except "Sauté." For Sauté mode keep the lid open.

f. Use Pressure release handle and Float Valve:

The pressure release handle loosely rests on the pressure release outlet and rotates between "sealing position" and "venting Position." The handle can even be removed for cleaning. For pressure cooking the "end" of this handle has to be pointed towards the "sealing position." Make sure to adjust the pressure handle right after locking the lid. Remember each mode except "Slow Cook", "Sauté", and "Keep Warm" requires sealing of the pressure release valve. Ensure that the float valve is also resting in the downward position. For Slow Cook and Keep Warm modes remember to turn the release valve to "Venting position" right after covering the lid. For Sauté mode, do not cover the lid.

g. Select the desired working mode/program:

As Instant Pot electric pressure cooker provides you with the range of cooking modes, and each mode has its own custom setting to adjust the pressure and time accordingly. To initiate cooking, simply press any of the operation keys for the desired program. Remember each operation has its own settings, but if you want to add changes to the time and pressure then use the timer and adjust keys to do so. A standard control panel gives you following options for cooking:

Soup	Meat/Stew	Bean/Chili	Porridge	Poultry
Steam	Rice	Multigrain	Sauté	Yogurt

After the mode selection, your Instant pot will automatically switch to the Preheating State within 10 seconds. During the preheating stage, the cooker will build up the internal pressure and then finally switch to the cooking state.

Working States:

Instant pot pressure cookers switch between three working states which are displayed on the led screen. These are Standby, Preheating, and Program operating states.

During Standby state, the LED display flashes "off" sign, whereas in a preheating state LED display changes to "on" symbol and function indicator lights up. However, during Program operating state, the LED display shows time as it counts down to the selected program.

Manual Operations:

Manual mode allows customized cooking settings. Using this key, you can set the time and pressure according to the demand of your recipe. However, "240 minutes" is the maximum cooking time limit it can offer. To use the manual option, press the designated key and then set the time through the timer key. Adjust pressure with operation keys.

Keep Warm/Cancel Key:

This key is used to change the state of the cooker. It can be used to cancel the ongoing operation or to switch to "Keep warm" mode from "standby" mode and vice versa.

h. Time and pressure Adjustment:

Either you are manually operating the system or selecting any particular cooking program, you can still adjust the time and pressure as needed. To adjust time and pressure, there are four different operational keys: "+", "-", "Pressure" and "Adjust".

To change the value for time, use the "+", "-" keys. To increase the cooking time press "+" or to decrease the cooking time press "-". Usually, the timer starts counting within 10 seconds of program selection. However, if you need to delay the cooking time, press "+" key within 10 seconds and then press "Timer" key. Now you can set the delay time as needed.

The pressure key allows you to switch between high and low pressures. This key can only be used for all the pressure cooking modes. For the Slow cook, Sauté, and Yogurt mode, the pressure key does not work. Adjustment key works for 3 types of adjustment settings:

1. To adjust the pressure during any selected program except for Rice and Manual functions.
2. To adjust the temperature for Sauté and Slow cook.
3. To select the program for "yogurt" preparation.

* Test run:

It is highly recommended to first test the appliance before you cook any meal. In this way, you can get familiar with the structure, components, basic functioning, and operation keys of the pressure cooker.

1. For initial testing, first open the lid, add about three measuring cups of water to the inner pot, and place it inside the base unit.
2. Cover the lid, lock it with a counterclockwise motion. Turn the pressure release handle to the "sealing position" and then select the "Steam" option from the given key in the control panel.
3. Now reduce the time limit to 2 minutes by pressing the "-" Key. After 10 seconds, it will switch to the preheating mode. Now, the cooker will start the operation.
4. Two minutes later, on the completion of the program, the device will automatically switch to "keep warm" mode.
5. Now turn the pressure release handle to "venting" position and then wait until the pressure is completely released.
6. Allow the cooker to cool down and then remove the water from the pot and wipe it dry. You are now ready to cook a delicious meal of your choice in your very own Instant Pot electric pressure cooker.

Instant Pot Safety Features

Safety is always the first priority while handling any electrical appliance. In case of any mishandling, a pressure cooker may cause scalding injuries. In order to ensure complete safety, instant pot pressure cookers come with 10 different safety features. This programmable instant device is installed with a highly secure electrical system which has a built-in monitoring mechanism. In addition to its powerful functionality, the product also offers the following safety measures.

1. Pressure Regulation:

Maintaining optimum pressure inside the vessel is most important in pressure cooking. Instant pot adjusts and regulates its working pressure according to the selected program. High and low-pressure options guarantee secure pressure mechanism.

2. Anti-Blockage Vent:

Steam must be completely released before lid opening. The anti-blockage vent in instant pot cooker prevents obstruction of the vent by food particles.

3. Lid Lock:

Instant pot pressure cookers have an efficient lid lock system that tightly binds it to the base unit during cooking. Lid lock prevents accidental lid opening even under high pressures.

4. Position sensors:

These sensors monitor the position of the lid. For each selected program, the sensors detect if the lid is placed in the right position. If not, then the display screen flashes "LID" symbol to indicate the wrong position.

5. Temperature Control:

For instant pot pressure cookers, every program requires an optimum temperature, which is mainly controlled by its temperature controller. It allows even distribution of heat to the inner pot and automatically changes the mode after cooking is completed.

6. High-Temperature monitoring:

To prevent burning of food, instant pot also monitors high temperatures. In certain cases, the temperature inside the cooker may reach beyond the safety limits. The cooker beeps instantly to indicate abnormally high temperature to ensure safety.

7. Pressure Controller:

The pressure controller maintains exact pressure for the selected program which guarantees safe cooking. It keeps the pressure in a suitable range and doesn't allow it to exceed beyond the safety limit.

8. Fuse cut off:

This security feature is a great relief for users. This feature immediately cuts off the power supply if the current or internal temperature reach or exceed a dangerous level.

9. Pressure Protection:

The base unit is provided with an internal chamber to endure extra pressure inside the vessel. When the pressure exceeds more than the safety limits, the cooker automatically releases the pressure to this internal chamber.

10. Smart detection:

Its smart detection system detects any leakage in the lid. This mechanism doesn't allow cooking operations until the lid is properly closed.

Safety Precautions

Besides these safety features, instant pot pressure cookers must be used with precaution and care. As mishandling can be dangerous, following recommendations will ensure more safety:

1. Always use the handles to touch the appliance, avoid touching it from its hot surface.
2. The appliance should not be used around children, disabled individuals, and people with no knowledge of pressure cookers.
3. Never keep the appliance in a hot oven or hot place.
4. Avoid moving the appliance when there is hot substance inside. If needed, move it with extreme care.
5. The device is built for indoor kitchen use only. Never use it outside.
6. As the device cooks under pressure, always make sure to keep at least 1 cup of liquid to pressurize the vessel. Before initiating any operation, make sure to secure the lid tightly.
7. Avoid overfilling the inner pot, as it may clog the pressure release valve. Keep all the ingredients to 2/3 full. For food that expands upon cooking, the inner pot must only be half filled.
8. Certain food items can produce froth and foam during cooking, and it can clog the pressure release valve. Make sure never to cook these items in this pressure cooker. These items include applesauce, pearl barley, cereals, split peas, cranberries, oatmeal, noodles, macaroni, spaghetti, and rhubarb.
9. Make sure to check anti-block shield, float valve, and pressure release valve before each use. Clean them if clogged.
10. During pressure cooking make sure that the pressure release handle is in the sealing position.
11. Open the pressure cooker only when it has cooled down and all of its pressure has been released completely. A pressurized cooker shows difficulty in moving the handles apart, thus do not force open the appliance until all the pressure is released.
12. Deep frying and pressure frying with oil are strictly prohibited for instant pot pressure cookers.
13. Never immerse the power plug and power cord in any liquid.
14. Make sure to unplug the device properly before cleaning its components. First, switch off the appliance and then unplug it from the power socket.
15. If any part of the appliance appears to be damaged or deformed, especially the power plug and cord then do not operate the device at all.

16. Always use the stainless steel inner pot for cooking. Do not place any other accessory inside the base unit.

17. Protect the power cord from touching any hot or sharp surfaces.

18. As this device supports only 110-120V~/60Hz, make sure to operate it on the same electrical system.

Troubleshooting

As instant pot pressure cooker is an advanced electrical device, it may need technical assistance and in-depth knowledge regarding all functions of the appliance. Certain issues may arise while using the product due to inappropriate handling, assembly mistakes or wrong command options. Following are the most common issues reported for instant pot pressure cookers. These problems may arise due to technical mishandling, but the following solutions may help resolve them:

1. **Difficulty in closing the lid**: The problem may arise if the "**Sealing ring**" is not installed properly or the "**float valve**" is in the popped-up position. Setting the sealing ring properly or pressing the float valve downward will resolve this problem instantly.

2. **Difficulty in opening the lid**: Either there is too much pressure inside the cooker or the float valve is stuck in the popped-up position. Use the release valve to reduce the internal pressure of the cooker or press the float valve lightly.

3. **Leaking Steam**: If the steam is leaking from the sides of the lid, then it means that either the sealing ring is absent, damaged or not fixed properly. Check the sealing ring and fix it properly, remove any food debris if stuck in the ring. Close the lid properly.

4. **Float Valve leaks steam over 2 minutes:** This problem occurs when something is wrong with the silicone seal of the float valve, either some food particle is stuck in the valve or the seal is worn out. Clean the silicone seal or replace if needed.

5. **Float Valve does not rise**: When there is little food or water inside the inner pot, the float valve may not rise. In such cases add more water as per the recipe. This problem may also arise if the valve is hindered by the lid locking pin. Close the lid completely in such cases.

6. **Nonstop steaming from Exhaust valve**: This problem occurs when the pressure release handle is not in the sealing position. Turn it carefully to the sealing position. If the same problem occurs due to control failure, then contact the support team.

7. **"LID" on LED display**: When the lid is not in the right position for any selected program, the display will flash "lid" on the screen. Close the lid properly for pressure cooking or leave it open to sauté.

8. **Display flashes "noPr"**: Cooker has not attained the working pressure during its preheating cycle. Check if the steam is leaking, if so follow step 3 and 4.

9. **Display flashes "Ovht":** it means that the inner pot is overheated. Push the cancel button to stop cooking immediately.

10. **"Blank display" after power connection**: After connecting the power cord if the display screen remains blank, it means the connection is faulty. So ensure proper

connection. It may also indicate that the electrical fuse has blown out, contact the support team in such a case.

11. **Error or CODES on the Display screen**:

C1 & C2 Code: It states fault in temperature sensor. Contact support team.

C5 code: When the temperature gets too high, either because of the absence of inner pot or there is no water in the inner pot. In such a case, place the inner pot or add more water to the pot.

C6 code: It states fault in the pressure sensor. Contact the support team.

12. **Half-cooked rice**: The premature opening of the lid or little water in the inner pot may result in half-cooked rice. Make sure to add more water or open the lid after the cooking time is complete.

13. **Rice too soft**: When there is too much water in the pot along with the rice, it may cause this problem. Check the proportion of water to dry rice.

14. **Constant Beeping during Cooking**: This indicates overheating, or that the pot has not gained appropriate cooking pressure. It occurs when starch deposits on the bottom of the inner pot and hinders even distribution of heat. Stop the process and check the bottom of the inner pot.

15. **Cracking sound**: This sound is produced when the pressure board expands in changing temperature, which is normal. But when the inner pot is wet from its bottom, the same sounds can be heard. In that case, clean the pot with a dry cloth and then place it inside the cooker.

Cleaning and Caring for your Instant Pot

As every electrical appliance needs constant care and maintenance, so does the instant pot pressure cooker. To ensure your personal safety, check all of its components at least once in a week. Regular maintenance will add up to the life of your cooker and will regulate its functionality. It is recommended that the product should be cleaned after each use. As instant pot consists of several different units, each part should be cleaned with extreme care.

1. Never clean the instant pot immediately after cooking. Unplug the appliance first, let it cool for 30 minutes, and then start the cleaning process.

2. The black inner housing rim has to be wiped using a piece of cloth. Avoid washing, as it can cause rusting of the exterior pot rim.

3. To clean the inner pot: First, remove the lid and take the pot out. Now wash it with any detergent or soap then rinse with clear water. Use a soft cloth to wipe dry the inner pot from inside out.

4. Wash the lid along with the sealing ring, anti-block shield, and exhaust valve with clear water. Wipe them dry using a soft cloth.

5. While washing the lid, make sure to leave the steam release pipe intact and do not remove it from the lid.

6. To clean the base unit: Remember not to immerse it completely in water. Use a wet cloth to wipe all the dirt out of it. Make sure that the device is completely unplugged while you are cleaning its pot.

7. To clean the power plug and the cord: Always use a dry brush to remove the dirt or dust from the surface.

Maintenance

Along with careful cleaning, an electric appliance also needs constant maintenance. To ensure personal safety, all the components of the product has to be checked at least once in a week. It is important to examine the power cord and its functionality. In case of following anomalies, contact the Instant pot support team immediately:

1. If the power plug and cord show any damage, deformation, discoloration, and expansion.
2. If a certain portion of the power plug and the cord feels hotter than usual.
3. If the instant pot shows abnormal heating or emits a burnt smell.
4. If the cooker produces any abnormal sounds or vibrations when its power is on.

Caution: Unplug the device immediately when you find any such anomalies. Do not try to repair anything by yourself. Contact the support team and discuss the issue in detail.

About the Recipes

The recipes in this book were chosen for appeal, ease of preparation, and speed.

With very few exceptions, you'll be ready in 35 minutes or less, start to finish. And almost every recipe requires no more than nine everyday ingredients to prepare.

All recipes include nutritional information, instructions for serving and the recipes in this book were tested with various instant pot. Where you might see instructions for cooking batches of food, you can probably save time and cook more at once. In addition, you might also find that you can shave a few minutes off the cooking time.

Each recipe had a set upper limit on the amount of fat and sodium – no more than 35 percent of calories from fat and no more than 140 milligrams of sodium per serving.

Regardless of what sizes instant pot you are using, understand that much like cooking in an oven or on the stovetop, timing may vary a little based on a number of factors – the size of your food, the size of the cuts of foods, etc....

Use your better judgment when cooking to determine when foods are cooked to your liking.

Let's Cook!

BREAKFAST

Creamy Peach Oatmeal

(**Serves**: 4 / **Prep time:** 5 minutes / **Cooking time**: 6 minutes)

Ingredients

- 2 cups old-fashioned oats
- 2 ¼ cups water
- 2 ¼ cups milk
- ½ teaspoon salt
- ½ teaspoon ground cinnamon
- ¼ cup sugar
- 2 peaches, peeled and sliced

How to

1. Add all the ingredients to the Instant Pot. Save a few peach slices for garnishing.
2. Secure the lid of the cooker and press the "Multigrain option."
3. Adjust the time to 6 minutes and let it cook.
4. After the beep, release the pressure naturally and remove the lid.
5. Serve with peach slices on top

Nutrition Values (Per Serving)

- Calories: 458
- Carbohydrate: 80.2g
- Protein: 15.2g
- Fat: 8.2g
- Sugar: 27.8g
- Sodium: 359mg

Coconut Cornmeal Porridge

(**Serves**: 6 / **Prep Time:** 15 minutes / **Cooking Time**: 6 minutes)

Ingredients

- 6 cups water
- 1 ¼ cups coconut milk
- 1 ¼ cups yellow cornmeal, fine
- 2 ½ sticks cinnamon
- 1 ¼ teaspoons vanilla extract
- ¾ teaspoon coconut flakes
- ¾ cup sweetened condensed milk

How to

1. Add 5 cups of water and all the coconut milk to the Instant Pot.
2. Mix the cornmeal with 1 cup of water and add the mixture to the pot.
3. Stir in vanilla extract, coconut flakes, and cinnamon sticks.
4. Secure the lid of the cooker and press the "Manual" function key.
5. Adjust the time to 6 minutes and cook at high pressure.
6. After the beep, release the pressure naturally and remove the lid.
7. Stir in sweetened condensed milk.
8. Serve and enjoy.

Nutrition Values (Per Serving)

- Calories: 253
- Carbohydrate: 46.2g
- Protein: 6.9g
- Fat: 3.1g
- Sugar: 17.2g
- Sodium: 179mg

Strawberry Cream Oatmeal

(**Serves**: 4 / **Prep time:** 5 minutes / **Cooking time**: 6 minutes)

Ingredients

- 2 cups old-fashioned oats
- 2 ¼ cups water
- 2 ¼ cups milk
- ½ teaspoon salt
- ½ teaspoon ground cinnamon
- ¼ cup sugar
- 8 strawberries, chopped

How to

1. Add all the ingredients to the Instant Pot. Save a few strawberry slices for garnishing.
2. Secure the lid of the cooker and press the "Multigrain option."
3. Adjust the time to 6 minutes and let it cook.
4. After the beep, release the pressure naturally and remove the lid.
5. Serve with the chopped strawberries on top.

Nutrition Values (Per Serving)

- Calories: 436
- Carbohydrate: 75g
- Protein: 14.7g
- Fat: 8g
- Sugar: 22g
- Sodium: 360mg

Coconut Rice Pudding

(**Serves**: 2 / **Prep Time:** 5 minutes / **Cooking Time**: 10 minutes)

Ingredients

- 1 cup coconut milk
- ¾ cup water
- ½ cup basmati rice, short grain
- ½ cup coconut cream
- 2 tablespoons maple syrup
- Pinch of sea salt
- Whipped cream and coconut flakes (garnish)

How to

1. Add all the ingredients to the Instant Pot.
2. Secure the lid of the cooker and press the "Manual" function key.
3. Adjust the time to 10 minutes and cook at high pressure.
4. After the beep, release the pressure naturally and remove the lid.
5. Stir the prepared pudding and serve in a bowl.
6. Add whipped cream and coconut flakes on top.

Nutrition Values (Per Serving)

- Calories: 476
- Carbohydrate: 36.5g
- Protein: 18.6g
- Fat: 27.9g
- Sugar: 9.8g
- Sodium: 887mg

Cranberry Apricot Steel-Cut Oats

(**Serves**: 4 / **Prep time:** 5 minutes / **Cooking time**: 10 minutes)

Ingredients

- 2 cups steel-cut oats
- 3 cups water
- 4 tablespoons butter
- 2 cups freshly squeezed orange juice
- 2 tablespoons dried cranberries
- 2 tablespoons raisins
- 2 tablespoons chopped dried apricots
- 2 tablespoons pure maple syrup
- ½ teaspoon ground cinnamon
- 4 tablespoons chopped pecans
- ¼ teaspoon salt

How to

1. Add all the ingredients to the Instant Pot.
2. Secure the lid of the cooker and press the "Manual" function key.
3. Adjust the time to 10 minutes and cook at high pressure.
4. After the beep, release the pressure naturally and remove the lid.
5. Stir the prepared oatmeal and serve in a bowl.
6. Garnish with fresh strawberries on top.

Nutrition Values (Per Serving)

- Calories: 351
- Carbohydrate: 45.3g
- Protein: 6.4g
- Fat: 16.8g
- Sugar: 14.5g
- Sodium: 238mg

Egg Stuffed Bell Pepper

(**Serves**: 4 / **Prep Time:** 5 minutes / **Cooking Time**: 6 minutes)

Ingredients

- 4 slices of whole wheat bread, toasted
- 4 slices of mozzarella
- 2 small bunches of arugula
- 4 fresh eggs, refrigerated
- 4 bell peppers, clean out the insides and ends cut off
- Aluminum foil.

For the Mock Hollandaise Sauce:

- 1 ½ cup mayonnaise
- 3 teaspoons Dijon mustard
- 6 tablespoons orange juice
- 2 teaspoons fresh lemon juice
- 2 tablespoons white wine vinegar
- 1 teaspoon salt
- 2 teaspoons of turmeric

How to

1. Add all the ingredients of Mock Hollandaise Sauce into a bowl and whisk them well. Set the sauce aside.
2. Add water to the pot and place the steamer trivet inside it.
3. Over the trivet, set the bell pepper cups, crack one egg into each cup, and then cover with aluminum foil.
4. Secure the lid of the cooker and press the "Manual" function key.
5. Adjust the time to 6 minutes and cook at low pressure.
6. After the beep, release the pressure naturally and remove the lid.
7. Remove the cooked bell peppers.
8. Stack the bread slices with cheese, arugula, and pepper cups.
9. Generously pour the sauce over the stacks and serve.

Nutrition Values (Per Serving)

- Calories: 614
- Carbohydrate: 46.4g
- Protein: 19.6g
- Fat: 40.4g
- Sugar: 15.6g
- Sodium: 1619mg

Creamy Latte Cut Oats

(**Serves**: 6/ **Prep Time**: 10 minutes / **Cooking Time**: 10 minutes)

Ingredients

- 5 cups water
- 2 cups milk
- 2 cups steel-cut oats
- 4 tablespoons sugar
- 2 teaspoons espresso powder
- ½ teaspoon salt
- 4 teaspoons vanilla extract
- Freshly whipped cream
- Finely grated chocolate

How to

1. Add all the ingredients to the Instant Pot.
2. Secure the lid of the cooker and press the "Manual" function key.
3. Adjust the time to 10 minutes and cook at high pressure.
4. After the beep, release the pressure naturally and remove the lid.
5. Stir the prepared oatmeal and serve in a bowl.
6. Garnish with whipped cream and grated chocolate on top.

Nutrition Values (Per Serving)

- Calories: 274
- Carbohydrate: 46.6g
- Protein: 9.4g
- Fat: 5.2g
- Sugar: 18.4g
- Sodium: 360mg

Breakfast Bacon Hash

(**Serves**: 3 / **Prep Time:** 20 minutes / **Cooking Time**: 20 minutes)

Ingredients

- 6 eggs
- 2 red potatoes, diced
- ½ package bacon, chopped
- ½ cup cheddar cheese
- ¼ cup green onions
- ¼ teaspoon black pepper
- ¼ teaspoon salt
- 1 tablespoon milk
- 6-inch springform pan

How to

1. Add bacon to the Instant Pot and select the "Sauté" function to cook for 3 minutes.
2. Transfer the crispy cooked bacon to the greased "spring pan."
3. Add the potatoes on top of bacon.
4. Crack all the eggs in a bowl and whisk them well with the milk.
5. Pour the egg mixture over the potatoes in the spring pan.
6. Sprinkle salt and pepper on top and cover with aluminum foil.
7. Pour some water into the Instant Pot, set the trivet inside and place the covered spring pan over the trivet.
8. Press the "Manual" key, adjust its settings to High pressure for 20 minutes.
9. After it is done, do a Natural release to release the steam.
10. Remove the lid and the spring pan. Transfer the hash to a plate.11. Sprinkle cheddar cheese on top then serve.

Nutrition Values (Per Serving)

- Calories: 400
- Carbohydrate: 24.8g
- Protein: 30.1g
- Fat: 20.7g
- Sugar: 3g
- Sodium: 533mg

Silver Almonds Oatmeal

(**Serves**: 6 / **Prep Time:** 10 minutes / **Cooking Time**: 10 minutes)

Ingredients

- 2 cups of steel-cut oats
- 1 cup Greek yogurt, plain
- 3 cups water
- 4 small apples, chopped
- ½ cup real maple syrup
- 1 teaspoon cinnamon
- 1 teaspoon cloves
- 4 tablespoons slivered almonds

How to

1. Add all the ingredients to the Instant Pot. Reserve some maple syrup, almonds, and Greek yogurt for garnishing
2. Secure the lid of the cooker and press the "Manual" function key.
3. Adjust the time to 10 minutes and cook at high pressure.
4. After the beep, release the pressure naturally and remove the lid.
5. Stir the prepared oatmeal and serve in a bowl.
6. Garnish with Greek yogurt, almonds, and maple syrup on top.

Nutrition Values (Per Serving)

- Calories: 299
- Carbohydrate: 59.3g
- Protein: 8.2g
- Fat: 4.8g
- Sugar: 32.9g
- Sodium: 21mg

3 Peppers Morning Hash

(**Serves**: 3 / **Prep Time:** 20 minutes / **Cooking Time**: 15 minutes)

Ingredients

- 6 eggs
- ½ green bell pepper, chopped
- 2 bacon slices, chopped
- ½ yellow bell pepper, chopped
- ½ cup cheddar cheese
- ½ red bell pepper, chopped
- ¼ teaspoon black pepper
- ¼ teaspoon salt
- 1 tablespoon milk
- 6-inch springform pan

How to

1. Add bacon to the Instant Pot and select the "Sauté" function to cook for 3 minutes.
2. Transfer the crispy cooked bacon to the greased "spring pan"
3. Add all the bell peppers on top of bacon.
4. Crack all the eggs in a bowl and whisk them well with the milk.
5. Pour the eggs mixture over the bell peppers in the spring pan.
6. Sprinkle salt and pepper on top and cover with aluminum foil.
7. Pour some water into the Instant Pot, set the trivet inside, and then place the covered spring pan over the trivet.
8. Press the "Manual" key, adjust its settings to High pressure for 15 minutes.
9. After it is done, do a Natural release to release the steam.
10. Remove the lid and the spring pan. Transfer the hash to a plate.
11. Sprinkle cheddar cheese on top then serve.

Nutrition Values (Per Serving)

- Calories: 406
- Carbohydrate: 23.1g
- Protein: 27.9g
- Fat: 19.2g
- Sugar: 2.9g
- Sodium: 512mg

Fresh Fruity Oatmeal

(**Serves**: 4 / **Prep Time:** 10 minutes / **Cooking Time**: 6 minutes)

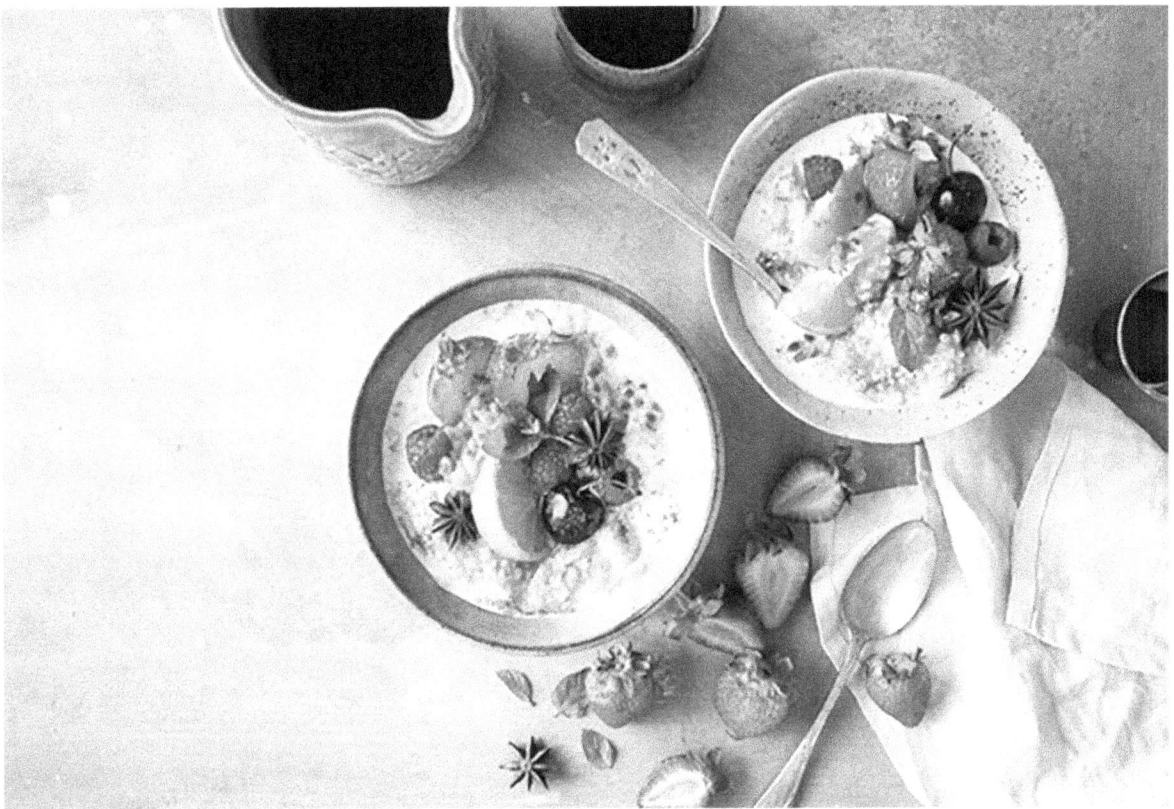

Ingredients

- 2 cups steel-cut oats
- 6 cups water
- ½ cup brown sugar
- 2 tablespoons cinnamon
- Sliced mixed fruits for topping

How to

1. Add all the ingredients to the Instant Pot.
2. Secure the lid of the cooker and press the "Manual" function key.
3. Adjust the time to 6 minutes and cook at high pressure.
4. After the beep, release the pressure naturally and remove the lid.
5. Stir the prepared oatmeal and serve in a bowl.
6. Garnish with sliced mixed fruits on top.

Nutrition Values (Per Serving)

- Calories: 232
- Carbohydrate: 48.2g
- Protein: 5.5g
- Fat: 2.7g
- Sugar: 18.1g
- Sodium: 19mg

Tasty Cornmeal Porridge

(**Serves**: 6 / **Prep Time:** 10 minutes / **Cooking Time**: 6 minutes)

Ingredients

- 6 cups water
- 1 ¼ cups milk
- 1 ¼ cups yellow cornmeal, fine
- 2 ½ sticks cinnamon
- 5 pimento berries
- 1 ¼ teaspoons vanilla extract
- ¾ teaspoon nutmeg, ground
- ¾ cup sweetened condensed milk

How to

1. Add 5 cups water and milk to the Instant Pot.
2. Mix the cornmeal with 1 cup of water and add it to the pot.
3. Stir in vanilla extract, pimento berries, nutmeg, and cinnamon sticks.
4. Secure the lid of the cooker and press the "Manual" function key.
5. Adjust the time to 6 minutes and cook at high pressure.
6. After the beep, release the pressure naturally and remove the lid.
7. Stir in sweetened condensed milk.
8. Serve and enjoy.

Nutrition Values (Per Serving)

- Calories: 247
- Carbohydrate: 43.5g
- Protein: 6.9g
- Fat: 5.4g
- Sugar: 23.7g
- Sodium: 90mg

Enriched Walnut Oatmeal

(**Serves**: 6 / **Prep Time:** 5 minutes / **Cooking Time**: 6 minutes)

Ingredients

- 2 cups steel-cut oats
- 4 cups water
- 2 cups unsweetened almond milk
- ½ cup walnuts, chopped fine
- 4 tablespoons ground flaxseeds
- 4 tablespoons chia seeds
- 2 large ripe bananas, mashed
- 4 tablespoons pure maple syrup
- 2 teaspoons ground cinnamon
- 2 teaspoons pure vanilla extract
- Pinch salt

How to

1. Add all the ingredients to the Instant Pot. Reserve some banana slices and walnuts for topping.
2. Secure the lid of the cooker and press the "Manual" function key.
3. Adjust the time to 6 minutes and cook at high pressure.
4. After the beep, release the pressure naturally and remove the lid.
5. Stir the prepared oatmeal and serve in a bowl.
6. Garnish with banana slices and chopped walnuts on top.

Nutrition Values (Per Serving)

- Calories: 284
- Carbohydrate: 37.2g
- Protein: 8.2g
- Fat: 12.4g
- Sugar: 10.6g
- Sodium: 55mg

Delicious Strawberry Compote

(**Serves**: 4 / **Prep Time:** 10 minutes / **Cooking Time**: 15 minutes)

Ingredients

- 2 lbs. fresh strawberries washed, trimmed, and cut in half
- ¼ cup sugar
- 2 oz. fresh orange juice
- 1 vanilla bean, chopped
- ½ teaspoon ground ginger

How to

1. Add all the ingredients to the Instant Pot.
2. Secure the lid of the cooker and press the "Manual" function key.
3. Adjust the time to 15 minutes and cook at high pressure.
4. After the beep, release the pressure naturally and remove the lid.
5. Stir the prepared compote, let it thicken as it cools.
6. Serve on toast and enjoy.

Nutrition Values (Per Serving)

- Calories: 152
- Carbohydrate: 35.5g
- Protein: 2.4g
- Fat: 1.6g
- Sugar: 27.6g
- Sodium: 14mg

Rice Pudding

(**Serves**: 3 / **Prep Time:** 5 minutes / **Cooking Time**: 10 minutes)

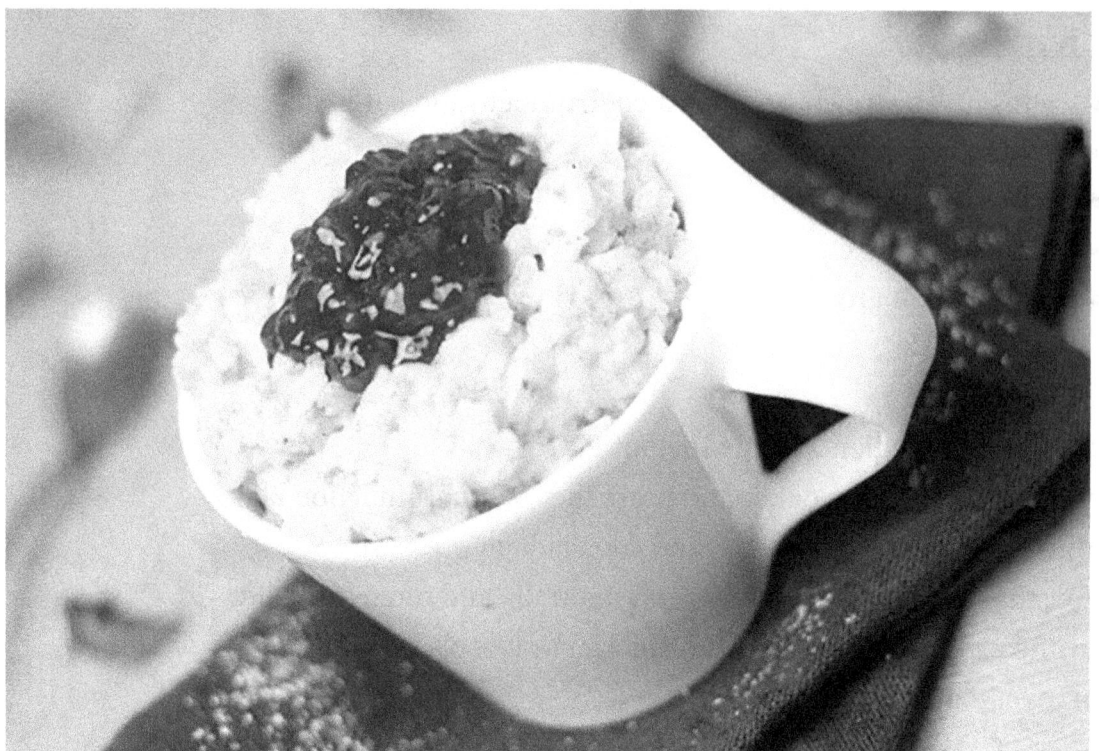

Ingredients

- 1 cup milk
- ¾ cup water
- ½ cup basmati rice
- ½ cup coconut cream
- 2 tablespoons maple syrup
- Pinch of sea salt
- 1 teaspoon vanilla extract
- Strawberry jam (garnish)

How to

1. Add all the ingredients to the Instant Pot.
2. Secure the lid of the cooker and press the "Manual" function key.
3. Adjust the time to 10 minutes and cook at high pressure.
4. After the beep, release the pressure naturally and remove the lid.
5. Stir the prepared pudding and serve in a bowl.
6. Add the strawberry jam on top.

Nutrition Values (Per Serving)

- Calories: 483
- Carbohydrate: 38.7g
- Protein: 19.1g
- Fat: 28.4g
- Sugar: 9.5g
- Sodium: 889mg

Super Healthy Oatmeal

(**Serves**: 2 / **Prep Time:** 5 minutes / **Cooking Time**: 3 minutes)

Ingredients

- 1 cup rolled oats
- 2 cups water
- 2 tablespoons honey
- 2 tablespoons wheat germ
- 2 teaspoons flaxseed oil
- ½ cup soy milk

How to

1. Add all the ingredients to the Instant Pot.
2. Secure the lid of the cooker and press the "Manual" function key.
3. Adjust the time to 3 minutes and cook at high pressure.
4. After the beep, release the pressure naturally and remove the lid.
5. Stir the prepared oatmeal and serve in a bowl.

Nutrition Values (Per Serving)

- Calories: 322
- Carbohydrate2: 52.4g
- Protein: 9.3g
- Fat: 9.6g
- Sugar: 20.4g
- Sodium: 42mg

Scrumptious Bread Pudding

(**Serves**: 4 / **Prep Time:** 5 minutes / **Cooking Time**: 11 minutes)

Ingredients

- 2 cups of challah bread, chopped & cubed
- 1 egg
- ¼ cup of milk
- ¼ cup sweetened condensed milk
- ½ teaspoon cinnamon
- 1 cup water
- 1/3 cup semi-sweet chocolate chunks
- 6-inch baking pan
- Aluminum foil

How to

1. Add egg along with all the wet ingredients to a bowl and mix well.
2. Grease a 6-inch baking pan and pour the egg mixture into it.
3. Add challah bread and chocolate chunks to the pan.
4. Add 1 cup water to the Instant Pot and place the trivet inside.
5. Arrange the spring pan over the trivet and cover with the aluminum foil.
6. Secure the lid of the cooker and press the "Manual" function key.
7. Adjust the time to 11 minutes and cook at high pressure.
8. After the beep, release the pressure naturally and remove the lid.
9. Remove the pudding from the pan.
10. Let it cool and serve.

Nutrition Values (Per Serving)

- Calories: 305
- Carbohydrate: 48.1g
- Protein: 8.7g
- Fat: 10.3g
- Sugar: 22.2g
- Sodium: 229mg

Blueberries Oatmeal

(**Serves**: 2 / **Prep Time:** 5 minutes / **Cooking Time**: 3 minutes)

Ingredients

- 1 cup old-fashioned rolled oats
- 2 cups water
- 1 cup blueberries
- 2 tablespoons sunflower seeds
- 2 tablespoons agave nectar

How to

1. Add all the ingredients except blueberries to the Instant Pot.
2. Secure the lid of the cooker and press the "Manual" function key.
3. Adjust the time to 3 minutes and cook at high pressure.
4. After the beep, release the pressure naturally and remove the lid.
5. Stir the prepared oatmeal and serve in a bowl.
6. Garnish with blueberries on top.

Nutrition Values (Per Serving)

- Calories: 268
- Carbohydrate: 54.1g
- Protein: 6.4g
- Fat: 4.3g
- Sugar: 22.7g
- Sodium: 10mg

Black Bean and Egg Casserole

(**Serves**: 3 / **Prep Time:** 10 minutes / **Cooking Time**: 25 minutes)

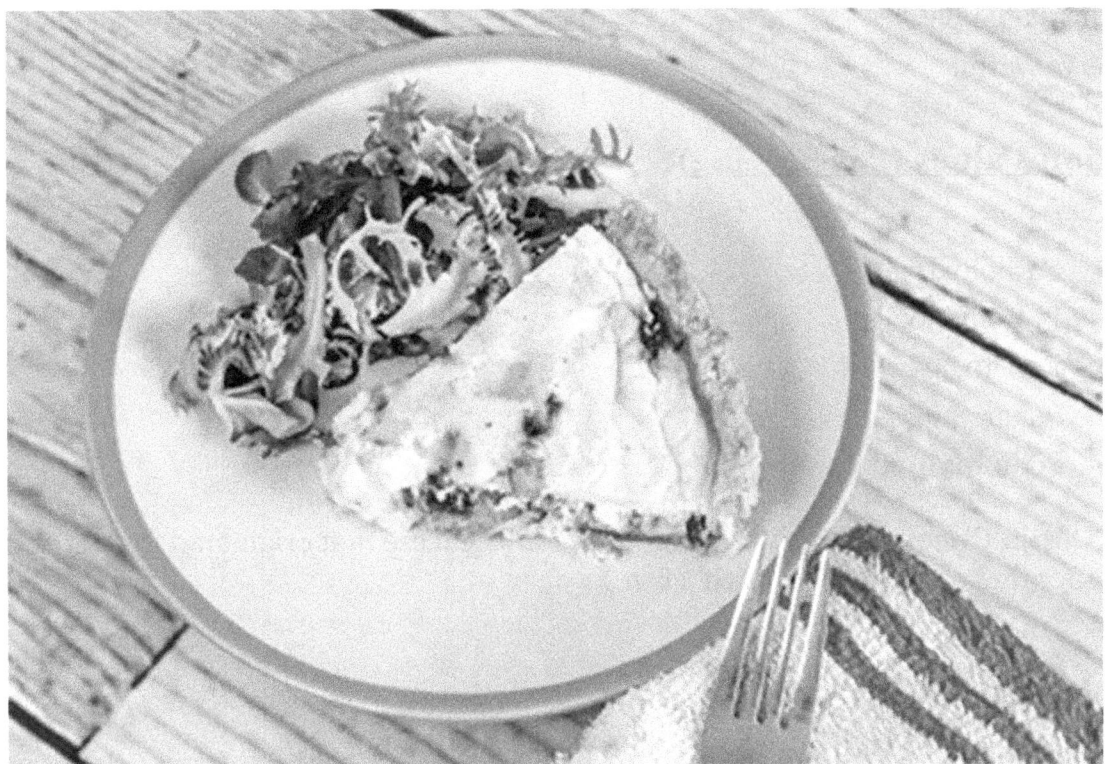

Ingredients

- 4 large eggs, well-beaten
- ½ lb. mild ground sausage
- ¼ large red onion, chopped
- ½ red bell pepper, chopped
- ½ can black beans, rinsed
- ¼ cup green onions
- ¼ cup flour
- ½ cup Cotija cheese*
- ½ cup mozzarella cheese
- sour cream, cilantro to garnish

How to

1. Add sausage and onion to the Instant Pot and select the "Sauté" function to cook for 3 minutes.
2. Combine flour with eggs and add this mixture to the sausages.
3. Add all the vegetables, cheeses, and beans.
4. Secure the lid of the cooker and press the "Manual" function key.

5. Adjust the time to 20 minutes and cook at high pressure.
6. After the beep, release the pressure naturally and remove the lid.
7. Remove the inner pot, place a plate on top then flip the pot to transfer the casserole to the plate.
8. Serve warm.

Nutrition Values (Per Serving)

- Calories: 564
- Carbohydrate: 33.4g
- Protein: 36.2g
- Fat: 30.7g
- Sugar: 4.3g
- Sodium: 1050mg

(**Note: Cotija Cheese*** - Cotija is a hard cow's milk cheese that originated from Mexico. It is named after the town of Cotija, Michoacán.)

Cashew Mango Oatmeal

(**Serves**: 2 / **Prep Time:** 5 minutes / **Cooking Time**: 3 minutes)

Ingredients

- 2 tablespoons unsweetened flaked coconut
- 1 cup old-fashioned rolled oats
- 2 tablespoons brown sugar
- 2 cups water
- ½ cup mango, chopped
- 2 tablespoons cashews, chopped

How to

1. Add all the ingredients to the Instant Pot. Reserve all the mango and cashews for the topping.
2. Secure the lid of the cooker and press the "Manual" function key.
3. Adjust the time to 3 minutes and cook at high pressure.
4. After the beep, release the pressure naturally and remove the lid.
5. Stir the prepared oatmeal and serve in a bowl.
6. Garnish with chopped mango and cashews on top.

Nutrition Values (Per Serving)

- Calories: 276
- Carbohydrate: 45.6g
- Protein: 7.1g
- Fat: 8.4g
- Sugar: 15.5g
- Sodium: 14mg

Morning Frittatas

(**Serves**: 2 / **Prep Time:** 10 minutes / **Cooking Time**: 5 minutes)

Ingredients

- 3 eggs
- 2 tablespoons almond milk
- Salt and pepper, to taste
- ¼ cup cheddar cheese
- ¼ cup red bell pepper, chopped
- ¼ cup onion, chopped
- 3 silicon baking molds

How to

1. Add 1 cup of water to the Instant Pot and place the trivet inside.
2. Now grease the silicon baking molds with oil and crack an egg into each mold.
3. Add all the vegetables, spices, and cheese on top.
4. Place the silicon baking molds over the trivet.
5. Secure the lid of the cooker and press the "Manual" function key.
6. Adjust the time to 5 minutes and cook at high pressure.
7. After the beep, release the pressure naturally and remove the lid.
8. Remove the stuffed molds and serve immediately.

Nutrition Values (Per Serving)

- Calories: 196
- Carbohydrate: 4g
- Protein: 12.5g
- Fat: 14.9g
- Sugar: 2.4g
- Sodium: 183mg

Spice Filled Oatmeal

(**Serves**: 2 / **Prep Time:** 15 minutes / **Cooking Time**: 3 minutes)

Ingredients

- 1 cup old-fashioned rolled oats
- ¼ cup grated extra-sharp cheddar
- ¼ teaspoon paprika
- kosher salt and black pepper
- 1 scallion, chopped
- 2 cups water

How to

1. Add all the ingredients to the Instant Pot, except cheese.
2. Secure the lid of the cooker and press the "Manual" function key.
3. Adjust the time to 3 minutes and cook at high pressure.
4. After the beep, release the pressure naturally and remove the lid.
5. Stir in shredded cheese and serve.

Nutrition Values (Per Serving)

- Calories: 210
- Carbohydrate: 27.9g
- Protein: 9g
- Fat: 7.3g
- Sugar: 0.7g
- Sodium: 98mg

Beans Rice Mix

(**Serves**: 4 / **Prep Time:** 12 minutes / **Cooking Time**: 15 minutes)

Ingredients

- 1 cup white basmati rice
- 1 cup whole mung beans
- ½ teaspoon turmeric powder
- ½ teaspoon sea salt
- 2 inches' ginger, grated or chopped
- 3 teaspoons shredded coconut
- bunch of cilantro, chopped
- 6 cups water
- ½ cup cremini mushrooms, sliced

How to

1. Add all the ingredients to the Instant Pot.
2. Secure the lid of the cooker and press the "Manual" function key.
3. Adjust the time to 15 minutes and cook at high pressure.
4. After the beep, release the pressure naturally and remove the lid.
5. Stir the prepared mixture and serve in a bowl.
6. Garnish with mushroom slices on top.

Nutrition Values (Per Serving)

- Calories: 202
- Carbohydrate: 41g
- Protein: 7g
- Fat: 1.3g
- Sugar: 0.4g
- Sodium: 255mg

Orange Marmalade Oatmeal

(**Serves**: 4 / **Prep Time:** 5 minutes / **Cooking Time**: 6 minutes)

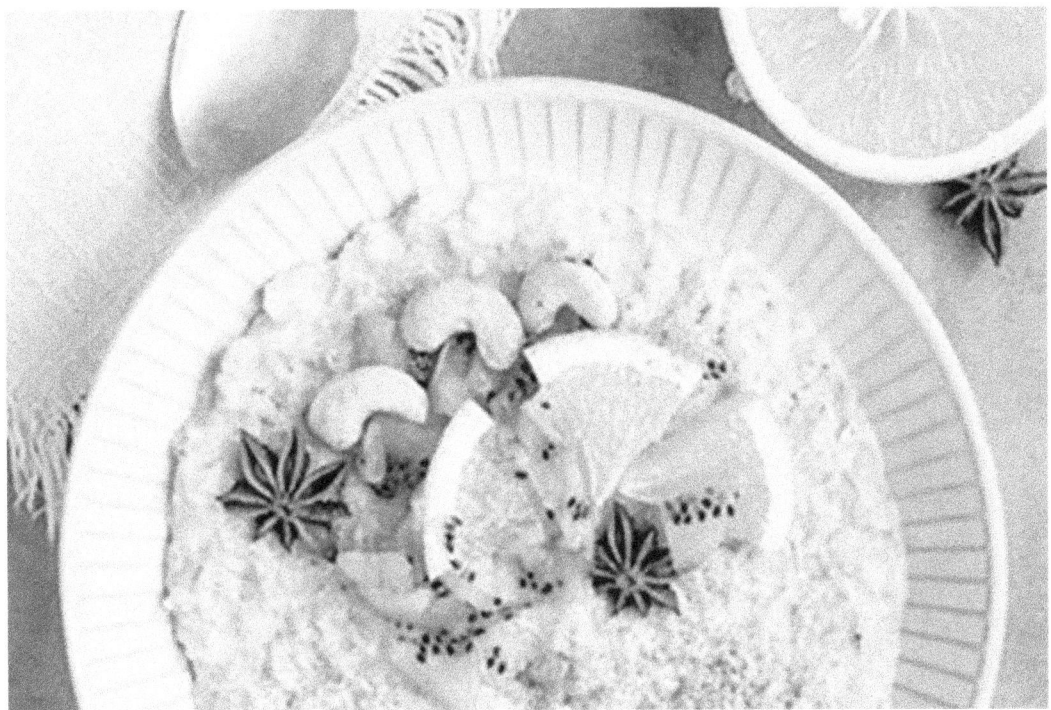

Ingredients

- 2 cups old-fashioned oats
- 2 ¼ cups water
- 2 ¼ cups milk
- ½ teaspoon salt
- ½ teaspoon ground cinnamon
- ¼ cup sugar
- 2 tablespoons plain low-fat Greek yogurt
- 2 tablespoons orange marmalade
- Orange and kiwi slices to garnish

How to

1. Add all the ingredients to the Instant Pot.
2. Secure the lid of the cooker and press the "Manual" function key.
3. Adjust the time to 6 minutes and cook at high pressure.
4. After the beep, release the pressure naturally and remove the lid.
5. Stir the prepared oatmeal and serve in a bowl.
6. Garnish with orange and kiwi slices on top.

Nutrition Values (Per Serving)

- Calories: 523
- Carbohydrate: 84.8g
- Protein: 26.5g
- Fat: 8.2g
- Sugar: 31.3g
- Sodium: 423mg

Garlic Eggs

(**Serves**: 4 / **Prep Time:** 10 minutes / **Cooking Time**: 30 minutes)

Ingredients

- 1 tablespoon olive oil
- 6 small tomatoes.
- 4 eggs
- 1 teaspoon garlic (minced)
- 1 teaspoon turmeric powder
- 1 green onion (chopped)
- Salt and pepper to taste.

How to

1. First, cut all the tomatoes in half or into three to four slices. Set them aside.
2. Pour one tablespoon of olive oil into the Instant Pot and Select "Sauté."
3. Now add the sliced tomatoes and sauté them with their cut side down.
4. Add minced garlic and powdered turmeric into the pot.
5. Add 4 eggs to the pot and stir them using a spatula. Scramble the eggs and mix them well with garlic and turmeric.
6. After cooking the egg scramble for 2 to 3 minutes on "Sauté" press "Cancel.
7. Sprinkle chopped green onions on top and serve.

Nutrition Values (Per Serving)

- Calories: 118
- Carbohydrate: 5.7g
- Protein: 6.7g
- Fat: 8.2g
- Sugar: 3.6g
- Sodium: 68mg

Oatmeal with Pistachios

(**Serves**: 4 / **Prep Time:** 5 minutes / **Cooking Time**: 6 minutes)

Ingredients

- 2 cups old-fashioned oats
- 2 ¼ cups water
- 2 ¼ cups milk
- ½ teaspoon salt
- ¼ teaspoon nutmeg
- 1 tablespoon honey
- 1 tablespoon dried cranberries
- 1 tablespoon dried cherries
- 1 tablespoon roasted pistachios

How to

1. Add all the ingredients to the Instant Pot, except for cranberries, cherries, and pistachios.
2. Secure the lid of the cooker and press the "Manual" function key.
3. Adjust the time to 6 minutes and cook at high pressure.
4. After the beep, release the pressure naturally and remove the lid.
5. Stir the prepared oatmeal and serve in a bowl.
6. Garnish with cranberries, cherries, and pistachios on top.

Nutrition Values (Per Serving)

- Calories: 415
- Carbohydrate: 66.8g
- Protein: 15g
- Fat: 8.9g
- Sugar: 12.9g
- Sodium: 369mg

Quinoa with Bananas

(**Serves**: 3 / **Prep Time:** 5 minutes / **Cooking Time**: 12 minutes)

Ingredients

- ¾ cup quinoa, soaked in water for at least 1 hour
- 1 (8 oz.) can almond milk
- ¾ cup water
- ½ cup banana, peeled and sliced
- 1 teaspoon vanilla extract
- 2 tablespoons honey
- 1 pinch of salt

Topping:

- 6 banana slices
- Grated chocolate

How to

1. Add all the ingredients for quinoa to the Instant Pot.
2. Secure the lid of the cooker and press "Rice" function key.
3. Adjust the time to 12 minutes and cook at low pressure.
4. After the beep, release the pressure naturally and remove the lid.
5. Stir the prepared quinoa well and serve in a bowl.
6. Add banana slices and grated chocolate on top.

Nutrition Values (Per Serving)

- Calories: 371
- Carbohydrate: 41.4g
- Protein: 7.3g
- Fat: 20.4g
- Sugar: 10.3g
- Sodium: 17.4mg

Korean Steamed Eggs

(**Serves**: 2 / **Prep Time:** 5 minutes / **Cooking Time**: 5 minutes)

Ingredients

- 3 large eggs
- ½ cup cold water
- 3 teaspoons chopped scallions
- Pinch of sesame seeds
- Pinch of garlic powder
- Salt and pepper to taste

How to

1. Add 1 cup water to the Instant Pot and place the trivet inside.
2. Add all the ingredients in a bowl and whisk well.
3. Take a heatproof bowl and pour the egg mixture into it.
4. Place the bowl over the trivet.
5. Secure the lid of the cooker and press the "Manual" function key.
6. Adjust the time to 5 minutes and cook at high pressure.
7. After the beep, release the pressure naturally and remove the lid.
8. Serve immediately with rice.

Nutrition Values (Per Serving)

- Calories: 443
- Carbohydrate: 26.5g
- Protein: 13.2g
- Fat: 14.2g
- Sugar: 3.4g
- Sodium: 214mg

Peanut Butter Oatmeal

(**Serves**: 4 / **Prep Time:** 5 minutes / **Cooking Time**: 6 minutes)

Ingredients

- 2 cups old-fashioned oats
- 2 ¼ cups water
- 2 ¼ cups milk
- ¼ cup dry fruits
- 1 tablespoon sugar
- 4 tablespoons peanut butter

How to

1. Add all the ingredients, except for dry fruits, to the Instant Pot.
2. Secure the lid of the cooker and press the "Manual" function key.
3. Adjust the time to 6 minutes and cook at high pressure.
4. After the beep, release the pressure naturally and remove the lid.
5. Stir the prepared oatmeal and serve in a bowl.
6. Garnish with dry fruits on top.

Nutrition Values (Per Serving)

- Calories: 512
- Carbohydrate: 73.3g
- Protein: 18.8g
- Fat: 16g
- Sugar: 18.6g
- Sodium: 143mg

Eggs with Herbs de Provence

(**Serves**: 3 / **Prep Time:** 10 minutes / **Cooking Time**: 10 minutes)

Ingredients

- 3 eggs
- ½ small onion chopped
- ½ cup cooked ham or bacon
- ¼ cup heavy cream
- ½ cup chopped kale leaves
- ½ cup cheddar cheese
- ½ teaspoon Herbs de Provence
- Sea salt and pepper, to taste

How to

1. Add 1 cup of water to the Instant Pot and place the trivet inside.
2. Add all the ingredients to a bowl except cheese and whisk well.
3. Take a heatproof container and pour the egg mixture into it.
4. Place the container over the trivet.
5. Secure the lid of the cooker and press the "Manual" function key.
6. Adjust the time to 10 minutes and cook at high pressure.
7. After the beep, release the pressure naturally and remove the lid.
8. Drizzle shredded cheese on top and serve hot.

Nutrition Values (Per Serving)

- Calories: 303
- Carbohydrate: 4.6g
- Protein: 19.7g
- Fat: 23.1g
- Sugar: 1.4g
- Sodium: 548mg

Nourishing Banana Oatmeal

(**Serves**: 4 / **Prep Time:** 5 minutes / **Cooking Time**: 6 minutes)

Ingredients

- 2 cups old-fashioned oats
- 2 ¼ cups water
- 2 ¼ cups milk
- 1 tablespoon sugar
- 2 bananas sliced
- 2 tablespoon molasses
- 4 tablespoons chopped toasted pecans

How to

1. Add oats, milk, water, and sugar into the Instant Pot.
2. Secure the lid of the cooker and press the "Manual" function key.
3. Adjust the time to 6 minutes and cook at high pressure.
4. After the beep, release the pressure naturally and remove the lid.
5. Stir the prepared oatmeal.
6. Serve with banana slices and pecans on top. Then drizzle molasses on it.

Nutrition Values (Per Serving)

- Calories: 518
- Carbohydrate: 72.9g
- Protein: 16g
- Fat: 18g
- Sugar: 17.4g
- Sodium: 72mg

Eggs Mushroom Casserole

(**Serves**: 3 / **Prep Time:** 5 minutes / **Cooking Time**: 10 minutes)

Ingredients

- 3 eggs
- ½ small onion chopped
- ½ cup cooked ham or bacon
- ¼ cup heavy cream
- ½ cup cheddar cheese
- ½ cup cremini mushrooms, cooked and sliced
- Sea salt and pepper, to taste

How to

1. Add 1 cup water to the Instant Pot and place the trivet inside.
2. Add all the ingredients to a bowl except cheese and whisk well.
3. Take a heatproof container and pour the egg mixture into it.
4. Place the container over the trivet.
5. Secure the lid of the cooker and press the "Manual" function key.
6. Adjust the time to 10 minutes and cook at high pressure.
7. After the beep, release the pressure naturally and remove the lid.
8. Drizzle the shredded cheese on top and serve hot.

Nutrition Values (Per Serving)

- Calories: 218
- Carbohydrate: 3.3g
- Protein: 14.6g
- Fat: 16.3g
- Sugar: 1.2g
- Sodium: 477mg

Almond Quinoa Meal

(**Serves**: 3 / **Prep Time:** 5 minutes / **Cooking Time**: 10 minutes)

Ingredients

- ¾ cup quinoa, soaked in water at least 1 hour
- 1 (8 oz.) can almond milk
- ¾ cup water
- ½ teaspoon crushed almonds
- 1 teaspoon vanilla extract
- 2 tablespoons honey
- 1 pinch of salt

Topping:

- ¼ cup almonds, soaked, peeled, and chopped

How to

1. Add all the ingredients for quinoa, to the Instant Pot.
2. Secure the lid of the cooker and press "Rice" function key.
3. Adjust the time to 10 minutes and press cook at low pressure.
4. After the beep, release the pressure naturally and remove the lid.
5. Stir the prepared quinoa well and serve in a bowl.
6. Add chopped almonds on top.

Nutrition Values (Per Serving)

- Calories: 376
- Carbohydrate 39.7g
- Protein: 7.9g
- Fat: 21.3g
- Sugar: 10.5g
- Sodium: 17.5 mg

Minty Pineapple Oatmeal

(**Serves**: 4 / **Prep Time:** 5 minutes / **Cooking Time**: 6 minutes)

Ingredients

- 2 cups old-fashioned oats
- 2 ¼ cups water
- 2 ¼ cups milk
- 1 tablespoon cinnamon sugar
- 2 cups pineapple, chopped
- 2 tablespoons fresh mint leaves

How to

1. Add oats, milk, water, and cinnamon sugar in the Instant Pot.
2. Secure the lid of the cooker and press the "Manual" function key.
3. Adjust the time to 6 minutes and cook at high pressure.
4. After the beep, release the pressure naturally and remove the lid.
5. Stir the prepared oatmeal.
6. Serve with fresh mint leaves and pineapple on top.

Nutrition Values (Per Serving)

- Calories: 434
- Carbohydrate: 73.7g
- Protein: 15g
- Fat: 8.1g
- Sugar: 16.4g
- Sodium: 71mg

Delicious Spinach Hash

(**Serves**: 3 / **Prep Time:** 20 minutes / **Cooking Time**: 20 minutes)

Ingredients

- 6 eggs
- 1 small onion, chopped
- 3 bacon strips, chopped
- ½ cup cheddar cheese
- 8 oz. baby spinach, chopped
- ¼ teaspoon black pepper
- 2 large sweet potatoes, diced
- ¼ teaspoon salt
- 1 tablespoon milk
- 6-inch springform pan

How to

1. Add bacon to the Instant Pot and select the "Sauté" function to cook for 3 minutes.
2. Transfer the crispy cooked bacon to the greased "spring pan."
3. Add sweet potatoes and spinach on top of bacon.
4. Crack all the eggs in a bowl and whisk them well with the milk.
5. Pour the eggs mixture over the bell peppers in the spring pan.
6. Sprinkle salt and pepper on top and cover with aluminum foil.
7. Pour some water into the Instant Pot, set the trivet inside, and then place the covered spring pan over the trivet.
8. Press the "Manual" key, adjust its settings to High pressure for 20 minutes.
9. After it is done, do a Natural release to release the steam.
10. Remove the lid and the spring pan. Transfer the hash to a plate.
11. Sprinkle cheddar cheese on top then serve.

Nutrition Values (Per Serving)

- Calories: 397
- Carbohydrate: 25.6g
- Protein: 31.1g
- Fat: 21.2g
- Sugar: 2.8g
- Sodium: 523mg

Vanilla Rice Pudding

(**Serves**: 4 / **Prep Time:** 5 minutes / **Cooking Time**: 25 minutes)

Ingredients

- 1 cup short grain brown rice
- 1 ½ cups water
- 1 tablespoon vanilla extract
- 1 cinnamon stick
- 1 tablespoon butter
- 1 cup raisins
- 3 tablespoons honey
- ½ cup heavy cream

How to

1. Add the water, rice, cinnamon stick, vanilla, and butter in the Instant Pot.
2. Secure the lid of the cooker and press the "Manual" function key.
3. Adjust the time to 20 minutes and cook at high pressure.
4. After the beep, release the pressure naturally and remove the lid.
5. Stir in honey, raisins, and cream.
6. Cook on "Sauté" function for 5 minutes.
7. Serve hot.

Nutrition Values (Per Serving)

- Calories: 438
- Carbohydrate: 83.5g
- Protein: 5g
- Fat: 11.4g
- Sugar: 36.6g
- Sodium: 67mg

Oeufs Cocotte

(**Serves**: 6 / **Prep Time:** 5 minutes / **Cooking Time**: 4 minutes)

Ingredients

- 6 eggs
- 6 slices of meat, fish or vegetables
- 6 slices of cheese
- 1 cup fresh herbs (garnish)
- 1 tablespoon avocado oil

How to

1. Add water to the Instant Pot and place the trivet inside.
2. Now grease the ramekin with oil and crack an egg into it.
3. Add meat, fish or vegetable slices to the ramekin, and then place the cheese slice on top.
4. Cover the ramekin with aluminum foil and place it over the trivet.
5. Secure the lid of the cooker and press the "Manual" function key.
6. Adjust the time to 4 minutes and cook at low pressure.
7. After the beep, release the pressure naturally and remove the lid.
8. Remove the stuffed ramekin and serve immediately.

Nutrition Values (Per Serving)

- Calories: 391
- Carbohydrate: 1g
- Protein: 53.2g
- Fat: 18.2g
- Sugar: 0.5g
- Sodium: 326mg

Nutritious Instant Porridge

(**Serves**: 4 / **Prep Time:** 5 minutes / **Cooking Time**: 3 minutes)

Ingredients

- 1 cup cashews (raw, unsalted)
- ½ cup Pepitas, shelled
- 1 cup Pecan halves
- 1 cup unsweetened dried coconut shreds
- 2 cups water
- 4 teaspoons coconut oil, melted
- 2 tablespoons maple syrup or honey

How to

1. Add all the ingredients to a blender, except water, maple syrup, and coconut oil. Blend well to form a smooth mixture.
2. Add the prepared mixture along with water, coconut oil, and maple syrup to the Instant Pot.
3. Secure the lid of the cooker and press "Porridge" option.
4. Adjust the time to 3 minutes and let it cook.
5. After the beep, release the pressure naturally and remove the lid.
6. Stir the prepared mixture and serve in a bowl.
7. Garnish with fresh fruits and cashews on top.

Nutrition Values (Per Serving)

- Calories: 615
- Carbohydrate: 29.4g
- Protein: 14.9g
- Fat: 53.4g
- Sugar: 9.5g
- Sodium: 22mg

Eggs & Red Beans Casserole

(**Serves**: 3 / **Prep Time:** 5 minutes / **Cooking Time**: 20 minutes)

Ingredients

- 3 eggs
- ½ small onion chopped
- ½ cup cooked ham or bacon
- ¼ cup heavy cream
- ½ cup cheddar cheese
- ½ cup red beans, boiled
- Sea salt and pepper, to taste

How to

1. Add 1 cup water to the Instant Pot and place the trivet inside.
2. Add all the ingredients to a bowl except cheese and whisk well.
3. Take a heatproof container and pour the egg mixture into it.
4. Place the container over the trivet.
5. Secure the lid of the cooker and press the "Manual" function key.
6. Adjust the time to 20 minutes and cook at high pressure.
7. After the beep, release the pressure naturally and remove the lid.
8. Drizzle the shredded cheese on top and serve hot.

Nutrition Values (Per Serving)

- Calories: 318
- Carbohydrate: 21.6g
- Protein: 21.2g
- Fat: 16.6g
- Sugar: 1.6g
- Sodium: 480mg

Cinnamon Quinoa Bowl

(**Serves**: 3 / **Prep Time:** 5 minutes / **Cooking Time**: 12 minutes)

Ingredients

- ¾ cup quinoa, soaked in water at least 1 hour
- 1 (8 oz.) can coconut milk
- ¾ cup water
- ½ teaspoon ground cinnamon
- 2 tablespoons pure maple syrup
- 1 teaspoon vanilla extract
- 1 pinch of salt

Toppings:
- Fresh fruits
- Coconut flakes

How to

1. Add all the ingredients for quinoa to the Instant Pot.
2. Secure the lid of the cooker and press "Rice" option.
3. Adjust the time to 12 minutes and cook at low pressure.
4. After the beep, release the pressure naturally and remove the lid.
5. Stir the prepared quinoa well and serve in a bowl.
6. Add fresh fruits and coconut flakes on top. Add more milk if needed.

Nutrition Values (Per Serving)

- Calories: 370
- Carbohydrate: 40.9g
- Protein: 7.8g
- Fat: 20.6g
- Sugar: 10.7g
- Sodium: 17mg

Egg Broccoli Casserole

(**Serves**: 3 / **Prep Time:** 10 minutes / **Cooking Time**: 20 minutes)

Ingredients

- 3 eggs
- ½ small onion chopped
- ½ cup cooked ham or bacon
- ¼ cup heavy cream
- ½ cup cheddar cheese
- ½ lb. broccoli florets
- Sea salt and pepper, to taste

How to

1. Add 1 cup water to the Instant Pot and place the trivet inside.
2. Add all the ingredients to a bowl except cheese and whisk well.
3. Take a heatproof container and pour the egg mixture into it.
4. Place the container over the trivet.
5. Secure the lid of the cooker and press the "Manual" function key.
6. Adjust the time to 20 minutes and cook at high pressure.
7. After the beep, release the pressure naturally and remove the lid.
8. Drizzle shredded cheese on top and serve hot.

Nutrition Values (Per Serving)

- Calories: 203
- Carbohydrate: 11.1g
- Protein: 6.2g
- Fat: 7.6g
- Sugar: 2.3g
- Sodium: 61mg

Coco Quinoa Bowl

(**Serves**: 3 / **Prep Time:** 5 minutes / **Cooking Time**: 10 minutes)

Ingredients

- ¾ cup quinoa, soaked in water at least 1 hour
- 1 (8 oz.) can milk,
- ¾ cup water
- ½ teaspoon cocoa powder
- 2 tablespoons honey
- 1 pinch of salt

Toppings:
- Chocolate chips
- Whipped cream

How to

1. Add all the ingredients for quinoa to the Instant Pot.
2. Secure the lid of the cooker and press the "Rice" function key.
3. Adjust the time to 10 minutes and cook at low pressure.
4. After the beep, release the pressure naturally and remove the lid.
5. Stir the prepared quinoa well and serve in a bowl.
6. Add chocolate chips and whipped cream on top.

Nutrition Values (Per Serving)

- Calories: 373
- Carbohydrate: 41.1g
- Protein: 7.9g
- Fat: 20.5g
- Sugar: 11.2g
- Sodium: 16mg

Brown Rice Pudding

(**Serves**: 2 / **Prep Time:** 5 minutes / **Cooking Time**: 10 minutes)

Ingredients

- 1 cups milk
- ¾ cup water
- ½ cup brown rice, short grain
- ½ cup heavy cream
- 2 tablespoons maple syrup
- Pinch of sea salt
- 1 teaspoon cocoa powder
- Whipped cream and grated chocolate (garnish)

How to

1. Add all the ingredients to the Instant Pot.
2. Secure the lid of the cooker and press the "Manual" function key.
3. Adjust the time to 10 minutes and cook at high pressure.
4. After the beep, release the pressure naturally and remove the lid.
5. Stir the prepared pudding and serve in a bowl.
6. Add whipped cream and grated chocolate on top.

Nutrition Values (Per Serving)

- Calories: 426
- Carbohydrate: 30.1g
- Protein: 15.2g
- Fat: 26.4g
- Sugar: 10.8g
- Sodium: 763mg

Potato Cornmeal Porridge

(**Serves**: 6 / **Prep Time:** 15 minutes / **Cooking Time**: 6 minutes)

Ingredients

- 6 cups water
- 1 ¼ cups milk
- 1 ¼ cups yellow cornmeal, fine
- ½ cup potatoes, shredded
- ¼ teaspoon salt
- ¼ teaspoon pepper
- ¼ cup corn kernels
- ¾ cup unsweetened condensed milk

How to

1. Add 5 cups of water and coconut milk to the Instant Pot.
2. Mix the cornmeal with 1 cup of water and add it to the pot.
3. Stir in potatoes, corns, salt, and pepper.
4. Secure the lid of the cooker and press the "Manual" function key.
5. Adjust the time to 6 minutes and cook at high pressure.
6. After the beep, release the pressure naturally and remove the lid.
7. Stir in unsweetened condensed milk.
8. Serve and enjoy.

Nutrition Values (Per Serving)

- Calories: 252
- Carbohydrate: 49.6g
- Protein: 7.2g
- Fat: 3.5g
- Sugar: 16.5g
- Sodium: 179mg

BEANS AND GRAINS

Black Bean Gravy

(**Serves:** 6 / **Prep time:** 5 minutes / **Cooking time:** 30 minutes)

Ingredients

- 1 lb. black beans, sorted and rinsed
- ½ teaspoon red pepper
- ½ teaspoon ground turmeric
- 1 tablespoon onion powder
- 2 teaspoons garlic powder
- 1 teaspoon salt
- 1 bay leaf
- 6 cups unsalted vegetable broth

How to

1. Add all the ingredients to the Instant Pot.
2. Cover and secure the lid. Turn its pressure release handle to the sealing position.
3. Cook on the "Beans/Chilli" function on the default settings.
4. After the beep, do a Natural release for 20 minutes.
5. Stir and serve hot with boiled white rice.

Nutrition Values (Per Serving)

- Calories: 289
- Carbohydrate: 53.7g
- Protein: 18 .7g
- Fat: 1.1g
- Sugar: 5.8g
- Sodium: 633mg

Chorizo Pinto Beans

(**Serves:** 3 / **Prep time:** 5 minutes / **Cooking time:** 47 minutes)

Ingredients

- ½ tablespoon cooking oil
- 2 oz. dry (Spanish) chorizo
- ½ yellow onion
- 1 ½ garlic cloves
- 1 cup dry pinto beans
- 1 bay leaf
- ½ teaspoon freshly cracked pepper
- 1 ½ cups chicken broth
- 7 ½ oz. can diced tomatoes

How to

1. Add oil, chorizo, garlic and onion to the Instant Pot. "Sauté" for 5 minutes.
2. Stir in beans, pepper and bay leaf. Cook for 1 minute, then add the broth.
3. Cover and secure the lid. Turn its pressure release handle to the sealing position.
4. Cook on the "Manual" function with high pressure for 35 minutes.
5. After the beep, do a Natural release for 20 minutes.
6. Stir in diced tomatoes and cook for 7 minutes on the "Sauté" setting.
7. Serve hot with boiled white rice or tortilla chips.

Nutrition Values (Per Serving)

- Calories: 337
- Carbohydrate: 50.5g
- Protein: 21.3g
- Fat: 5.7g
- Sugar: 5.4g
- Sodium: 671mg

Spinach Chickpea Curry

(**Serves:** 4 / **Prep Time:** 10 minutes / **Cooking Time:** 24 minutes)

Ingredients

- ½ cup raw chickpeas
- 1 ½ tablespoons cooking oil
- ½ cup chopped onions
- 1 bay leaf
- ½ tablespoon grated garlic
- ¼ tablespoon grated ginger
- ¾ cup water
- 1 cup fresh tomato puree
- ½ green chili, finely chopped
- ¼ teaspoon turmeric
- ½ teaspoon coriander powder
- 1 teaspoon chili powder
- 1 cup chopped baby spinach
- Salt, to taste
- Fistful of chopped fresh cilantro

How to

1. Add oil and onions to the Instant Pot. "Sauté" for 5 minutes.
2. Stir ginger, garlic paste, green chili and bay leaf. Cook for 1 minute, then add all the spices.
3. Add chickpeas, tomato puree and water to the pot.
4. Cover and secure the lid. Turn its pressure release handle to the sealing position.
5. Cook on the "Manual" function with high pressure for 15 minutes.
6. After the beep, do a Natural release for 20 minutes.
7. Stir in spinach and cook for 3 minutes on the "Sauté" setting.
8. Serve hot with boiled white rice.

Nutrition Values (Per Serving)

- Calories: 180
- Carbohydrate: 25.3g
- Protein: 6.7g
- Fat: 7g
- Sugar: 6.9g
- Sodium: 79mg

Almond Risotto

(Serves: 3 / **Prep Time:** 10 minutes / **Cooking Time:** 5 minutes)

Ingredients

- 2 cups vanilla almond milk
- ½ cup Arborio (short-grain Italian) rice
- 2 tablespoons agave syrup
- 1 teaspoon vanilla extract
- ¼ cup toasted almond flakes

How to

1. Add all the ingredients to the Instant Pot.
2. Cover and secure the lid. Turn its pressure release handle to the sealing position.
3. Cook on the "Manual" function with high pressure for 5 minutes.
4. After the beep, do a Natural release for 20 minutes.
5. Garnish with almond flakes and serve.

Nutrition Values (Per Serving)

- Calories: 116
- Carbohydrate: 22.5g
- Protein: 2g
- Fat: 2.1g
- Sugar: 0.2g
- Sodium: 82mg

Spinach Lentils Stew

(**Serves:** 4 / **Prep Time:** 10 minutes / **Cooking Time:** 24 minutes)

Ingredients

- ½ cup raw lentils
- 1 ½ tablespoons cooking oil
- ½ cup chopped onions
- 1 bay leaf
- ½ tablespoon grated garlic
- ¼ tablespoon grated ginger
- ¾ cup water
- 1 cup fresh tomato puree
- ½ green chili, finely chopped
- ¼ teaspoon turmeric
- ½ teaspoon coriander powder
- 1 teaspoon chili powder
- 1 cup chopped baby spinach
- Salt, to taste
- ½ cup fresh cilantro

How to

1. Add oil and onions to the Instant Pot. "Sauté" for 5 minutes.
2. Stir ginger, garlic paste and bay leaf. Cook for 1 minute, then add all the spices.
3. Add lentils, tomato puree and water to the pot.
4. Cover and secure the lid. Turn its pressure release handle to the sealing position.
5. Cook on the "Manual" function with high pressure for 15 minutes.
6. After the beep, do a Natural release for 20 minutes.
7. Stir in spinach and cook for 3 minutes on the "Sauté" setting.
8. Serve hot with boiled white rice.

Nutrition Values (Per Serving)

- Calories: 169
- Carbohydrate: 23.2g
- Protein: 7.9g
- Fat: 5.7g
- Sugar: 4.4g
- Sodium: 75mg

Spicy Red Bean Curry

(**Serves:** 4 / **Prep Time:** 10 minutes / **Cooking Time:** 24 minutes)

Ingredients

- ½ cup raw red beans
- 1 ½ tablespoons cooking oil
- ½ cup chopped onions
- 1 bay leaf
- ½ tablespoon grated garlic
- ¼ tablespoon grated ginger
- ¾ cup water
- 1 cup fresh tomato puree
- ½ green chili, finely chopped
- ¼ teaspoon turmeric
- ½ teaspoon coriander powder
- 1 teaspoon chili powder
- 1 cup chopped baby spinach
- Salt, to taste
- ½ cup fresh cilantro

How to

1. Add oil and onions to the Instant Pot. "Sauté" for 5 minutes.
2. Stir ginger, garlic paste, green chili and bay leaf. Cook for 1 minute, then add all the spices.
3. Add red beans, tomato puree and water to the pot.
4. Cover and secure the lid. Turn its pressure release handle to the sealing position.
5. Cook on the "Manual" function with high pressure for 15 minutes.
6. After the beep, do a Natural release for 20 minutes.
7. Stir in spinach and cook for 3 minutes on the "Sauté" setting.
8. Serve hot with boiled white rice.

Nutrition Values (Per Serving)

- Calories: 163
- Carbohydrate: 22.8g
- Protein: 7g
- Fat: 5.7g
- Sugar: 4.4g
- Sodium: 78mg

Inviting Butternut Squash Risotto

(**Serves:** 3 / **Prep Time:** 10 minutes / **Cooking Time:** 12 minutes)

Ingredients

- ½ (2 lbs.) butternut squash, diced
- 1 tablespoon olive oil
- 1 sprig sage, leaves removed
- 2 garlic cloves, whole
- 1 cup Arborio (short-grain Italian) rice
- 2 tablespoons white wine
- 2 cups water
- 1 teaspoon sea salt
- ½ teaspoon nutmeg, freshly ground

How to

1. Add oil, sage and garlic to the Instant Pot and "Sauté" for 2 minutes.
2. Add diced butternut squash and stir fry for 5 minutes.
3. Add all the remaining ingredients to the cooker.
4. Cover and secure the lid. Turn its pressure release handle to the sealing position.
5. Cook on the "Manual" function with high pressure for 5 minutes.
6. After the beep, do a Natural release and remove the lid.
7. Stir and serve.

Nutrition Values (Per Serving)

- Calories: 323
- Carbohydrate: 62.4g
- Protein: 5.3g
- Fat: 5.2g
- Sugar: 2.3g
- Sodium: 638mg

Split Pea Curry

(**Serves:** 3 / **Prep Time:** 10 minutes / **Cooking Time:** 14 minutes)

Ingredients

- ½ tablespoon olive oil
- ½ medium white onion, diced
- ½ medium carrot, diced into small cubes
- ½ celery stick, diced into cubes
- 3 garlic cloves, diced finely
- 1 bay leaf
- ½ teaspoon paprika powder
- ¾ teaspoon cumin powder
- ¼ teaspoon salt
- ⅛ teaspoon cinnamon powder
- ⅛ teaspoon chili powder or cayenne pepper
- 1 cup split yellow peas, rinsed well
- ¼ cup chopped tinned tomatoes
- 2 tablespoons lemon juice
- 2 cups vegetable stock

How to

1. Add oil, onion, celery and garlic to the Instant Pot and "Sauté" for 4 minutes.
2. Add all the remaining ingredients to the cooker.
3. Cover and secure the lid. Turn its pressure release handle to the sealing position.
4. Cook on the "Manual" function with high pressure for 10 minutes.
5. After the beep, do a Natural release and remove the lid.
6. Stir and serve.

Nutrition Values (Per Serving)

- Calories: 206
- Carbohydrate: 33.5g
- Protein: 11g
- Fat: 3.4g
- Sugar: 3.4g
- Sodium: 246mg

Fried Beans Mix

(**Serves:** 6 / **Prep Time:** 15 minutes / **Cooking Time:** 45 minutes)

Ingredients

- 1 lb. pinto beans, soaked and rinsed
- ¾ cup chopped onion
- 2 garlic cloves, roughly chopped
- ½ jalapeno, seeded and chopped
- 1 teaspoon dried oregano
- ¾ teaspoon ground cumin
- ¼ teaspoon ground black pepper
- 1 ½ tablespoons lard
- 2 cups vegetable broth
- 2 cups water
- ½ teaspoon sea salt

How to

1. Add all the ingredients to the Instant Pot.
2. Cover and secure the lid. Turn its pressure release handle to the sealing position.
3. Cook on the "Bean/Chilli" function for 45 minutes.
4. After the beep, do a Natural release for 20 minutes.
5. Let it cool, then use an immersion blender to puree the mixture.
6. Stir well and serve.

Nutrition Values (Per Serving)

- Calories: 314
- Carbohydrate: 49.6g
- Protein: 18.1g
- Fat: 4.7g
- Sugar: 2.5g
- Sodium: 423mg

Fennel Risotto

(**Serves:** 3 / **Prep Time:** 15 minutes / **Cooking Time:** 14 minutes)

Ingredients

- ½ medium brown onion, finely diced
- 1 tablespoon olive oil
- ¼ medium fennel, diced
- ¼ bunch of asparagus, diced
- ¼ teaspoon salt
- 1 garlic clove, chopped
- 1 cup Arborio risotto rice
- 3 tablespoons white wine
- Zest of ¼ lemon
- 1 cup vegetable stock
- 1 cup chicken stock
- 1 tablespoon butter
- ¼ cup grated Parmesan cheese

How to

1. Add oil, onion, fennel and asparagus to the Instant Pot and "Sauté" for 4 minutes.
2. Add all the remaining ingredients (except the cheese) to the cooker.
3. Cover and secure the lid. Turn its pressure release handle to the sealing position.
4. Cook on the "Manual" function with high pressure for 10 minutes.
5. After the beep, do a Natural release and remove the lid.
6. Stir in cheese and serve.

Nutrition Values (Per Serving)

- Calories: 238
- Carbohydrates: 24.1g
- Protein: 6.9g
- Fat: 17.5g
- Sugar: 1.8g
- Sodium: 528mg

Comforting Mexican Black Beans

(**Serves:** 3 / **Prep Time:** 10 minutes / **Cooking Time:** 22 minutes)

Ingredients

- ½ (15 oz.) can black beans, rinsed and drained
- ¼ cup brown rice
- ¾ cup water
- ¼ cup picante sauce
- 1 bay leaf
- ½ teaspoon cumin
- ½ teaspoon garlic salt
- Lime juice

How to

1. Add all the ingredients to the Instant Pot.
2. Cover and secure the lid. Turn its pressure release handle to the sealing position.
3. Cook on the "Manual" function with high pressure for 22 minutes.
4. After the beep, do a Natural release for 20 minutes.
5. Stir and serve hot with boiled white rice.

Nutrition Values (Per Serving)

- Calories: 103
- Carbohydrates: 20g
- Protein: 4.5g
- Fat: 0.6g
- Sugar: 1.4g
- Sodium: 155mg

Cilantro Rice

(**Serves:** 6 / **Prep Time:** 10 minutes / **Cooking Time:** 11 minutes)

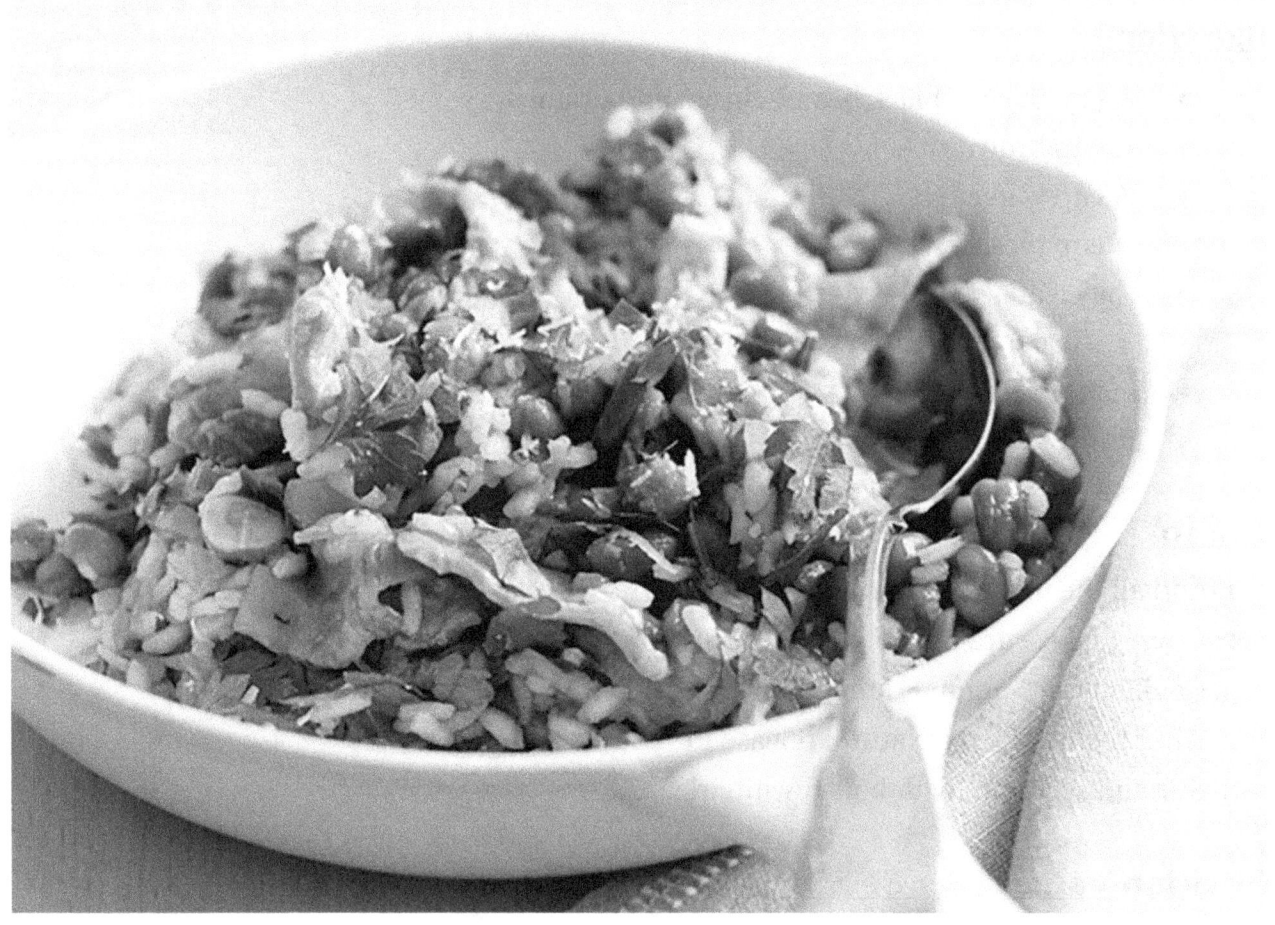

Ingredients

- ½ tablespoon butter
- ½ yellow onion, diced
- 1 garlic clove, minced
- 2 cups water
- 1 ⅓ cup white rice
- ½ tablespoon chicken bouillon
- ½ cup peas
- ½ teaspoon cumin
- 2 oz. can green chilies
- ¼ bunch cilantro, chopped
- ¾ teaspoon fresh lime juice
- Salt, to taste

How to

1. Add oil, onion and garlic to the Instant Pot and "Sauté" for 4 minutes.
2. Add all the remaining ingredients to the cooker.
3. Cover and secure the lid. Turn its pressure release handle to the sealing position.
4. Cook on the "Manual" function with high pressure for 7 minutes.
5. After the beep, do a Natural release and remove the lid.
6. Garnish with fresh cilantro and serve.

Nutrition Values (Per Serving)

- Calories: 167
- Carbohydrate: 34.8g
- Protein: 3.1g
- Fat: 1.3g
- Sugar: 0.9g
- Sodium: 84mg

Mung Bean Risotto

(**Serves:** 6 / **Prep Time:** 20 minutes / **Cooking Time:** 30 minutes)

Ingredients

- 1 ½ cup green mung beans
- 1 cup brown basmati rice
- 1 teaspoon coconut oil
- 1 teaspoon cumin seeds
- 1 red onion, chopped
- 2 cans crushed tomatoes
- 3 cloves of garlic
- 2-inch ginger, peeled and chopped
- 2 teaspoons turmeric
- 2 teaspoons ground coriander
- 1 teaspoon cayenne
- ½ teaspoon black pepper
- 8 cups water
- 2 teaspoons lemon juice
- 2 teaspoons salt

How to

1. Add tomatoes, garlic, onions, spices and 2 tablespoons water to a food processor and blend to form a puree.
2. Pour some oil into the Instant Pot and heat it on the "Sauté" setting.
3. "Sauté" the cumin seeds in the heated oil and stir in the tomato puree. Let it cook for 15 minutes.
4. Add the green mung beans and rice. Secure the lid.
5. Cook on the "Manual" function for 15 minutes at high pressure.
6. After the beep, do a Natural release and remove the lid.
7. Stir and serve with crackers.

Nutrition Values (Per Serving)

- Calories: 205
- Carbohydrate: 41g
- Protein: 7.2g
- Fat: 1.4g
- Sugar: 4.3g
- Sodium: 214mg

Bean Barley Stew

(**Serves:** 4 / **Prep Time:** 10 minutes / **Cooking Time:** 20 minutes)

Ingredients

- ½ cup chickpeas, soaked and rinsed
- ½ cup Cannellini beans, soaked and rinsed
- ¼ cup barley, soaked and rinsed
- 1 garlic clove, chopped
- ½ tablespoon olive oil
- 1 clove
- 4 pepper kernels
- 3 coriander seeds
- 2 cups water
- Salt and pepper to taste
- Tea infuser (to hold the spices)

How to

1. Add oil, water, garlic, barley, salt, chickpeas and the tea infuser (filled with all the spices) to the Instant Pot.
2. Set a steamer trivet above it and place the cannellini beans into it.
3. Secure the lid and select the "Manual" function with high pressure for 15 minutes.
4. After the beep, do a Natural release and remove the lid.
5. Remove the steamer trivet and transfer the beans to the pot.
6. Remove the tea infuser. Stir well and cook for 5 minutes on the "Sauté" setting.
7. Serve hot.

Nutrition Values (Per Serving)

- Calories: 196
- Carbohydrate: 32.1g
- Protein: 10.5g
- Fat: 3.5g
- Sugar: 3.2g
- Sodium: 161mg

Coconut Risotto

(**Serves:** 3 / **Prep Time:** 10 minutes / **Cooking Time:** 5 minutes)

Ingredients

- 2 cups coconut milk
- ½ cup Arborio (short-grain Italian) rice
- 2 tablespoons coconut sugar
- 1 teaspoon vanilla extract
- ¼ cup toasted coconut flakes

How to

1. Add all the ingredients to the Instant Pot.
2. Cover and secure the lid. Turn its pressure release handle to the sealing position.
3. Cook on the "Manual" function with high pressure for 5 minutes.
4. After the beep, do a Natural release for 20 minutes.
5. Garnish with coconut flakes and serve.

Nutrition Values (Per Serving)

- Calories: 532
- Carbohydrate: 42.1g
- Protein: 5.9g
- Fat: 40.4g
- Sugar: 13.9g
- Sodium: 25mg

Instant Black Bean Burrito

(**Serves:** 4 / **Prep Time:** 10 minutes / **Cooking Time:** 12 minutes)

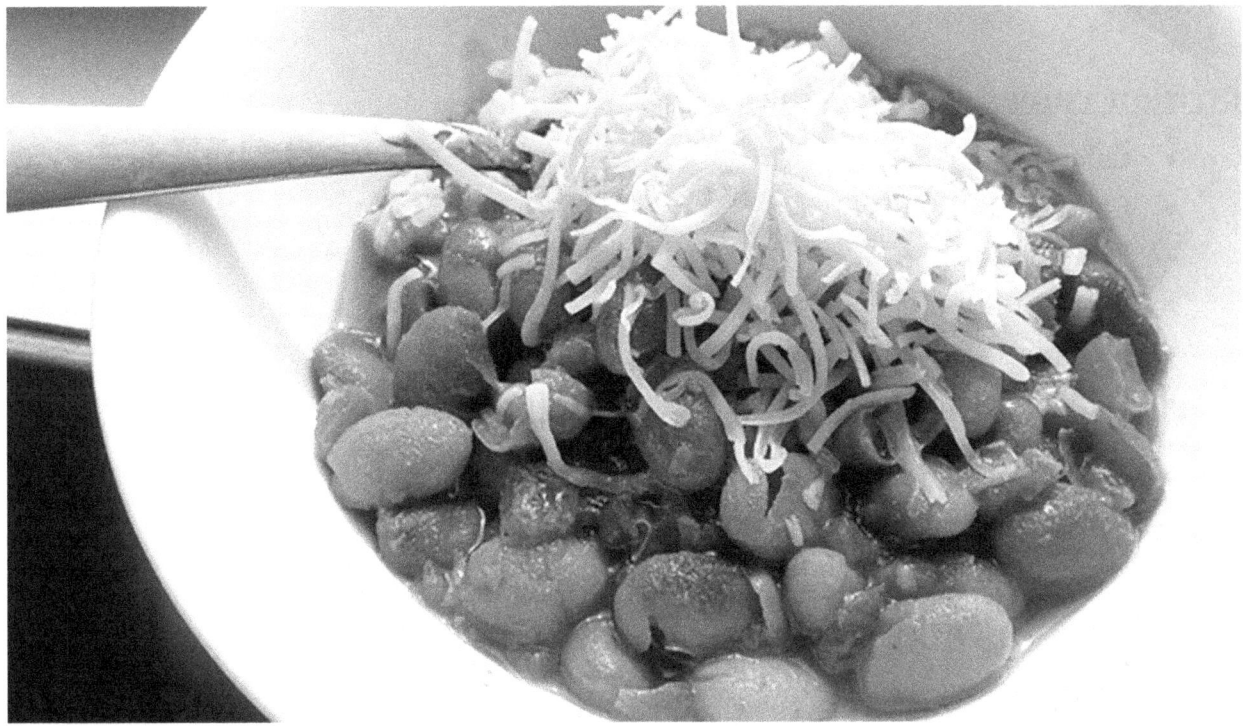

Ingredients

- ½ tablespoon olive oil
- ½ small onion, diced
- ½ garlic clove, minced
- ½ teaspoon chili powder
- ¼ teaspoon Kosher salt
- ¾ lb. boneless, skinless chicken thighs, cut into 1-inch pieces
- ½ can black beans, rinsed
- ½ cup long-grain white rice, uncooked
- ½ cup salsa
- 1 cup chicken broth
- 2 tablespoons chopped cilantro
- 2 tablespoons Cheddar cheese

How to

1. Add oil with onion and garlic to the Instant Pot and select "Sauté" to cook for 2 minutes.
2. Add all the remaining ingredients and secure the lid.
3. Cook on the "Manual" function for 10 minutes on high pressure.

4. After the beep, do a Natural release for 10 minutes, then release the remaining steam with a Quick release.
5. Garnish with chopped cilantro and shredded Cheddar.
6. Serve.

Nutrition Values (Per Serving)

- Calories: 320
- Carbohydrate: 23.5g
- Protein: 33.1g
- Fat: 33.1g
- Sugar: 2.1g
- Sodium: 633mg

Chipotle Lentil Curry

(**Serves:** 3 / **Prep Time:** 5 minutes / **Cooking Time:** 15 minutes)

Ingredients

- ½ medium onion, chopped
- ½ medium green bell pepper, chopped
- ½ tablespoon canola oil
- 1 garlic clove, chopped
- 1 ½ tablespoons chili powder
- 1 can (¼ oz.) diced tomatoes
- 2 cups vegetable broth
- 1 cup brown lentils, rinsed and picked over
- 1 chipotle in adobo sauce, seeded and chopped
- ¼ cup sun-dried tomatoes, chopped
- ½ teaspoon ground cumin
- Salt, to taste

How to

1. Add oil with onion and bell pepper to the Instant Pot and select "Sauté" to cook for 2 minutes.
3. Stir in garlic and chili powder, then sauté for 1 minute.
4. Add all the remaining ingredients and secure the lid.
5. Cook on the "Manual" function for 12 minutes on high pressure.
6. After the beep, do a Natural release for 10 minutes, then release the remaining steam with a Quick release.
7. Garnish with chopped cilantro and shredded Cheddar cheese.
8. Serve.

Nutrition Values (Per Serving)

- Calories: 204
- Carbohydrate: 29.8g
- Protein: 13.4g
- Fat: 5.2g
- Sugar: 10.8g
- Sodium: 687mg

Delicious Lentil Risotto

(**Serves:** 2 / **Prep Time:** 10 minutes / **Cooking Time:** 20 minutes)

Ingredients

- ½ cup dry lentils, soaked overnight
- ½ tablespoon olive oil
- ½ medium onion, chopped
- ½ celery stalk, chopped
- 1 sprig parsley, chopped
- ½ cup Arborio (short-grain Italian) rice
- 1 garlic clove, lightly mashed
- 2 cups vegetable stock

How to

1. Add oil and onions to the Instant Pot and "Sauté" for 5 minutes.
2. Add all the remaining ingredient to the Instant Pot.
3. Cover and secure the lid. Turn its pressure release handle to the sealing position.
4. Cook on the "Manual" function with high pressure for 15 minutes.
5. After the beep, do a Natural release for 20 minutes.
6. Stir and serve hot with boiled white rice.

Nutrition Values (Per Serving)

- Calories: 260
- Carbohydrate: 47.2g
- Protein: 10.7g
- Fat: 3.5g
- Sugar: 2.2g
- Sodium: 247mg

Bean Mustard Curry

(**Serves:** 4 / **Prep Time:** 10 minutes / **Cooking Time:** 14 minutes)

Ingredients

- ½ cup ketchup
- 2 tablespoons molasses
- 2 teaspoons mustard powder
- ¼ teaspoon ground black pepper
- 1 ½ slices bacon, chopped
- ½ medium onion, chopped
- ½ small green bell pepper, chopped
- 1 ½ cans navy beans, rinsed and drained
- 1 teaspoon apple cider vinegar

How to

1. Select the "Sauté" function on your Instant Pot and add the oil with onion, bacon and bell pepper. Cook for 6 minutes.
2. Add all the remaining ingredients and secure the lid.
3. Cook on the "Manual" function for 8 minutes on high pressure.
4. After the beep, do a Natural release for 10 minutes, then release the remaining steam with a Quick release.
5. Garnish with chopped cilantro on top.
6. Serve.

Nutrition Values (Per Serving)

- Calories: 373
- Carbohydrate: 64.5g
- Protein: 21.2g
- Fat: 4.7g
- Sugar: 16.1g
- Sodium: 507mg

Lime Rich Rice

(Serves: 8 / **Prep Time:** 5 minutes / **Cooking Time:** 5 minutes)

Ingredients

- 2 ½ cups vegetable broth
- 2 cups long-grain white rice, rinsed
- 2 tablespoons lemon juice
- Freshly ground black pepper, to taste
- 4 tablespoons Parmesan cheese, grated freshly
- 2 teaspoons fresh lemon zest, grated finely
- 4 tablespoons fresh mint leaves, chopped

How to

1. Add rice, broth, black pepper and lemon juice to the Instant Pot.
2. Cover and secure the lid. Turn its pressure release handle to the sealing position.
3. Cook on the "Manual" function with high pressure for 5 minutes.
4. After the beep, do a Natural release for 7 minutes.
5. Stir in lemon zest and cheese. Mix well.
6. Garnish with fresh mint and serve.

Nutrition Values (Per Serving)

- Calories: 228
- Carbohydrate: 38.2g
- Protein: 9.5g
- Fat: 3.8g
- Sugar: 0.4g
- Sodium: 372mg

White Bean Curry

(**Serves:** 6 / **Prep time:** 5 minutes / **Cooking time:** 30 minutes)

Ingredients

- 1 lb. white beans, soaked and rinsed
- ½ teaspoon red pepper
- ½ teaspoon ground turmeric
- 1 tablespoon onion powder
- 2 teaspoons garlic powder
- 1-2 teaspoons salt
- 1 bay leaf
- 6 cups unsalted vegetable broth

How to

1. Add all the ingredients to the Instant Pot.
2. Cover and secure the lid. Turn its pressure release handle to the sealing position.
3. Cook on the "Bean/Chilli" function on the default settings.
4. After the beep, do a Natural release for 20 minutes.
5. Stir and serve hot with boiled white rice.

Nutrition Values (Per Serving)

- Calories: 286
- Carbohydrate: 54.1g
- Protein: 19.1g
- Fat: 1.2g
- Sugar: 5.2g
- Sodium: 612mg

Delectable Rice Pilaf

(**Serves:** 8 / **Prep Time:** 5 minutes / **Cooking Time:** 10 minutes)

Ingredients

- 4 cups raw short-grain white rice, rinsed
- 5 cups chicken stock
- 2 rice wine
- 2 tablespoons vegetable oil
- 2 cups leftover meat, chopped
- 4 potatoes, cubed
- 4 carrots, chopped
- 2 lbs. white mushrooms, halved
- 2 lbs. green beans, chopped
- 4 kale greens, chopped
- 2 tablespoons soy sauce
- 2 tablespoons oyster sauce
- Chopped green onion for garnish

How to

1. Add all the ingredients to the Instant Pot, except green onions and oyster sauce.
2. Cover and secure the lid. Turn its pressure release handle to the sealing position.
3. Cook on the "Bean/Chilli" function for 10 minutes.
4. After the beep, do a Natural release for 10 minutes.
5. Stir in oyster sauce and green onions. Let it sit for 5 minutes.
6. Serve hot.

Nutrition Values (Per Serving)

- Calories: 567
- Carbohydrate: 105.9g
- Protein: 24.7g
- Fat: 5.8g
- Sugar: 6.6g
- Sodium: 881mg

Pea & Corn Rice

(**Serves:** 3 / **Prep Time:** 5 minutes / **Cooking Time:** 8 minutes)

Ingredients

- 1 cup basmati rice, rinsed
- 1 ½ tablespoons olive oil
- ½ large onion, diced small
- Salt, to taste
- 1 ½ tablespoons chopped cilantro stalks
- 1 large garlic clove, finely diced
- ½ teaspoon turmeric powder
- ½ cup frozen sweet corn kernels
- ½ cup frozen garden peas
- ¾ cup chicken stock
- 1 dollop of butter

How to

1. Add oil and onions to the Instant Pot and "Sauté" for 5 minutes.
2. Stir in all the remaining ingredients except the butter.
3. Cover and secure the lid. Turn its pressure release handle to the sealing position.
4. Cook on the "Manual" function with high pressure for 3 minutes.
5. After the beep, do a Natural release for 7 minutes.
6. Stir in butter and let it melt into the rice.
7. Serve warm.

Nutrition Values (Per Serving)

- Calories: 356
- Carbohydrate: 61.3g
- Protein: 7.1g
- Fat: 9.2g
- Sugar: 3.6g
- Sodium: 363mg

Spanish Chorizo Red Beans

(**Serves:** 3 / **Prep time:** 5 minutes / **Cooking time:** 47 minutes)

Ingredients

- ½ tablespoon cooking oil
- 2 oz. dry (Spanish) chorizo
- ½ yellow onion
- 1 ½ garlic cloves
- 1 cup red beans, soaked and rinsed
- 1 bay leaf
- Freshly cracked pepper
- 1 ½ cups reduced sodium chicken broth
- 7 ½ oz. can diced tomatoes

How to

1. Add oil, chorizo, garlic and onion to the Instant Pot. "Sauté" for 5 minutes.
2. Stir in beans, pepper and bay leaf. Cook for 1 minute, then add the broth.
3. Cover and secure the lid. Turn its pressure release handle to the sealing position.
4. Cook on the "Manual" function with high pressure for 35 minutes.
5. After the beep, do a Natural release for 20 minutes.
6. Stir in diced tomatoes and cook for 7 minutes on the "Sauté" setting.
7. Serve hot with boiled white rice or tortilla chips.

Nutrition Values (Per Serving)

- Calories: 321
- Carbohydrate: 49.1g
- Protein: 21.4g
- Fat: 5.4g
- Sugar: 5.3g
- Sodium: 647mg

Vegetable Rice

(**Serves:** 3 / **Prep Time:** 15 minutes / **Cooking Time:** 12 minutes)

Ingredients

- 3 tablespoons olive oil
- ½ large onion, diced small
- ½ cup green bell pepper, chopped
- 1 cup basmati rice, rinsed
- ½ cup carrots, chopped
- ½ cup green onion, chopped
- 1 large garlic clove, finely diced
- ½ cup frozen garden peas
- ¾ cup vegetable stock
- Salt, to taste
- Black pepper, to taste

How to

1. Add oil and all the vegetables to the Instant Pot and "Sauté" for 7 minutes.
2. Stir in all the remaining ingredients except the butter.
3. Cover and secure the lid. Turn its pressure release handle to the sealing position.
4. Cook on the "Manual" function with high pressure for 5 minutes.
5. After the beep, do a Natural release for 7 minutes.
6. Stir and serve warm.

Nutrition Values (Per Serving)

- Calories: 423
- Carbohydrate: 61.2g
- Protein: 7.8g
- Fat: 12.9g
- Sugar: 5.9g
- Sodium: 298mg

Shrimp & Rice Paella

(**Serves:** 8 / **Prep Time:** 10 minutes / **Cooking Time:** 5 minutes)

Ingredients

- 32 oz. frozen wild-caught shrimp
- 16 oz. jasmine rice
- 4 oz. butter
- 4 oz. chopped fresh parsley
- 2 teaspoons sea salt
- ½ teaspoon black pepper
- 2 pinches crushed red pepper
- 2 medium lemons, juiced
- 2 pinches saffron
- 24 oz. chicken broth
- 8 garlic cloves, minced

How to

1. Add all the ingredients to the Instant Pot.
2. Place the shrimp on top.
3. Cover and secure the lid. Turn its pressure release handle to the sealing position.
4. Cook on the "Manual" function with high pressure for 5 minutes.
5. After the beep, do a Natural release for 7 minutes.
6. If needed, remove the shells of the shrimp and then add the shrimp back to the rice.
7. Stir and serve warm.

Nutrition Values (Per Serving)

- Calories: 437
- Carbohydrate: 49.1g
- Protein: 30.6g
- Fat: 13.7g
- Sugar: 0.8g
- Sodium: 1086mg

Coconut Rice

(**Serves:** 6 / **Prep Time:** 10 minutes / **Cooking Time:** 3 minutes)

Ingredients

- 1 ½ cups jasmine rice
- 1 can coconut milk
- ½ cup water
- 1 teaspoon sugar
- ¼ teaspoon salt

How to

1. Add all the ingredients to the Instant Pot.
2. Cover and secure the lid. Turn its pressure release handle to the sealing position.
3. Cook on the "Manual" function with high pressure for 3 minutes.
4. After the beep, do a Natural release for 7 minutes.
5. Serve warm.

Nutrition Values (Per Serving)

- Calories: 255
- Carbohydrate: 38.9g
- Protein: 3.9g
- Fat: 9.5g
- Sugar: 2g
- Sodium: 103mg

Black Beans with Chorizo

(**Serves:** 3 / **Prep time:** 5 minutes / **Cooking time:** 47 minutes)

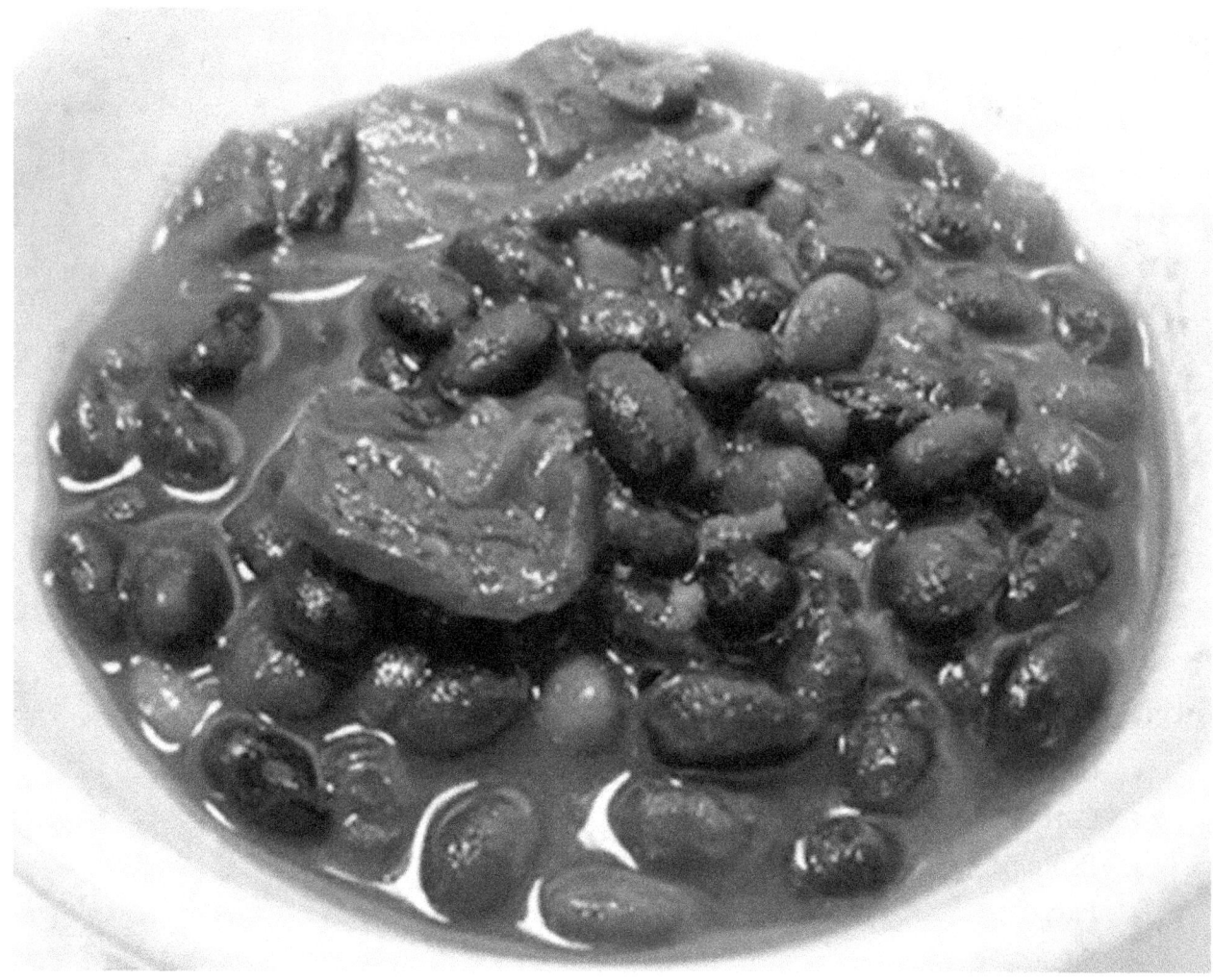

Ingredients

- ½ tablespoon cooking oil
- 2 oz. dry (Spanish) chorizo
- ½ yellow onion
- 1 ½ garlic cloves
- 1 cup black beans, soaked and rinsed
- 1 bay leaf
- ½ teaspoon cracked pepper
- 1 ½ cups reduced sodium chicken broth
- 7 ½ oz. can diced tomatoes

How to

1. Add oil, chorizo, garlic and onion to the Instant Pot. "Sauté" for 5 minutes.
2. Stir in beans, pepper and bay leaf. Cook for 1 minute, then add the broth.
3. Cover and secure the lid. Turn its pressure release handle to the sealing position.
4. Cook on the "Manual" function with high pressure for 35 minutes.
5. After the beep, do a Natural release in 20 minutes.
6. Stir in diced tomatoes and cook for 7 minutes on the "Sauté" setting.
7. Serve hot with boiled white rice or tortilla chips.

Nutrition Values (Per Serving)

- Calories: 324
- Carbohydrate: 48.8g
- Protein: 21.3g
- Fat: 5.6g
- Sugar: 5.3g
- Sodium: 647mg

Cumin Rice

(**Serves:** 3 / **Prep Time:** 10 minutes / **Cooking Time:** 5 minutes)

Ingredients

- 1 ½ cups jasmine rice
- 2 cups water
- ½ teaspoon salt
- 2 teaspoons cumin seeds
- 1 tablespoon butter

How to

1. Add butter and cumin seeds to the Instant Pot. "Sauté" for 2 minutes.
2. Add all the remaining ingredients to the cooker.
3. Cover and secure the lid. Turn its pressure release handle to the sealing position.
4. Cook on the "Manual" function with high pressure for 3 minutes.
5. After the beep, do a Natural release for 7 minutes.
6. Serve warm.

Nutrition Values (Per Serving)

- Calories: 359
- Carbohydrate: 72.6g
- Protein: 6.3g
- Fat: 4.2g
- Sugar: 0g
- Sodium: 422mg

Brown Chicken Rice

(**Serves:** 6 / **Prep Time:** 10 minutes / **Cooking Time:** 33 minutes)

Ingredients

- 1 medium onion
- 3 garlic cloves
- 2 cups baby carrots
- 2 cups cremini mushrooms
- 2 cups brown rice, raw
- 1 tablespoon olive oil
- 2 ¼ cups chicken broth
- 2 lbs. chicken thigh, boneless, skinless
- ⅛ teaspoon salt
- ⅛ teaspoon ground black pepper
- 10 oz. soup, cream of chicken, canned, condensed
- 2 tablespoons Worcestershire sauce
- 1 tablespoon fresh thyme

How to

1. Add oil, garlic, vegetables and onions to the Instant Pot. "Sauté" for 2 minutes.
2. Add all the remaining ingredients to the cooker. Place the chicken pieces on top.
3. Cover and secure the lid. Turn its pressure release handle to the sealing position.
4. Cook on the "Manual" function with high pressure for 31 minutes.
5. After the beep, do a Natural release for 7 minutes.
6. Remove the chicken and shred its meat. Add the meat back to the rice.
7. Stir and serve warm.

Nutrition Values (Per Serving)

- Calories: 606
- Carbohydrate: 58.8g
- Protein: 52.4g
- Fat: 16.6g
- Sugar: 4.7g
- Sodium: 897mg

Mushroom Risotto

(**Serves:** 2 / **Prep Time:** 10 minutes / **Cooking Time:** 20 minutes)

Ingredients

- ½ cup cremini mushrooms, sliced
- ½ tablespoon olive oil
- ½ medium onion, chopped
- ½ celery stalk, chopped
- 1 sprig parsley, chopped
- ½ cup Arborio (short-grain Italian) rice
- 1 garlic clove, lightly mashed
- 2 cups vegetable stock

How to

1. Add oil and onions to the Instant Pot and "Sauté" for 5 minutes.
2. Add all the remaining ingredients to the Instant Pot.
3. Cover and secure the lid. Turn its pressure release handle to the sealing position.
4. Cook on the "Manual" function with high pressure for 15 minutes.
5. After the beep, do a Natural release for 20 minutes.
6. Stir and serve hot with boiled white rice.

Nutrition Values (Per Serving)

- Calories: 226
- Carbohydrate: 42.7g
- Protein: 4.4g
- Fat: 3.9g
- Sugar: 2.3g
- Sodium: 59mg

Mexican-Style Rice

(**Serves:** 3 / **Prep Time:** 10 minutes / **Cooking Time:** 11 minutes)

Ingredients

- 1 tablespoon avocado oil
- ¼ cup onion, chopped
- 2 garlic cloves, finely chopped
- 1 cup long-grain white rice
- ½ teaspoon salt
- 2 tablespoons crushed tomatoes
- 2 cups chicken stock
- ¼ teaspoon cumin
- ¼ teaspoon garlic powder
- ¼ teaspoon smoked paprika
- 2 tablespoons cilantro, chopped
- 2 tablespoons sun-dried tomatoes

How to

1. Add oil, onion and garlic to the Instant Pot. "Sauté" for 3 minutes.
2. Stir in rice and mix well with the onion.
3. Add all the remaining ingredients to the cooker.
4. Cover and secure the lid. Turn its pressure release handle to the sealing position.
5. Cook on the "Manual" function with high pressure for 8 minutes.
6. After the beep, do a Natural release.
7. Stir and serve warm.

Nutrition Values (Per Serving)

- Calories: 252
- Carbohydrate: 53.1g
- Protein: 5.6g
- Fat: 1.5g
- Sugar: 1.9g
- Sodium: 922mg

Sausage Mushroom Rice

(**Serves:** 8 / **Prep Time:** 10 minutes / **Cooking Time:** 38 minutes)

Ingredients

- 1 cup dried shrimp, soaked
- 8 Chinese dried mushrooms, soaked
- 6 Chinese sausages, diced
- 4 tablespoons cooking oil
- 2 onions, minced
- 4 ½ cups brown rice, rinsed and drained
- 6 cups chicken or vegetable broth
- ½ cup chopped cilantro

How to

1. Add oil and onion to the Instant Pot. "Sauté" for 3 minutes.
2. Stir in mushrooms, sausages and shrimp. Sauté for 5 minutes.
3. Add all the remaining ingredients to the cooker.
4. Cover and secure the lid. Turn its pressure release handle to the sealing position.
5. Cook on the "Manual" function with high pressure for 30 minutes.
6. After the beep, do a Natural release and remove the lid.
7. Stir and serve warm.

Nutrition Values (Per Serving)

- Calories: 768
- Carbohydrate: 95.8g
- Protein: 51.4g
- Fat: 19.3g
- Sugar: 1.5g
- Sodium: 303mg

Saucy Red Beans

(**Serves:** 6 / **Prep time:** 5 minutes / **Cooking time:** 30 minutes)

Ingredients

- 1 lb. red beans, soaked and rinsed
- ½ teaspoon red pepper
- ½ teaspoon ground turmeric
- 1 tablespoon onion powder
- 2 teaspoons garlic powder
- 1-2 teaspoons salt
- 1 bay leaf
- 6 cups unsalted vegetable broth

How to

1. Add all the ingredients to the Instant Pot.
2. Cover and secure the lid. Turn its pressure release handle to the sealing position.
3. Cook on the "Beans/Chilli" function on default settings.
4. After the beep, do a Natural release for 20 minutes.
5. Stir and serve hot with boiled white rice.

Nutrition Values (Per Serving)

- Calories: 282
- Carbohydrate: 54.1g
- Protein: 18.2g
- Fat: 1.3g
- Sugar: 5.4g
- Sodium: 634mg

Beef Rice

(Serves: 3 / **Prep Time:** 5 minutes / **Cooking Time:** 16 minutes**)**

Ingredients

- ½ tablespoon olive oil
- ½ lb. lean ground beef
- ½ cup diced red onion
- ½ teaspoon chili powder
- ¼ teaspoon ground cumin
- ¼ teaspoon salt
- ½ cup long-grain white rice, rinsed well and drained
- 1 cup water
- 1 cup chunky salsa
- 1 cup black beans, rinsed and drained
- ½ cup cooked corn kernels
- 1 tablespoon chopped fresh cilantro
- ½ cup shredded Cheddar cheese

How to

1. Add oil and onion to the Instant Pot. "Sauté" for 3 minutes.
2. Stir in beef, cumin, salt and chili powder. Sauté for 5 minutes.
3. Add all the remaining ingredients to the cooker.
4. Cover and secure the lid. Turn its pressure release handle to the sealing position.
5. Cook on the "Manual" function with high pressure for 8 minutes.
6. After the beep, do a Natural release and remove the lid.
7. Stir and serve warm.

Nutrition Values (Per Serving)

- Calories: 378
- Carbohydrate: 43.5g
- Protein: 31.6g
- Fat: 8.8g
- Sugar: 5g
- Sodium: 868mg

Cauliflower Risotto

(**Serves:** 8 / **Prep Time:** 10 minutes / **Cooking Time:** 33 minutes)

Ingredients

- 2 small heads of cauliflower, cut in chunks
- 6 tablespoons olive oil, divided
- Salt and freshly ground black pepper, to taste
- 1 cup freshly grated Parmesan, divided
- 2 tablespoons olive oil
- 2 large onions, diced
- 4 garlic cloves, minced
- 2 cups pearl barley
- 6 cups vegetable or chicken broth
- 4 sprigs thyme
- 2 tablespoons butter
- 4 tablespoons chopped fresh parsley

How to

1. Add oil, garlic and onion to the Instant Pot. "Sauté" for 3 minutes.
2. Stir in cauliflower chunks and "Sauté" for 5 minutes.
3. Add all the remaining ingredients to the cooker, except the cheese and butter.
4. Cover and secure the lid. Turn its pressure release handle to the sealing position.
5. Cook on the "Manual" function with high pressure for 25 minutes.
6. After the beep, do a Natural release and remove the lid.
7. Stir in butter and cheese.
8. Serve warm.

Nutrition Values (Per Serving)

- Calories: 372
- Carbohydrate: 48.2g
- Protein: 8.4g
- Fat: 18.8g
- Sugar: 1g
- Sodium: 69mg

Vegetable & Corn Rice

(**Serves:** 3 / **Prep Time:** 5 minutes / **Cooking Time:** 9 minutes)

Ingredients

- 1 cup basmati rice, rinsed
- 1 ½ tablespoons olive oil
- ½ large onion, diced small
- Salt, to taste
- 1 ½ tablespoons chopped cilantro stalks
- 1 large garlic clove, finely diced
- ½ heaped teaspoon turmeric powder
- ½ cup frozen sweet corn kernels
- ½ cup carrots, chopped
- ¼ cup green onions, chopped
- ¼ cup bell peppers, chopped
- ½ cup frozen garden peas
- 1 cup chicken stock
- Dollop of butter, to finish

How to

1. Add oil and all the vegetables to the Instant Pot and "Sauté" for 5 minutes.
2. Stir in all the remaining ingredients except the butter.
3. Cover and secure the lid. Turn its pressure release handle to the sealing position.
4. Cook on the "Manual" function with high pressure for 4 minutes.
5. After the beep, do a Natural release for 7 minutes.
6. Stir in butter and let it melt into the rice.
7. Serve warm.

Nutrition Values (Per Serving)

- Calories: 423
- Carbohydrate: 66g
- Protein: 7.8g
- Fat: 14.9g
- Sugar: 5.9g
- Sodium: 298mg

Yellow Potato Rice

(**Serves:** 3 / **Prep Time:** 5 minutes / **Cooking Time:** 10 minutes)

Ingredients

- 1 cup basmati rice, rinsed
- 1 ½ tablespoons olive oil
- ½ large onion, diced small
- Salt, to taste
- 3 medium-sized potatoes, diced
- 1 ½ tablespoons chopped cilantro stalks
- 1 large garlic clove, finely diced
- ½ teaspoon turmeric powder
- 1 cup chicken stock
- 1 teaspoon butter

How to

1. Add oil and all the vegetables to the Instant Pot and "Sauté" for 5 minutes.
2. Stir in all the remaining ingredients except the butter.
3. Cover and secure the lid. Turn its pressure release handle to the sealing position.
4. Cook on the "Manual" function with high pressure for 5 minutes.
5. After the beep, do a Natural release for 7 minutes.
6. Stir in butter and let it melt into the rice.
7. Serve warm.

Nutrition Values (Per Serving)

- Calories: 466
- Carbohydrate: 86.1g
- Protein: 9g
- Fat: 9.2g
- Sugar: 3.9g
- Sodium: 339mg

Mung Bean Curry

(**Serves:** 4 / **Prep Time:** 10 minutes / **Cooking Time:** 25 minutes)

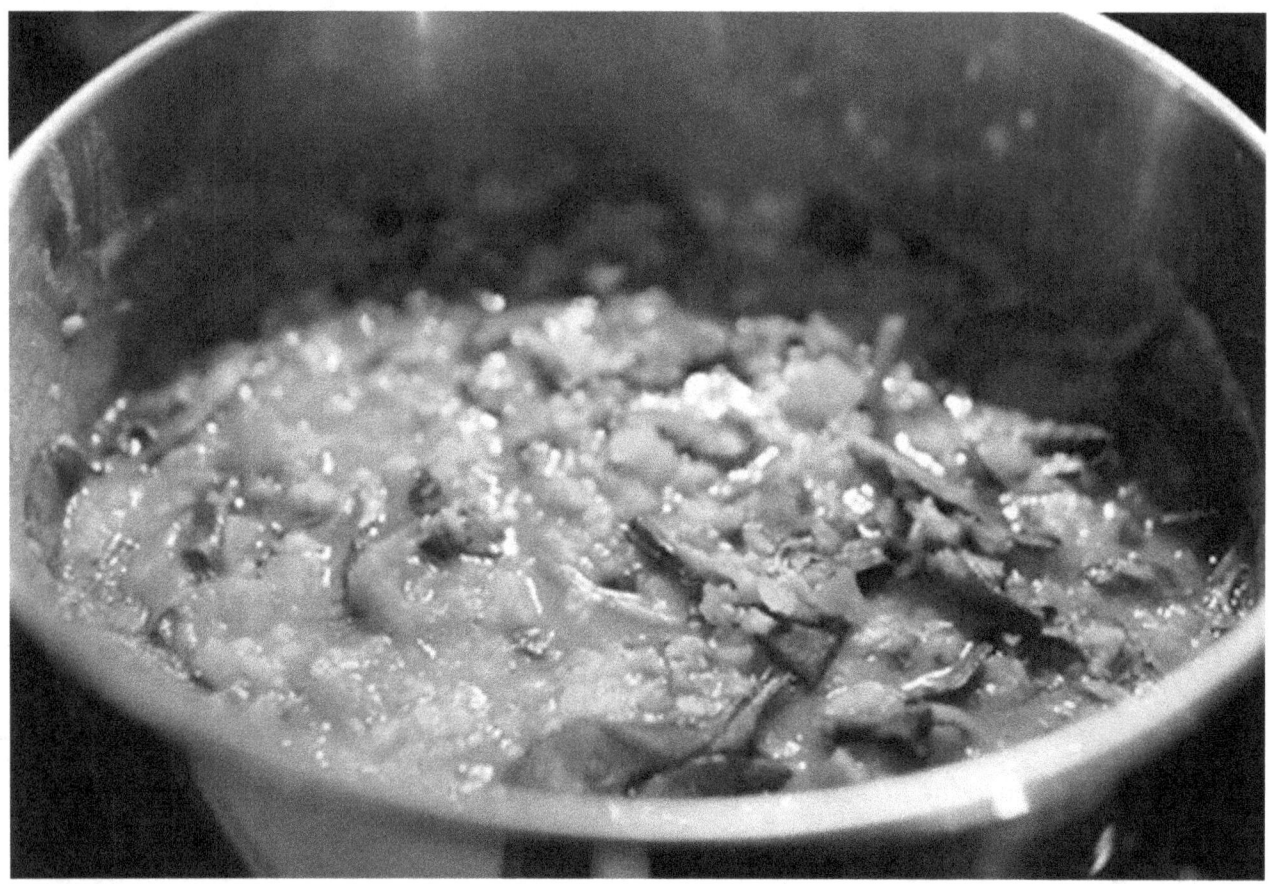

Ingredients

- ½ cup raw mung beans
- 1 ½ tablespoons cooking oil
- ½ cup chopped onions
- 1 bay leaf
- ½ tablespoon grated garlic
- ¼ tablespoon grated ginger
- ¾ cup water
- 1 cup vegetable broth
- ¼ teaspoon turmeric
- ½ teaspoon coriander powder
- 1 teaspoon chili powder
- 1 cup chopped baby spinach
- Salt, to taste

How to

1. Add the oil and onions to the Instant Pot. "Sauté" for 5 minutes.
2. Stir ginger, garlic paste and bay leaf. Cook for 1 minute, then add all the spices.
3. Put the mung beans, broth and water to the pot.
4. Cover and secure the lid. Turn its pressure release handle to the sealing position.
5. Cook on the "Manual" function with high pressure for 15 minutes.
6. After the beep, do a Natural release for 20 minutes.
7. Stir in spinach and cook for 3 minutes on the "Sauté" setting.
8. Serve hot with boiled white rice.

Nutrition Values (Per Serving)

- Calories: 158
- Carbohydrate: 19.2g
- Protein: 8g
- Fat: 5.9g
- Sugar: 2.6g
- Sodium: 248mg

Flavorsome Bacon Rice

(**Serves:** 8 / **Prep Time:** 10 minutes / **Cooking Time:** 38 minutes)

Ingredients

- 8 bacon strips, chopped
- 8 dried mushrooms, soaked
- 4 tablespoons cooking oil
- 2 onions, minced
- 4 ½ cups brown rice, rinsed and drained
- 6 cups vegetable broth
- ½ cup chopped cilantro

How to

1. Add oil and onion to the Instant Pot. "Sauté" for 3 minutes.
2. Stir in mushrooms and bacon. "Sauté" for 5 minutes.
3. Add all the remaining ingredients to the cooker.
4. Cover and secure the lid. Turn its pressure release handle to the sealing position.
5. Cook on the "Manual" function with high pressure for 30 minutes.
6. After the beep, do a Natural release and remove the lid.
7. Stir and serve warm.

Nutrition Values (Per Serving)

- Calories: 594
- Carbohydrate: 85.6g
- Protein: 19.6g
- Fat: 18.6g
- Sugar: 2g
- Sodium: 1018mg

Scrumptious Black-Eyed Peas

(**Serves:** 4 / **Prep Time:** 10 minutes / **Cooking Time:** 14 minutes)

Ingredients

- ½ cup ketchup
- 2 tablespoons molasses
- 2 teaspoons mustard powder
- ¼ teaspoon ground black pepper
- 1 ½ slices thick-cut bacon, chopped
- ½ medium onion, chopped
- ½ small green bell pepper, chopped
- 1 ½ cans black-eyed peas, soaked and rinsed
- 1 teaspoon apple cider vinegar

How to

1. Select the "Sauté" function on your Instant Pot and add oil with onion, bacon and bell pepper. Cook for 6 minutes.
2. Add all the remaining ingredients and secure the lid.
3. Cook on the "Manual" function for 8 minutes on high pressure.
4. After the beep, do a Natural release for 10 minutes, then release the remaining steam with a Quick release.
5. Garnish with chopped cilantro on top.
6. Serve.

Nutrition Values (Per Serving)

- Calories: 512
- Carbohydrate: 15g
- Protein: 44.2g
- Fat: 13.7g
- Sugar: 9.3g
- Sodium: 194mg

Chickpea Tacos

(**Serves:** 6 / **Prep Time:** 10 minutes / **Cooking Time:** 31 minutes)

Ingredients

- ½ cup raw chickpeas
- 1 ½ tablespoons cooking oil
- ½ cup chopped onions
- ½ tablespoon grated garlic
- ¼ tablespoon grated ginger
- ¾ cup water
- ½ cup fresh tomato puree
- ½ green chili, finely chopped
- ¼ teaspoon turmeric
- ½ teaspoon coriander powder
- 1 teaspoon chili powder
- ½ carrot, shredded
- ½ cup green bell pepper, sliced
- Salt, to taste
- 1 tablespoon fresh cilantro
- 6 tortillas

How to

1. Add oil and onions to the Instant Pot. "Sauté" for 5 minutes.
2. Stir ginger, garlic paste and green chili. Cook for 1 minute, then add all the spices.
3. Add chickpeas, tomato puree and water to the pot.
4. Cover and secure the lid. Turn its pressure release handle to the sealing position.
5. Cook on the "Manual" function with high pressure for 15 minutes.
6. After the beep, do a Natural release in 20 minutes.
7. Stir in shredded carrots and bell pepper. Cook for 10 minutes on the "Sauté" setting.
8. Fill the tortillas with prepared filling and serve.

Nutrition Values (Per Serving)

- Calories: 165
- Carbohydrate: 25.7g
- Protein: 5.3g
- Fat: 5.3g
- Sugar: 4.3g
- Sodium: 58mg

Enticing Three-Bean Stew

(**Serves:** 3 / **Prep Time:** 10 minutes / **Cooking Time:** 14 minutes)

Ingredients

- ½ tablespoon olive oil
- ½ medium white onion, diced
- ½ medium carrot, diced into small cubes
- ½ celery stick, diced into cubes
- 3 garlic cloves, diced finely
- 1 bay leaf
- ½ teaspoon paprika powder
- ¾ teaspoon cumin powder
- ¼ teaspoon salt
- ⅛ teaspoon cinnamon powder
- ⅛ teaspoon chili powder or cayenne pepper
- ¼ cup black beans, soaked and rinsed
- ¼ cup red beans, soaked and rinsed
- ¼ cup white beans, soaked and rinsed
- ¼ cup chopped tinned tomatoes
- 2 tablespoons lemon juice
- 2 cups vegetable stock

How to

1. Add oil, onion, celery and garlic to the Instant Pot and "Sauté" for 4 minutes.
2. Add all the remaining ingredients to the cooker.
3. Cover and secure the lid. Turn its pressure release handle to the sealing position.
4. Cook on the "Manual" function with high pressure for 10 minutes.
5. After the beep, do a Natural release and remove the lid.
6. Stir and serve.

Nutrition Values (Per Serving)

- Calories: 213
- Carbohydrate: 35.6g
- Protein: 12g
- Fat: 3.3g
- Sugar: 3.6g
- Sodium: 251mg

Chickpea Rice

(**Serves:** 8 / **Prep Time:** 10 minutes / **Cooking Time:** 38 minutes)

Ingredients

- 8 bacon strips, chopped
- ½ cup chickpeas, soaked
- 4 tablespoons cooking oil
- 2 onions, minced
- 4 ½ cups brown rice, rinsed and drained
- 6 cups vegetable broth
- ½ cup chopped cilantro

How to

1. Add oil and onion to the Instant Pot. "Sauté" for 3 minutes.
2. Stir in bacon. Sauté for 5 minutes.
3. Add all the remaining ingredients to the cooker.
4. Cover and secure the lid. Turn its pressure release handle to the sealing position.
5. Cook on the "Manual" function with high pressure for 30 minutes.
6. After the beep, do a Natural release and remove the lid.
7. Stir and serve warm.

Nutrition Values (Per Serving)

- Calories: 637
- Carbohydrate: 92.6g
- Protein: 21.4g
- Fat: 19.4g
- Sugar: 3g
- Sodium: 1020mg

Corn Lentil Stew

(**Serves:** 3 / **Prep Time:** 10 minutes / **Cooking Time:** 14 minutes)

Ingredients

- ½ medium onion, chopped
- 1 medium carrot, sliced
- 3 ½ cups water
- ⅓ cup dried lentils
- 1 medium tomato
- ½ cup fresh or frozen corn
- 1 tablespoon tamari or soy sauce
- ½ cup cooked brown rice
- Salt and pepper, to taste

How to

1. Add oil, onion and carrots to the Instant Pot and "Sauté" for 4 minutes.
2. Add water, lentils, tomatoes and corn to the cooker.
3. Cover and secure the lid. Turn its pressure release handle to the sealing position.
4. Cook on the "Manual" function with high pressure for 10 minutes.
5. After the beep, do a Natural release and remove the lid.
6. Stir in cooked rice, tamari sauce, salt and pepper.
7. Serve warm.

Nutrition Values (Per Serving)

- Calories: 239
- Carbohydrate: 47.4g
- Protein: 10.1g
- Fat: 1.5g
- Sugar: 4.2g
- Sodium: 367mg

VEGETABLES & SIDE DISHES

Spaghetti Squash

(**Serves**: 2 / **Prep time:** 5 minutes / **Cooking time**: 20 minutes)

Ingredients

- 1 (2 lbs.) spaghetti squash
- 1 cup water
- Cilantro to serve

How to

1. Slice the squash in half. Remove the seeds from its center.
2. Pour a cup of water into the insert of the Instant Pot and place the trivet inside.
3. Arrange the two halves of the squash over the trivet, with the skin side down.
4. Secure the lid and select "Manual" with high pressure for 20 minutes.
5. After the beep, do a Natural release and remove the lid.
6. Remove the squash and use two forks to shred it from inside.
7. Serve with fresh cilantro or spicy pork filling if needed.

Nutrition Values (Per Serving)

- Calories: 146
- Carbohydrate: 32.2g
- Protein: 3.4g
- Fat: 2.6g
- Sugar: 0.5g
- Sodium: 93mg

Cucumber Quinoa Salad

(**Serves**: 4 / **Prep Time:** 10 minutes / **Cooking Time**: 1 minute)

Ingredients

- ½ cup quinoa, rinsed
- ¾ cup water
- ¼ teaspoon salt
- ½ carrot, peeled and shredded
- ½ cucumber, chopped
- ½ cup frozen edamame, thawed
- 3 green onions, chopped
- 1 cup shredded red cabbage
- ½ tablespoon soy sauce
- 1 tablespoon lime juice
- 2 tablespoons sugar
- 1 tablespoon vegetable oil
- 1 tablespoon freshly grated ginger
- 1 tablespoon sesame oil
- pinch of red pepper flakes
- ½ cup peanuts, chopped
- ¼ cup freshly chopped cilantro
- 2 tablespoons chopped basil

How to

1. Add the quinoa, salt, and water to the Instant Pot.
2. Secure the lid and select the "Manual" function with high pressure for 1 minute.
3. After the beep, do a quick release and remove the lid.
4. Meanwhile, add the remaining ingredients to a bowl and mix well.
5. Add the cooked quinoa to the prepared mixture and mix well.
6. Serve as a salad.

Nutrition Values (Per Serving)

- Calories: 320
- Carbohydrate: 31.2g
- Protein: 12.1g
- Fat: 18.5g
- Sugar: 9.1g
- Sodium: 279mg

Saucy Baked Beans

(**Serves**: 4 / **Prep time:** 10 minutes / **Cooking time**: 1 hour)

Ingredients

- 1 cup dry Navy beans (soaked for 8 hours and rinsed)
- ½ cup bacon, diced
- ¼ medium onion, diced
- ½ teaspoon sea salt
- ½ teaspoon pepper
- ½ teaspoon dry mustard
- ½ tablespoon Worcestershire sauce
- ½ tablespoon balsamic vinegar
- 1 tablespoon tomato paste
- 3 tablespoons dark brown sugar
- 3 tablespoons molasses
- ½ cup chicken stock
- ½ cup water

How to

1. Add the bacon to the Instant Pot and "Sauté" for 3 minutes until it turns crispy.
2. Remove the bacon and add onions to cook for 5 minutes with occasional stirring.
3. Stir in all the remaining ingredients.
4. Secure the lid and select the "Bean" function with 30 minutes cooking time.
5. After the beep, do a Natural release for 10 minutes, then remove the lid.
6. Stir in cooked bacon and cook for another 10 minutes on "Sauté" setting.
7. Serve hot.

Nutrition Values (Per Serving)

- Calories: 269
- Carbohydrate: 51.7g
- Protein: 13g
- Fat: 2g
- Sugar: 18.2g
- Sodium: 420mg

Quinoa Brussels Sprout Salad

(**Serves**: 4 / **Prep Time:** 10 minutes / **Cooking Time**: 1 minute)

Ingredients

- ½ cup cabbage, chopped
- ½ cup quinoa, rinsed
- ½ carrot, peeled and shredded
- ¾ cup water
- ¼ teaspoon salt
- 1 cup Brussels sprout, diced
- ½ cup red onions, sliced
- 1 tablespoon brown sugar
- 2 tablespoons, balsamic vinegar
- 1 tablespoon vegetable oil
- 1 tablespoon sunflower seeds
- 1 teaspoon ginger, grated
- 1 garlic clove, minced
- Black pepper to taste

How to

1. Add quinoa, salt, and water to the Instant Pot.
2. Secure the lid and select the "Manual" function with high pressure for 1 minute.
3. After the beep, do a quick release and remove the lid.
4. Meanwhile, add the remaining ingredients to a bowl and mix well.
5. Add the cooked quinoa to the prepared mixture and stir.
6. Serve as a salad.

Nutrition Values (Per Serving)

- Calories: 151
- Carbohydrate: 22.5g
- Protein: 4.4g
- Fat: 5.2g
- Sugar: 5.2g
- Sodium: 165mg

Mushrooms with Butternut Squash

(**Serves**: 4 / **Prep time:** 10 minutes / **Cooking time**: 40 minutes)

Ingredients

- 1 tablespoon olive oil
- ½ cup onion, chopped
- 3 garlic cloves, minced
- 1 red bell pepper, diced
- 2 cups butternut squash, peeled and diced
- 1 ½ cups Arborio rice*
- 3 ½ cup vegetable broth
- ½ cup dry white wine
- 8 oz. white mushrooms, sliced
- 1 teaspoon salt
- 1 teaspoon black pepper
- ¼ teaspoon oregano
- 1 ½ a tablespoon nutritional yeast

How to

1. Add the oil to the insert of the Instant Pot and select the "Sauté" function.
2. Put the onion, bell pepper, butternut squash, and garlic to the oil and sauté for 5 minutes.
3. Now stir in rice, broth, salt, pepper, mushrooms, oregano, coriander, and wine.
4. Secure the lid and select the "Bean" function with 30 minutes cooking time.
5. After the beep, do a Natural release for 10 minutes then remove the lid.
6. Add nutritional yeast, cook for another 5 minutes on "Sauté" setting.
7. Serve warm.

Nutrition Values (Per Serving)

- Calories: 422
- Carbohydrate: 72g
- Protein: 14.5g
- Fat: 5.5g
- Sugar: 5.5g
- Sodium: 1296g

(**Note: Arborio rice*** - Arborio rice is an Italian short-grain rice. It is named after the town of Arborio, in the Po Valley, which is situated in the main growing region. Arborio is also grown in Arkansas, California, and Missouri in the United States.)

Seasoned Potatoes

(**Serves**: 6 / **Prep Time:** 10 minutes / **Cooking Time**: 20 minutes)

Ingredients

- ½ cup avocado oil
- 3 lbs. russet potatoes
- 1 teaspoon onion powder
- 2 teaspoons garlic powder
- 2 teaspoons sea salt
- ½ teaspoon paprika
- ½ teaspoon ground black pepper
- 2 cups chicken broth

How to

1. Add oil to the insert of the Instant Pot and select "Sauté" function on it.
2. Add diced potatoes to the oil and sauté for 8 minutes.
3. Now stir in all the remaining ingredients.
4. Secure the lid and select the "Manual" function with 10 minutes cooking time.
5. After the beep, do a "Quick release" and remove the lid.
6. Sprinkle additional seasoning on top and serve.

Nutrition Values (Per Serving)

- Calories: 200
- Carbohydrate: 38.2g
- Protein: 5.9g
- Fat: 3.1g
- Sugar: 3.3g
- Sodium: 893mg

Maple-glazed Brussel Sprouts

(**Serves**: 4 / **Prep Time:** 10 minutes / **Cooking Time**: 4 minutes)

Ingredients

- 1 lb. Brussels sprouts (trimmed)
- 2 tablespoons freshly squeezed orange juice
- ½ teaspoon grated orange zest
- ½ tablespoon Earth Balance buttery spread
- 1 tablespoon maple syrup
- Black pepper, or to taste
- Salt, or to taste

How to

1. Add all the ingredients to the Instant Pot.
2. Secure the lid and select the "Manual" function for 4 minutes with high pressure.
3. Do a quick release after the beep then, remove the lid.
4. Stir well and serve immediately.

Nutrition Values (Per Serving)

- Calories: 166
- Carbohydrate: 14.5g
- Protein: 3.9g
- Fat: 11.4g
- Sugar: 6.1g
- Sodium: 149mg

Mayo Potato Salad

(**Serves**: 3 / **Prep Time:** 10 minutes / **Cooking Time**: 5 minutes)

Ingredients

- 3 medium russet potatoes, peeled and cubed
- 1 cup water
- 3 large eggs
- 1/8 cup finely chopped onion
- ½ cup mayonnaise
- 1 tablespoon finely chopped fresh parsley
- ½ tablespoon dill pickle juice
- ½ tablespoon mustard
- Salt and pepper to taste

How to

1. Pour a cup of water into the insert of the Instant Pot and place the steamer trivet inside.
2. Arrange the potatoes and eggs over the trivet.
3. Secure the lid and select the "Manual" function with high pressure for 4 minutes.
4. After the beep, do a Quick release and remove the lid.
5. Meanwhile, in a separate bowl combine onion, mayo, mustard, parsley, and pickle juice.
6. Add cooked potatoes and mix gently with the mixture.
7. Peel all the eggs and dice two to add to the mixture.
8. Serve with egg slices and sprinkled seasoning on top.

Nutrition Values (Per Serving)

- Calories: 383
- Carbohydrate: 44.7g
- Protein: 10.8g
- Fat: 18.8g
- Sugar: 5.7g
- Sodium: 638mg

Black Beans with Chorizo

(**Serves**: 4 / **Prep Time:** 5 minutes / **Cooking Time**: 32 minutes)

Ingredients

- ½ tablespoon vegetable oil
- 3 oz. Spanish-style chorizo, split
- ½ lb. dried black beans
- ½ medium onion, sliced
- 3 whole garlic cloves
- ½ orange, split in half
- 1 bay leaf
- 4 cups chicken stock
- Kosher salt to taste
- Chopped fresh cilantro, for serving

How to

1. Add oil and chorizo to the Instant Pot and "Sauté" for 2 minutes
2. Add all the remaining ingredients into the cooker.
3. Secure the lid and select the "Manual" function for 30 minutes with high pressure.
4. Do a quick release after the beep then remove the lid.
5. Remove and discard onion, bay leaf, and orange from the beans.
6. Stir and serve with fresh cilantro on top.

Nutrition Values (Per Serving)

- Calories: 336
- Carbohydrate: 60.6g
- Protein: 16.4g
- Fat: 3.8g
- Sugar: 4.1g
- Sodium: 1061mg

Quinoa Mushroom Salad

(**Serves**: 4 / **Prep Time:** 10 minutes / **Cooking Time**: 1 minute)

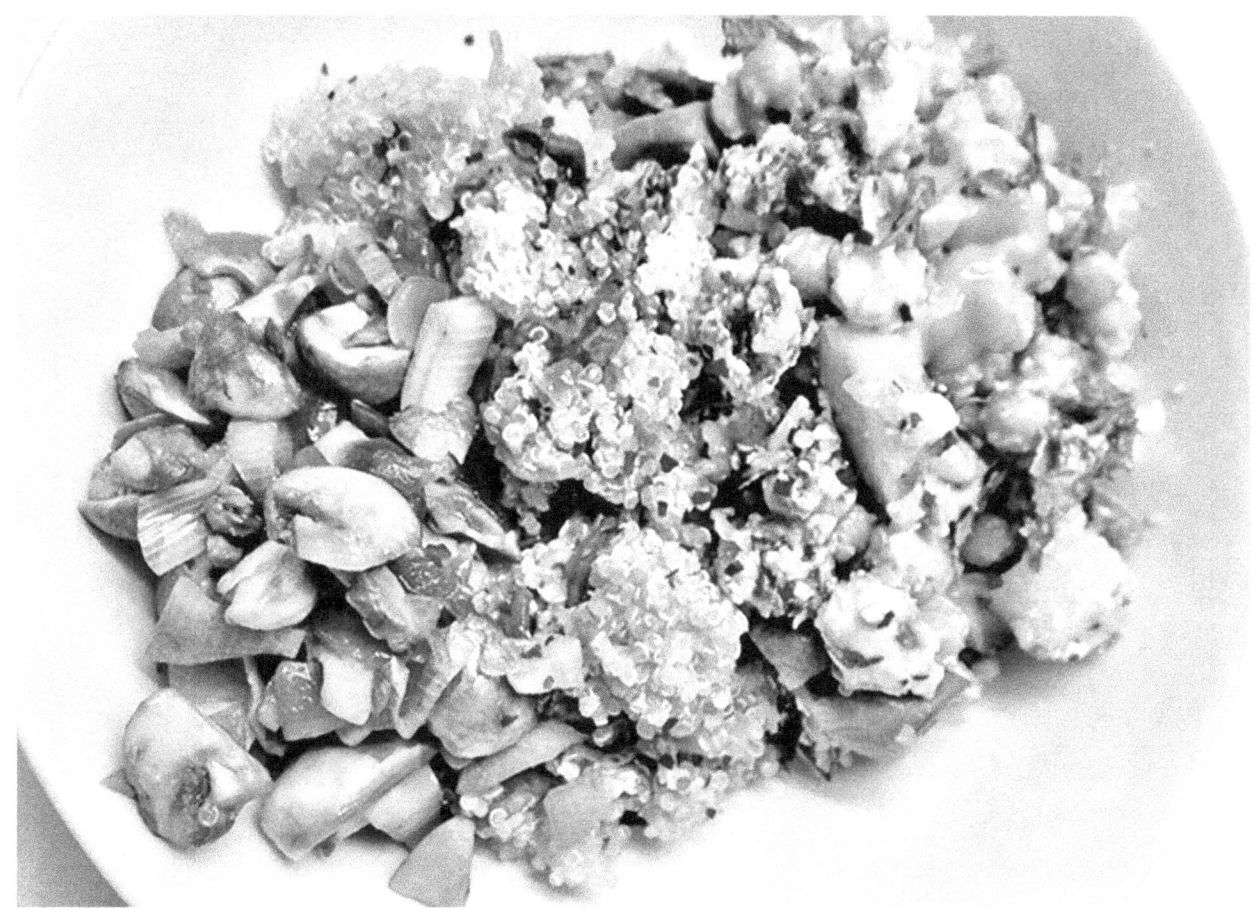

Ingredients

- ½ cup quinoa, rinsed
- ¾ cup water
- ¼ teaspoon salt
- ½ carrot, peeled and shredded
- ½ cup green onions
- ½ cup cremini mushrooms, diced
- 1 tablespoon lime juice
- 1 tablespoon vegetable oil
- 1 tablespoon freshly grated ginger
- 1 tablespoon sesame oil
- Pinch of red pepper flakes

How to

1. Add the quinoa, salt, and water to the Instant Pot.
2. Secure the lid and select the "Manual" function with high pressure for 1 minute.
3. After the beep, do a quick release and remove the lid.
4. Meanwhile, add the remaining ingredients to a bowl and mix well.
5. Add the cooked quinoa to the prepared mixture and mix well.
6. Serve as a salad.

Nutrition Values (Per Serving)

- Calories: 156
- Carbohydrate: 17.6g
- Protein: 3.7g
- Fat: 8.2g
- Sugar: 1.1g
- Sodium: 158mg

Tasty Cauliflower Rice

(**Serves**: 8 / **Prep Time:** 5 minutes / **Cooking Time**: 7 minutes)

Ingredients

- 2 medium heads of cauliflower, cut into chunks
- 4 tablespoons olive oil
- ½ teaspoon salt
- 1 teaspoon dried parsley
- ½ teaspoon cumin
- ½ teaspoon turmeric
- ½ teaspoon paprika
- Fresh cilantro

How to

1. Pour a cup of water into the insert of the Instant Pot.
2. Place the steamer trivet inside.
3. Arrange the cauliflower chunks over the trivet.
4. Secure the lid and select the "Manual" function with high pressure for 2 minutes.
5. After the beep, do a Quick release and remove the lid.
6. Remove the chunks and empty the Instant Pot.
7. Add the oil and cooked cauliflower into the cooker. Press the "Sauté" function key.
8. Use a potato masher to mash the cauliflower well.
9. Stir in all the remaining ingredients and "Sauté" for 5 minutes.
10. Serve with cilantro on top.

Nutrition Values (Per Serving)

- Calories: 161
- Carbohydrate: 4.2g
- Protein: 3.1g
- Fat: 16.1g
- Sugar: 2g
- Sodium: 378mg

Instant Sweet Potato

(**Serves**: 2 / **Prep Time:** 5 minutes / **Cooking Time**: 10 minutes)

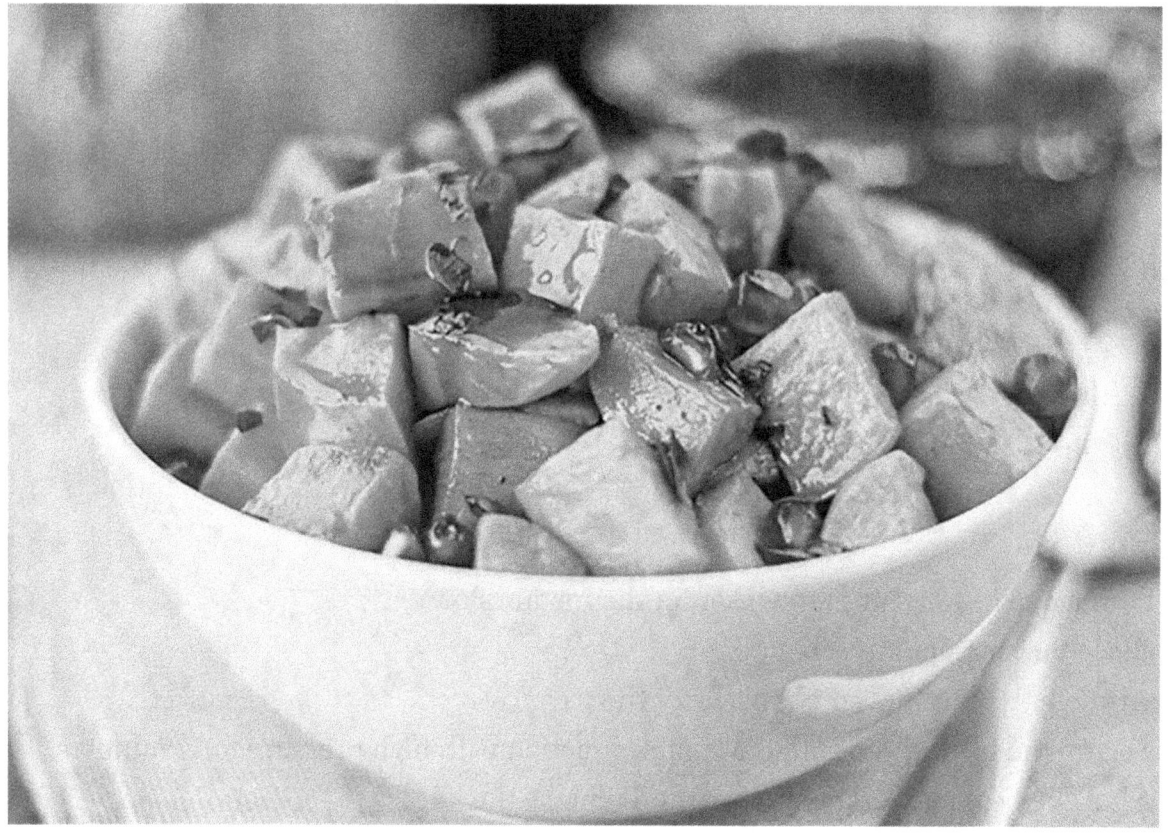

Ingredients

- 1 cup water
- 2 medium sweet potatoes, peeled
- Salt and pepper to taste
- 1 tablespoon olive oil

How to

1. Pour a cup of water into the insert of the Instant Pot.
2. Place the steamer trivet inside.
3. Arrange the sweet potatoes over the trivet.
4. Secure the lid and select "Steam" function for 10 minutes.
5. After the beep, do a Natural release and remove the lid.
6. Remove the potatoes and cut them into cubes.
7. Add oil and potatoes into the Instant Pot and "Sauté" for 5 minutes while stirring.
8. Garnish with parsley and pomegranate seeds.
9. Serve

Nutrition Values (Per Serving)

- Calories: 100
- Carbohydrate: 23g
- Protein: 2g
- Fat: 0g
- Sugar: 7g
- Sodium: 74mg

Instant Pot Mac & Cheese

(**Serves**: 4 / **Prep Time:** 5 minutes / **Cooking Time**: 4 minutes)

Ingredients

- ½ lb. pasta
- ½ teaspoon hot sauce
- 1 tablespoon butter
- ½ tablespoon dry mustard powder
- 2 cups water
- ½ cup of milk
- ½ lb. cheddar cheese
- ½ cup Monterey Jack cheese

How to

1. Add water, pasta, hot sauce, and dry mustard to the Instant Pot
2. Secure the lid and select the "Manual" function for 4 minutes with high pressure.
3. Do a quick release after the beep then remove the lid.
4. Strain the pasta and return it back to the pot. Select the "Sauté" function to cook.
5. Add cheese, milk, and butter to the pasta and let it melt.
6. Stir and serve.

Nutrition Values (Per Serving)

- Calories: 492
- Carbohydrate: 33.9g
- Protein: 25.4g
- Fat: 28.3g
- Sugar: 1.8g
- Sodium: 497mg

Quinoa Tomato Salad

(**Serves**: 4 / **Prep Time:** 10 minutes / **Cooking Time**: 1 minute)

Ingredients

- ½ cup quinoa, rinsed
- ¾ cup water
- ½ cup cherry tomatoes, sliced
- ¼ teaspoon salt
- ½ carrot, peeled and shredded
- ½ cucumber, chopped
- 3 green onions, chopped
- ½ tablespoon soy sauce
- 1 tablespoon lime juice
- 2 tablespoons sugar
- 1 tablespoon vegetable oil
- 1 tablespoon sesame oil
- pinch of red pepper flakes
- ½ cup peanuts, chopped
- ¼ cup freshly chopped cilantro
- 2 tablespoons chopped basil

How to

1. Add quinoa, salt, and water to the Instant Pot.
2. Secure the lid and select the "Manual" function with high pressure for 1 minute.
3. After the beep, do a quick release and remove the lid.
4. Meanwhile, add the remaining ingredients to a bowl and mix well.
5. Add the cooked quinoa to the prepared mixture and mix well.
6. Serve as a salad.

Nutrition Values (Per Serving)

- Calories: 285
- Carbohydrate: 27.6g
- Protein: 8.7g
- Fat: 17.2g
- Sugar: 8.8g
- Sodium: 275mg

Flavorsome Brussels Sprout Salad

(**Serves**: 8 / **Prep Time:** 05 minutes / **Cooking Time**: 5 minutes)

Ingredients

- 2 lbs. Brussels sprouts, trimmed and halved
- 1 tablespoon unsalted butter, melted
- 2 cup pomegranate seeds
- ½ cup almonds, chopped

How to

1. Pour a cup of water into the insert of the Instant Pot.
2. Place the steamer trivet inside.
3. Arrange the Brussel sprouts over the trivet.
4. Secure the lid and select the "Manual" function with high pressure for 5 minutes.
5. After the beep, do a Natural release and remove the lid.
6. Transfer the sprouts in a platter and pour melted butter on top.
7. Sprinkle almonds and pomegranate seeds on top and serve.

Nutrition Values (Per Serving)

- Calories: 196
- Carbohydrate: 35.6g
- Protein: 5.1g
- Fat: 4.8g
- Sugar: 14.7g
- Sodium: 39mg

Lime Potatoes

(**Serves**: 2 / **Prep Time:** 05 minutes / **Cooking Time**: 10 minutes)

Ingredients

- ½ tablespoon olive oil
- 2 ½ medium potatoes, scrubbed and cubed
- 1 tablespoon fresh rosemary, chopped
- Freshly ground black pepper to taste
- ½ cup vegetable broth
- 1 tablespoon fresh lemon juice

How to

1. Put the oil, potatoes, pepper, and rosemary to the Instant Pot.
2. "Sauté" for 4 minutes with constant stirring.
3. Add all the remaining ingredients into the Instant Pot.
4. Secure the lid and select the "Manual" function for 6 minutes with high pressure.
5. Do a quick release after the beep then remove the lid.
6. Give a gentle stir and serve warm.

Nutrition Values (Per Serving)

- Calories: 225
- Carbohydrate: 43.3g
- Protein: 5.1g
- Fat: 4.1g
- Sugar: 3.2g
- Sodium: 36mg

Sauce Dipped Spinach

(**Serves**: 2 / **Prep Time:** 5 minutes / **Cooking Time**: 11 minutes)

Ingredients

- 1 tablespoon olive oil
- ½ medium onion, chopped
- ½ tablespoon garlic, minced
- ¼ teaspoon red pepper flakes, crushed
- 4 cups fresh spinach, chopped
- ½ cup tomatoes, chopped
- ¼ cup homemade tomato puree
- ¼ cup white wine
- 2/3 cup vegetable broth

How to

1. Add oil and onion to the Instant Pot. "Sauté" for 3 minutes with constant stirring.
2. Now add pepper, garlic and spinach and cook for another 3 minutes.
3. Add all the remaining ingredients to the Pot.
4. Secure the lid and select the "Manual" function for 5 minutes with high pressure.
5. Do a quick release after the beep then remove the lid.
6. Give a gentle stir and serve warm.

Nutrition Values (Per Serving)

- Calories: 142
- Carbohydrate: 9.9g
- Protein: 4.5g
- Fat: 7.9g
- Sugar: 4.1g
- Sodium: 312mg

Honey-glazed Carrots

(**Serves**: 3 / **Prep Time:** 5 minutes / **Cooking Time**: 5 minutes)

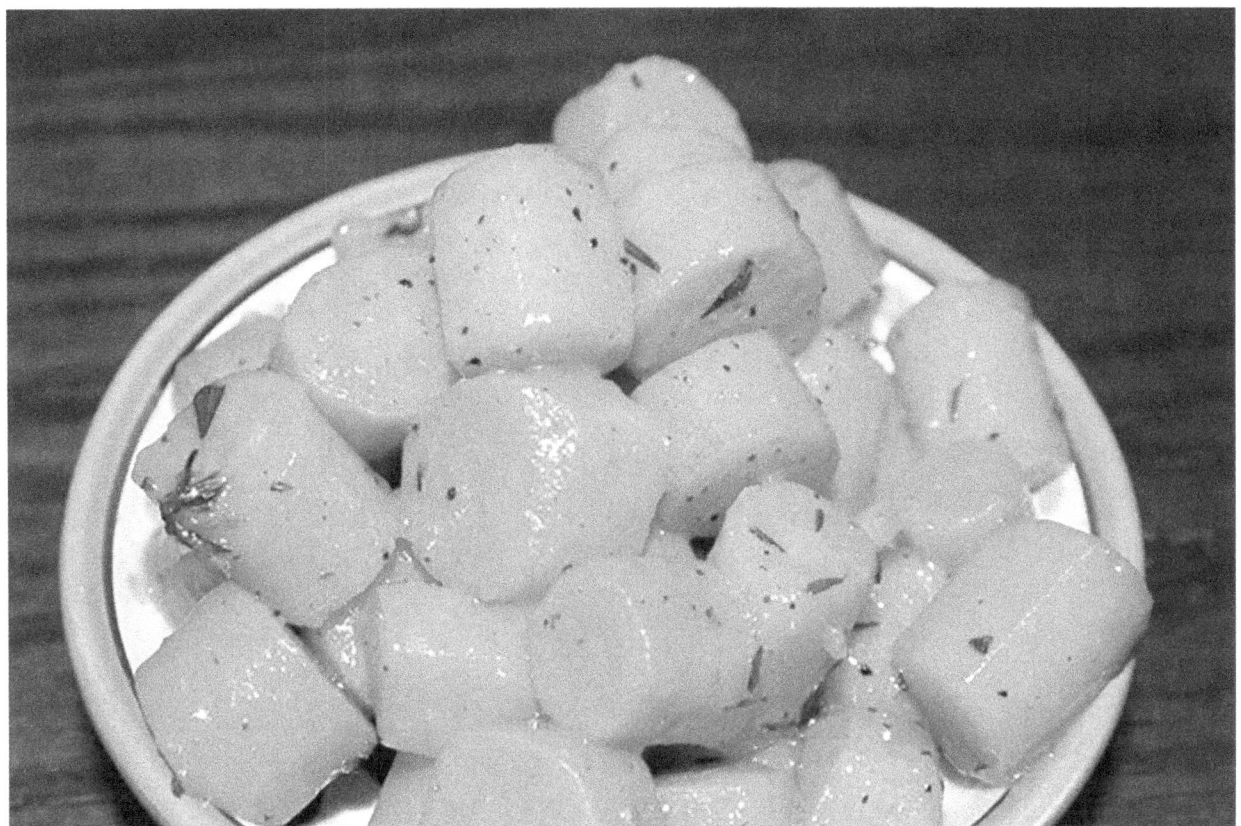

Ingredients

- 1 lb. carrots, peeled and cut into chunks
- 2 tablespoons golden raisins
- ½ cup water
- ½ tablespoon unsalted butter, melted
- ½ tablespoon honey
- 2/3 teaspoon red pepper flakes, crushed
- Salt to taste

How to

1. Add raisins, water, and carrots to the Instant Pot
2. Secure the lid and select the "Manual" function for 5 minutes with low pressure.
3. After the beep, do a quick release then remove the lid.
4. Strain the carrots and transfer them to a large bowl.
5. Put the remaining ingredients into the bowl and mix well.
6. Serve warm.

Nutrition Values (Per Serving)

- Calories: 109
- Carbohydrate: 22.8g
- Protein: 1.5g
- Fat: 2g
- Sugar: 13.9g
- Sodium: 170mg

Nutritious Chickpea Bowl

(**Serves**: 3 / **Prep Time:** 10 minutes / **Cooking Time**: 25 minutes)

Ingredients

- ½ tablespoon olive oil
- ½ onion, chopped
- ½ tablespoon fresh ginger, minced
- ½ tablespoon garlic, minced
- ½ teaspoons curry powder
- ½ teaspoon ground cumin
- ½ teaspoon ground coriander
- 1 medium tomato, chopped finely
- ½ cup dried chickpeas, rinsed, soaked, and drained
- ½ cup water
- Pinch of salt
- Freshly ground black pepper to taste
- 1 tablespoon fresh parsley, chopped

How to

1. Add oil and onion to the Instant Pot and Select the "Sauté" function to cook for 3 minutes.
2. Now add the garlic, ginger, and spices to cook for another 2 minutes.
3. Add water and chickpeas to the pot then secure the lid.
4. Switch the cooker to the Manual function with high pressure and 20 minutes cooking time.
5. After it is done, do a Quick release then remove the lid.
6. Sprinkle some salt and black pepper on top and garnish with parsley.
7. Serve hot.

Nutrition Values (Per Serving)

- Calories: 211
- Carbohydrate: 26.2g
- Protein: 7.8g
- Fat: 9.4g
- Sugar: 4.8g
- Sodium: 65mg

Fresh Kale Salad

(**Serves**: 4 / **Prep Time:** 10 minutes / **Cooking Time**: 1 minute)

Ingredients

- ½ bunch kale, chopped
- ½ cup quinoa, rinsed
- ½ carrot, peeled and shredded
- ¾ cup water
- ¼ teaspoon salt
- ½ beets, cooked and diced
- ½ cup red onions, sliced
- 1 tablespoon Dijon mustard
- 2 tablespoons, balsamic vinegar
- 1 tablespoon vegetable oil
- 1 tablespoon sunflower seeds
- 1 garlic clove, minced
- Salt and pepper to taste

How to

1. Add quinoa, salt, and water to the Instant Pot.
2. Secure the lid and select the "Manual" function with high pressure for 1 minute.
3. After the beep, do a quick release and remove the lid.
4. Meanwhile, add the remaining ingredients to a bowl and mix well.
5. Add the cooked quinoa to the prepared mixture and stir.
6. Serve as a salad.

Nutrition Values (Per Serving)

- Calories: 140
- Carbohydrate: 19.5g
- Protein: 4.1g
- Fat: 5.3g
- Sugar: 3.1g
- Sodium: 213mg

Steamed Garlic Broccoli

(**Serves**: 6 / **Prep Time:** 5 minutes / **Cooking Time**: 10 minutes)

Ingredients

- 6 cups broccoli florets
- 1 cup water
- ½ garlic cloves, minced
- 2 tablespoons peanut oil
- 2 tablespoons Chinese rice wine
- Fine Sea Salt to taste

How to

1. Pour a cup of water into the insert of the Instant Pot.
2. Place the steamer trivet inside.
3. Arrange the broccoli florets over the trivet.
4. Secure the lid and select the "Manual" function with low pressure for 5 minutes.
5. After the beep, do a Natural release and remove the lid.
6. Strain the florets and return them back to the pot. Add the remaining ingredients to the broccoli.
7. Select "Sauté" and stir-fry for 5 minutes.
8. Garnish with lemon slices and serve.

Nutrition Values (Per Serving)

- Calories: 72
- Carbohydrate: 6.1g
- Protein: 2.6g
- Fat: 4.8g
- Sugar: 1.6g
- Sodium: 73mg

Wine-glazed Mushrooms

(**Serves**: 6 / **Prep Time:** 5 minutes / **Cooking Time**: 6 minutes)

Ingredients

- 2 tablespoons olive oil
- 6 garlic cloves, minced
- 2 lbs. fresh mushrooms, sliced
- 1/3 cup balsamic vinegar
- 1/3 cup white wine
- Salt to taste
- Black pepper to taste

How to

1. Add the oil and garlic to the Instant Pot and Select the "Sauté" function to cook for 1 minute.
2. Now add all the remaining ingredients to the cooker.
3. Switch the cooker to the "Manual" function with high pressure and 5 minutes cooking time.
4. After it is done, do a Quick release then remove the lid.
5. Sprinkle some salt and black pepper if desired then serve.

Nutrition Values (Per Serving)

- Calories: 91
- Carbohydrate: 6.5g
- Protein: 5g
- Fat: 5.1g
- Sugar: 2.8g
- Sodium: 38mg

Steamed Artichoke

(**Serves**: 4 / **Prep Time:** 5 minutes / **Cooking Time**: 10 minutes)

Ingredients

- 4 artichokes, trimmed
- 2 lemons, one juiced and one sliced
- ½ tablespoon peppercorns, whole
- 1 ½ garlic cloves, chopped
- ½ tablespoons olive oil
- 2 cups water
- Salt to taste
- Pepper to taste

How to

1. Pour the water and peppercorns into the insert of the Instant Pot.
2. Place the steamer trivet inside.
3. Arrange the artichokes over the trivet.
4. Secure the lid and select the "Manual" function with low pressure for 5 minutes.
5. After the beep, do a Natural release and remove the lid.
6. Strain the artichokes and return them back to the pot.
7. Add oil and all the remaining ingredients back into the Instant Pot, and then "Sauté" for 5 minutes while stirring.
8. Serve hot.

Nutrition Values (Per Serving)

- Calories: 103
- Carbohydrate: 20.5g
- Protein: 5.7g
- Fat: 2.1g
- Sugar: 2.4g
- Sodium: 201mg

Green Beans with Tomatoes

(**Serves**: 8 / **Prep Time:** 05 minutes / **Cooking Time**: 6 minutes)

Ingredients

- 2 tablespoons olive oil
- 2 garlic cloves, crushed
- 4 cups fresh tomatoes, diced
- 2 lbs. green beans
- Salt to taste

How to

1. Add oil and garlic to the Instant Pot and "Sauté" for 1 minute.
2. Stir in tomatoes and sauté for another minute.
3. Set the steamer trivet in the pot and arrange green beans over it.
4. Secure the lid and select the "Manual" function with high pressure for 5 minutes.
5. After it is done, do a Natural release to release the steam.
6. Remove the lid and the trivet along with green beans.
7. Add the beans to tomatoes in the pot.
8. Sprinkle salt and stir well. Serve hot.

Nutrition Values (Per Serving)

- Calories: 82
- Carbohydrate: 11.8g
- Protein: 2.9g
- Fat: 3.8g
- Sugar: 4g
- Sodium: 31mg

Avocado Quinoa Salad

(**Serves**: 4 / **Prep Time:** 5 minutes / **Cooking Time**: 1 minute)

Ingredients

- ½ cup quinoa, rinsed
- ¾ cup water
- ¼ teaspoon salt
- ½ carrot, peeled and shredded
- ½ cup avocados, diced
- ½ cup green onions
- ½ cup cabbage, chopped
- 1 tablespoon lime juice
- 1 tablespoon avocado oil
- 1 tablespoon freshly grated ginger
- 1 pinch of red pepper flakes

How to

1. Add quinoa, salt, and water to the Instant Pot.
2. Secure the lid and select the "Manual" function with high pressure for 1 minute.
3. After the beep, do a quick release and remove the lid.
4. Meanwhile, add the remaining ingredients to a bowl and mix well.
5. Add the cooked quinoa to the prepared mixture and mix well.
6. Garnish with avocado slices on top and serve as a salad.

Nutrition Values (Per Serving)

- Calories: 163
- Carbohydrate: 19.3g
- Protein: 3.9g
- Fat: 8.5g
- Sugar: 1.3g
- Sodium: 160mg

3 Pepper Salad

(**Serves**: 4 / **Prep Time:** 5 minutes / **Cooking Time**: 10 minutes)

Ingredients

- 2 red peppers, thinly sliced into strips
- 2 yellow peppers, thinly sliced
- 1 green pepper, thinly sliced
- 2 cups tomato puree
- 1 red onion, thinly sliced into strips
- 2 garlic cloves
- 1 bunch parsley, chopped
- 1 tablespoon olive oil
- Salt to taste
- Black pepper to taste

How to

1. Add oil and all the vegetables to the Instant Pot.
2. Select "Sauté" and stir-fry for 5 minutes with constant stirring.
3. Stir in tomato puree, salt, and pepper.
4. Secure the lid and select the "Manual" function for 5 minutes at high pressure.
5. After the beep, do a quick release and remove the lid.
6. Stir well and serve.

Nutrition Values (Per Serving)

- Calories: 132
- Carbohydrate: 23.7g
- Protein: 4.1g
- Fat: 4.2g
- Sugar: 9.2g
- Sodium: 81mg

Asparagus Sticks

(**Serves**: 3 / **Prep Time:** 10 minutes / **Cooking Time**: 3 minutes)

Ingredients

- 1 cup water
- 8 oz. thinly sliced Prosciutto*
- 1lb. thick Asparagus sticks
- Salt to taste
- Pepper to taste

How to

1. Wrap each prosciutto slice over the asparagus sticks.
2. Pour a cup of water into the Instant Pot.
3. Arrange a steamer trivet inside.
4. Place the wrapped asparagus sticks over the trivet.
5. Secure the lid and select "Manual" with high pressure for 3 minutes.
6. After the beep, do a natural release then remove the lid.
7. Transfer the steamed asparagus sticks to the platter.
8. Sprinkle salt and pepper then serve.

Nutrition Values (Per Serving)

- Calories: 164
- Carbohydrate: 9.6g
- Protein: 17.6g
- Fat: 5.7g
- Sugar: 3g
- Sodium: 1337mg

(**Note: Prosciutto*** - Prosciutto is an Italian dry-cured ham that is usually thinly sliced and served uncooked; this style is called prosciutto crudo in Italian and is distinguished from cooked ham, prosciutto cotto.)

Instant Mashed Potato

(**Serves**: 4 / **Prep Time:** 5 minutes / **Cooking Time**: 18 minutes)

Ingredients

- 2 cups water
- 6-8 medium potatoes (peeled)
- 1 teaspoon coarse rock salt
- 2 tablespoons full cream
- Additional salt and pepper to taste

How to

1. Add water, potatoes, and salt to the Instant Pot.
2. Secure the lid and select the "Manual" function for 18 minutes with high pressure.
3. After the beep, do a Natural release in 10 minutes and remove the lid.
4. Drain the water from the pot and leave the potatoes inside.
5. Use a potato masher to mash the potatoes in the pot.
6. Stir in cream, pepper, and additional salt. Mix well.
7. Serve and enjoy.

Nutrition Values (Per Serving)

- Calories: 394
- Carbohydrate: 62.5g
- Protein: 10.3g
- Fat: 9.9g
- Sugar: 8.5g
- Sodium: 216mg

Cheesy Jacket Potato

(**Serves**: 5 / **Prep Time:** 10 minutes / **Cooking Time**: 20 minutes)

Ingredients

- 5 medium potatoes
- 2 cups water
- 1 ½ tablespoons butter
- Salt and Pepper to taste
- ¼ cup cheddar cheese, shredded
- ¼ cup mozzarella cheese, shredded
- 1 teaspoon red pepper flakes

How to

1. Prick all the potatoes in the center and create a slit on top.
2. Top the potatoes with cheese, butter, salt, pepper, and pepper flakes.
3. Add water to the Instant Pot and place a steamer trivet inside.
4. Arrange the stuffed potatoes over the trivet with their pricked side up.
5. Secure the lid and cook on "Manual" function for 20 minutes with high pressure.
6. When the timer goes off, do a Natural release and remove the lid.
7. Transfer the potatoes to the platter and sprinkle with some salt and pepper.
8. Serve and enjoy.

Nutrition Values (Per Serving)

- Calories: 205
- Carbohydrate: 33.8g
- Protein: 5.5g
- Fat: 5.9g
- Sugar: 2.5g
- Sodium: 84mg

Chickpea Hummus

(**Serves**: 4 / **Prep Time:** 5 minutes / **Cooking Time**: 20 minutes)

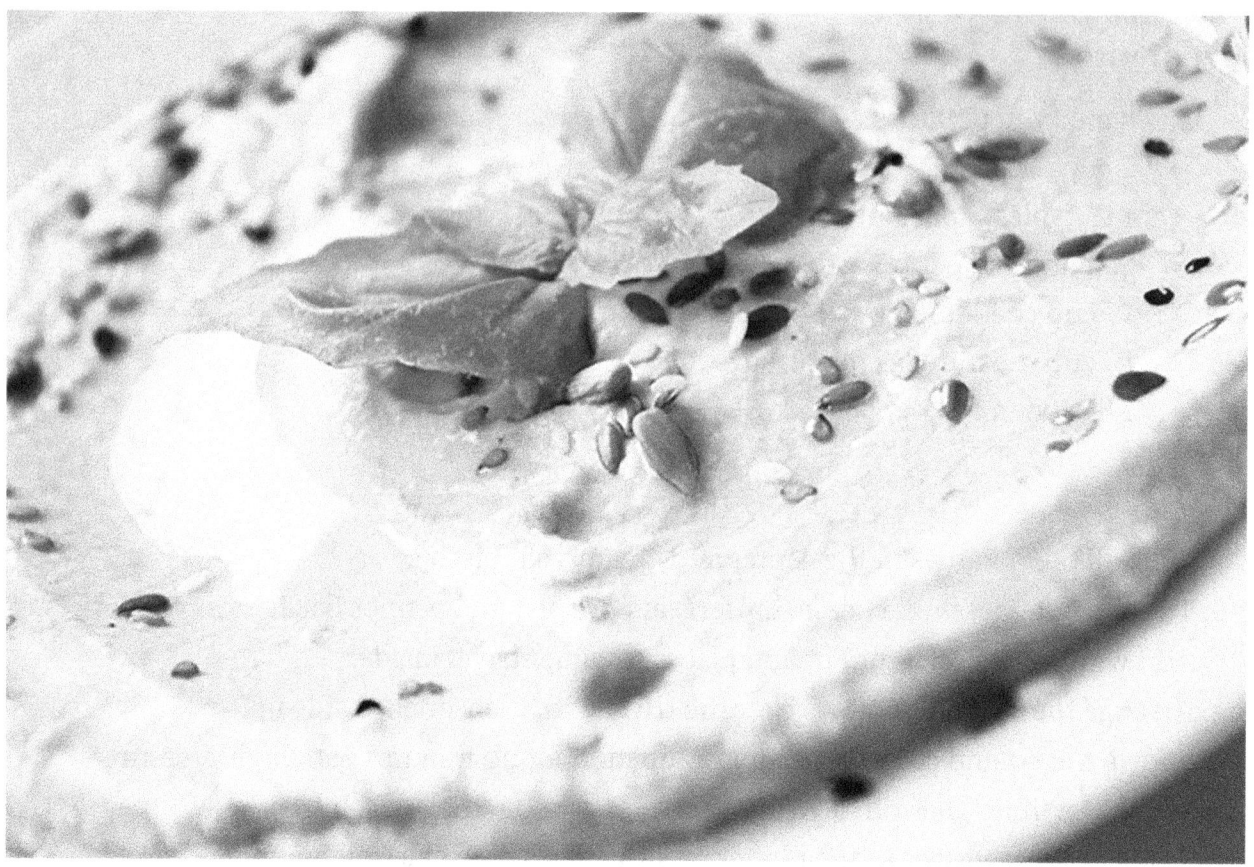

Ingredients

- ½ cup dry chickpeas, soaked
- 1 bay leaf
- 2 garlic cloves
- 1 tablespoon tahini
- ½ lemon, juiced
- ¼ teaspoon powdered cumin
- ¼ teaspoon sea salt
- ¼ bunch Parsley, chopped
- ¼ teaspoon paprika
- 1 tablespoon olive oil

How to

1. Add 3 cups of water, chickpeas, bay leaf and garlic cloves to the Instant Pot.
2. Secure the lid and select the "Manual" function for 18 minutes with high pressure.
3. After the beep, do a Natural release and remove the lid.
4. Strain and rinse the cooked chickpeas. Discard the bay leaf.
5. Add oil and all the remaining ingredients to the Instant Pot and "Sauté" for 2 minutes.
6. Return the chickpeas to the pot and use an immerse blender to form a smooth puree.
7. Stir and serve.

Nutrition Values (Per Serving)

- Calories: 149
- Carbohydrate: 17.4g
- Protein: 5.7g
- Fat: 7.1g
- Sugar: 2.9g
- Sodium: 128mg

Potato & Cauliflower Mash

(**Serves**: 8 / **Prep Time:** 5 minutes / **Cooking Time**: 25 minutes)

Ingredients

- 3 cups water
- 4 lbs. potatoes (peeled)
- 16 oz. cauliflower florets
- 1 teaspoon coarse rock salt
- 2 tablespoons full cream
- additional salt and pepper to taste

How to

1. Add water, potatoes, cauliflower, and salt to the Instant Pot.
2. Secure the lid and select the "Manual" function for 25 minutes with high pressure.
3. After the beep, do a Natural release in 10 minutes and remove the lid.
4. Drain the water from the pot and leave the potatoes and cauliflower inside.
5. Use a potato masher to mash the cauliflower and potatoes in the pot.
6. Stir in cream, pepper, and additional salt. Mix well.
7. Serve and enjoy.

Nutrition Values (Per Serving)

- Calories: 204
- Carbohydrate: 38.7g
- Protein: 6.6g
- Fat: 2.1g
- Sugar: 6.4g
- Sodium: 62mg

Green Beans Salad

(**Serves**: 4 / **Prep Time:** 5 minutes / **Cooking Time**: 7 minutes)

Ingredients

- ½ oz. dry porcini mushrooms, soaked
- 1 cup water
- 1 lb. green beans, trimmed
- 1 lb. potatoes, quartered
- ½ teaspoon sea salt, divided
- Black pepper ground to taste

How to

1. Add water, potatoes, mushrooms, and salt to the Instant Pot.
2. Place the steamer trivet over the potatoes. Arrange all the green beans in the steamer.
3. Secure the lid and select the "Manual" function for 7 minutes with high pressure.
4. After the beep, do a Natural release in 10 minutes and remove the lid.
5. Transfer the greens to a platter. Strain the potatoes and mushrooms.
6. Add the potatoes and mushroom to the green beans.
7. Mix gently and serve. Sprinkle some pepper and salt on top.

Nutrition Values (Per Serving)

- Calories: 127
- Carbohydrate: 27.7g
- Protein: 4.9g
- Fat: 0.3g
- Sugar: 2.9g
- Sodium: 249mg

Tasty Corn Cobs

(**Serves**: 4 / **Prep Time:** 10 minutes / **Cooking Time**: 2 minutes)

Ingredients

- 4 ears corn
- 2 cups water
- Salt and pepper to taste
- 1 tablespoon lemon juice
- 1 tablespoon melted butter

How to

1. Add water and arrange the corn ears vertically in the Instant Pot.
2. Keep the larger end of the corn ears dipped in the water or arrange diagonally.
3. Secure the lid and select the "Manual" function with high pressure for 2 minutes.
4. After the beep, do a Natural release then remove the lid carefully.
5. Strain the corn ears and transfer them to a platter.
6. Drizzle some lemon juice along with melted butter on top.
7. Sprinkle salt and pepper then serve hot.

Nutrition Values (Per Serving)

- Calories: 158
- Carbohydrate: 29.1g
- Protein: 5.1g
- Fat: 4.7g
- Sugar: 5.1g
- Sodium: 48mg

Vegetable Chickpea Salad

(**Serves**: 4 / **Prep Time:** 10 minutes / **Cooking Time**: 20 minutes)

Ingredients

- ½ bunch kale, chopped
- ½ cup chickpeas, soaked and rinsed
- ½ carrot, peeled and shredded
- 1 cup water
- ¼ teaspoon salt
- ½ cup cabbage, sliced
- ½ cup green onions, chopped
- ½ cup red onions, sliced
- 1 tablespoon brown sugar
- 2 tablespoons, balsamic vinegar
- 1 tablespoon vegetable oil
- 1 tablespoon ginger, grated
- 1 tablespoon sunflower seeds
- 1 garlic clove, minced
- Black pepper to taste

How to

1. Add chickpeas, salt, and water to the Instant Pot.
2. Secure the lid and select the "Manual" function with high pressure for 20 minutes.
3. After the beep, do a quick release and remove the lid.
4. Meanwhile, add the remaining ingredients to a bowl and mix well.
5. Strain the cooked chickpeas and add to the prepared mixture and stir.
6. Serve as a salad.

Nutrition Values (Per Serving)

- Calories: 164
- Carbohydrate: 24.1g
- Protein: 6g
- Fat: 5.4g
- Sugar: 7.5g
- Sodium: 169mg

Boiled Bok Choy

(**Serves**: 2 / **Prep Time:** 05 minutes / **Cooking Time**: 7 minutes)

Ingredients

- 1 garlic clove, smashed
- 1 bunch bok choy*, trimmed
- 1 cup or more water
- Salt and pepper to taste

How to

1. Add water, garlic, and bok choy to the Instant Pot.
2. Secure the lid and select the "Manual" function for 7 minutes with high pressure.
3. After the beep, do a Quick release and remove the lid.
4. Strain the cooked bok choy and transfer it to a platter.
5. Sprinkle some salt and pepper on top.
6. Serve.

Nutrition Values (Per Serving)

- Calories: 27
- Carbohydrate: 5g
- Protein: 3.1g
- Fat: 0.5g
- Sugar: 1g
- Sodium: 135mg

(**Note: Bok Choy*** - Bok choy or pak choi is a type of Chinese cabbage. Chinensis varieties do not form heads and have smooth, dark green leaf blades instead, forming a cluster reminiscent of mustard greens or celery.)

Garlic with White Beets

(**Serves**: 4 / **Prep Time:** 10 minutes / **Cooking Time**: 10 minutes)

Ingredients

- 6 whole white beets
- 4 cups water
- 2 teaspoons salt
- 2 tablespoons olive oil
- 4 cloves garlic, minced
- 2 tablespoons lime juice

How to

1. Separate the white part of the beets from the green ones. Wash and rinse.
2. Cut the white parts into cubes and add them to the Instant Pot along with water.
3. Secure the lid and select the "Manual" function for 10 minutes with high pressure.
4. After the beep, do a Natural release and remove the lid.
5. Now add the green parts of the beets to the Instant Pot and let it stay for 5 minutes.
6. Strain the beets and set them aside.
7. Add oil and garlic to the Instant Pot and "Sauté" for 2 minutes.
8. Return the beets to the pot and sauté for a minute.
9. Drizzle lime juice and salt then serve.

Nutrition Values (Per Serving)

- Calories: 133
- Carbohydrate: 17.4g
- Protein: 2.3g
- Fat: 7.3g
- Sugar: 9g
- Sodium: 1323mg

Italian Potato Salad

(**Serves**: 4 / **Prep Time:** 10 minutes / **Cooking Time**: 5 minutes)

Ingredients

- 2 cups water
- 1 ½ lbs. red potatoes, large dice
- ½ bunch parsley, finely chopped
- ¼ medium red onion, finely chopped
- 2 tablespoons white wine vinegar
- 2 tablespoons Olive Oil
- ½ teaspoon salt
- a dash of freshly ground pepper

How to

1. Pour water into the insert of the Instant Pot. Add potatoes to the water.
2. Secure the lid and select the "Manual" function for 5 minutes with high pressure.
3. After the beep, do a Quick release and remove the lid.
4. Strain the potatoes and transfer them to a bowl.
5. Add all the remaining ingredients and mix gently.
6. Serve.

Nutrition Values (Per Serving)

- Calories: 184
- Carbohydrate: 27.9g
- Protein: 3.3g
- Fat: 7.3g
- Sugar: 2g
- Sodium: 306mg

Cabbage with Bacon

(**Serves**: 4 / **Prep Time:** 10 minutes / **Cooking Time**: 8 minutes)

Ingredients

- 2 tablespoons butter
- 2 small onions, sliced into strips
- 6 oz. bacon, chopped
- 2 medium savoy cabbages, sliced into strips
- 2 cups vegetable broth

How to

1. Add the butter, bacon, and onions to the Instant Pot and "Sauté" for 5 minutes.
2. Stir in cabbage and cook for another minute.
3. Pour the vegetable broth into the pot and secure the lid.
4. Select the "Manual" function with high pressure for 3 minutes.
5. After the beep, do a Quick release and remove the lid.
6. Serve and enjoy.

Nutrition Values (Per Serving)

- Calories: 428
- Carbohydrate: 30.7g
- Protein: 34.4g
- Fat: 24.7g
- Sugar: 16.4g
- Sodium: 1488mg

Milk-Soaked Fennels

(**Serves**: 2 / **Prep Time:** 10 minutes / **Cooking Time**: 4 minutes)

Ingredients

- 1 acorn squash, cut in half and cleaned
- 1 tablespoon butter
- 1 cup water
- 1 tablespoon maple syrup
- ¼ teaspoon ground cinnamon
- Kosher salt to taste
- Freshly ground black pepper to taste

How to

1. Add half of the seasoning to one half of the squash and rest of the seasoning to the other half.
2. Add water to the Instant Pot and set a trivet inside.
3. Place the seasoned acorn squash over the trivet with its skin side down.
4. Secure the lid and cook for 4 minutes at high pressure on the "Manual" function.
5. After the beep, do a Quick release and remove the lid.
6. Sprinkle some nutmeg and serve.

Nutrition Values (Per Serving)

- Calories: 108
- Carbohydrate: 14.5g
- Protein: 0.6g
- Fat: 5.8g
- Sugar: 6g
- Sodium: 125mg

Fresh Red Beets

(**Serves**: 3 / **Prep Time:** 5 minutes / **Cooking Time**: 7 minutes)

Ingredients

- 3 red beets, red part only, quartered
- ½ oz. water
- Salt and pepper to taste

How to

1. Pour a cup of water into the insert of the Instant Pot.
2. Place the steamer trivet inside.
3. Arrange the beets over the trivet.
4. Secure the lid and select the "Manual" function with high pressure for 7 minutes.
5. After the beep, do a Natural release and remove the lid.
6. Transfer the beets to the platter, sprinkle salt and water on to
7. Serve.

Nutrition Values (Per Serving)

- Calories: 44
- Carbohydrate: 10g
- Protein: 1.7g
- Fat: 0.2g
- Sugar: 8g
- Sodium: 77mg

Quinoa Lime Salad

(**Serves**: 4 / **Prep Time:** 10 minutes / **Cooking Time**: 1 minute)

Ingredients

- ½ cup quinoa, rinsed
- ¾ cup water
- ¼ teaspoon salt
- ½ carrot, peeled and shredded
- 1 tablespoon lime juice
- 1 tablespoon vegetable oil
- 1 tablespoon freshly grated ginger
- 1 tablespoon sesame oil
- Pinch of red pepper flakes

How to

1. Add quinoa, salt, and water to the Instant Pot.
2. Secure the lid and select the "Manual" function with high pressure for 1 minute.
3. After the beep, do a quick release and remove the lid.
4. Meanwhile, add the remaining ingredients to a bowl and mix well.
5. Add the cooked quinoa to the prepared mixture and mix well.
6. Serve as a salad.

Nutrition Values (Per Serving)

- Calories: 149
- Carbohydrate: 16.3g
- Protein: 3.2g
- Fat: 8.2g
- Sugar: 0.6g
- Sodium: 156mg

Creamy Rich Sweet Potatoes

(**Serves**: 4 / **Prep Time:** 10 minutes / **Cooking Time**: 25 minutes)

Ingredients

- ½ egg
- 1 cup water
- 1 large sweet potato, sliced
- ¼ cup brown sugar
- 1 tablespoon butter, melted
- ¼ teaspoon vanilla
- ¼ teaspoon ground cinnamon
- 1 tablespoon heavy cream
- 1 pinch ground nutmeg
- ½ tablespoon flour
- 2 tablespoons pecans, chopped

How to

1. Pour water into the Instant Pot. Place the steamer trivet inside.
2. Arrange the sweet potato slices over the trivet.
3. Secure the lid and select the "Manual" function with high pressure for 8 minutes.
4. After the beep, do a Natural release and remove the lid.
5. Transfer the slices to a bowl, add butter, vanilla, nutmeg, and cinnamon. Use an electric mixer to form a smooth mixture.
6. Stir in egg and cream then transfer the mixture to a baking dish.
7. Mix butter with sugar, nuts, and flour then pour this mixture over the sweet potato mix.
8. Place this baking dish over the trivet in the Instant Pot. Secure the lid.
9. Cook for 15 minutes at high pressure using the "Manual" function.
10. After the beep, do a Natural release then remove the lid.
11. Serve hot.

Nutrition Values (Per Serving)

- Calories: 151
- Carbohydrate: 19.8g
- Protein: 3.3g
- Fat: 7.4g
- Sugar: 11.9g
- Sodium: 50mg

Juicy Quinoa Olives

(**Serves**: 4 / **Prep Time:** 10 minutes / **Cooking Time**: 1 minute)

Ingredients

- ½ cup quinoa, rinsed
- ¾ cup water
- ¼ teaspoon salt
- ½ carrot, peeled and shredded
- ½ cup green onions
- ¼ cup black olives, sliced
- 1 tablespoon lime juice
- 1 tablespoon olive oil
- 1 tablespoon freshly grated ginger
- 1 pinch of red pepper flakes

How to

1. Add quinoa, salt, and water to the Instant Pot.
2. Secure the lid and select the "Manual" function with high pressure for 1 minute.
3. After the beep, do a quick release and remove the lid.
4. Meanwhile, add the remaining ingredients to a bowl and mix well.
5. Add the cooked quinoa to the prepared mixture and mix well.
6. Serve as a salad.

Nutrition Values (Per Serving)

- Calories: 133
- Carbohydrate: 17.8g
- Protein: 3.5g
- Fat: 5.8g
- Sugar: 0.9g
- Sodium: 231mg

Cheese-filled Sweet Potatoes

(**Serves**: 3 / **Prep Time:** 10 minutes / **Cooking Time**: 20 minutes)

Ingredients

- 3 medium sweet potatoes
- 2 cups water
- Salt & Pepper
- ¼ cup cheddar cheese, shredded
- ¼ cup mozzarella cheese, shredded
- 1 teaspoon red pepper flakes

How to

1. Prick all the sweet potatoes in the center and create a slit on top.
2. Top the sweet potatoes with cheese, salt, pepper, and pepper flakes.
3. Add water to the Instant Pot and place a steamer trivet inside.
4. Arrange the stuffed potatoes over the trivet with their pricked side up.
5. Secure the lid and cook on "Manual" function for 20 minutes with high pressure.
6. When the timer goes off, do a Natural release and remove the lid.
7. Transfer the sweet potatoes to the platter and sprinkle some salt and pepper.
8. Serve and enjoy.

Nutrition Values (Per Serving)

- Calories: 247
- Carbohydrate: 24.8g
- Protein: 15.1g
- Fat: 9.9g
- Sugar: 7.1g
- Sodium: 360mg

Mayo Mushroom Salad

(**Serves**: 3 / **Prep Time:** 10 minutes / **Cooking Time**: 5 minutes)

Ingredients

- 3 medium russet potatoes, peeled and cubed
- ½ cup cremini mushroom, diced
- 1 cup water
- 1/8 cup finely chopped onion
- ½ cup mayonnaise
- 1 tablespoon finely chopped fresh parsley
- ½ tablespoon dill pickle juice
- ½ tablespoon mustard
- Salt and pepper to taste

How to

1. Pour water into the insert of the Instant Pot and place the steamer trivet inside.
2. Arrange the potatoes and mushrooms over the trivet.
3. Secure the lid and select "Manual" with high pressure for 4 minutes.
4. After the beep, do a Quick release and remove the lid.
5. Meanwhile, in a separate bowl combine onion, mayo, mustard, parsley and pickle juice.
6. Add cooked mushrooms and potatoes, mix gently together with the mixture.
7. Serve with mushroom slices and additional seasoning on top.

Nutrition Values (Per Serving)

- Calories: 315
- Carbohydrate: 44.8g
- Protein: 4.8g
- Fat: 13.9g
- Sugar: 5.6g
- Sodium: 569mg

SOUPS, STEWS AND CHILIES

Nutritious Tomato Soup

(**Serves**: 4 / **Prep time:** 6 minutes / **Cooking time**: 13 minutes)

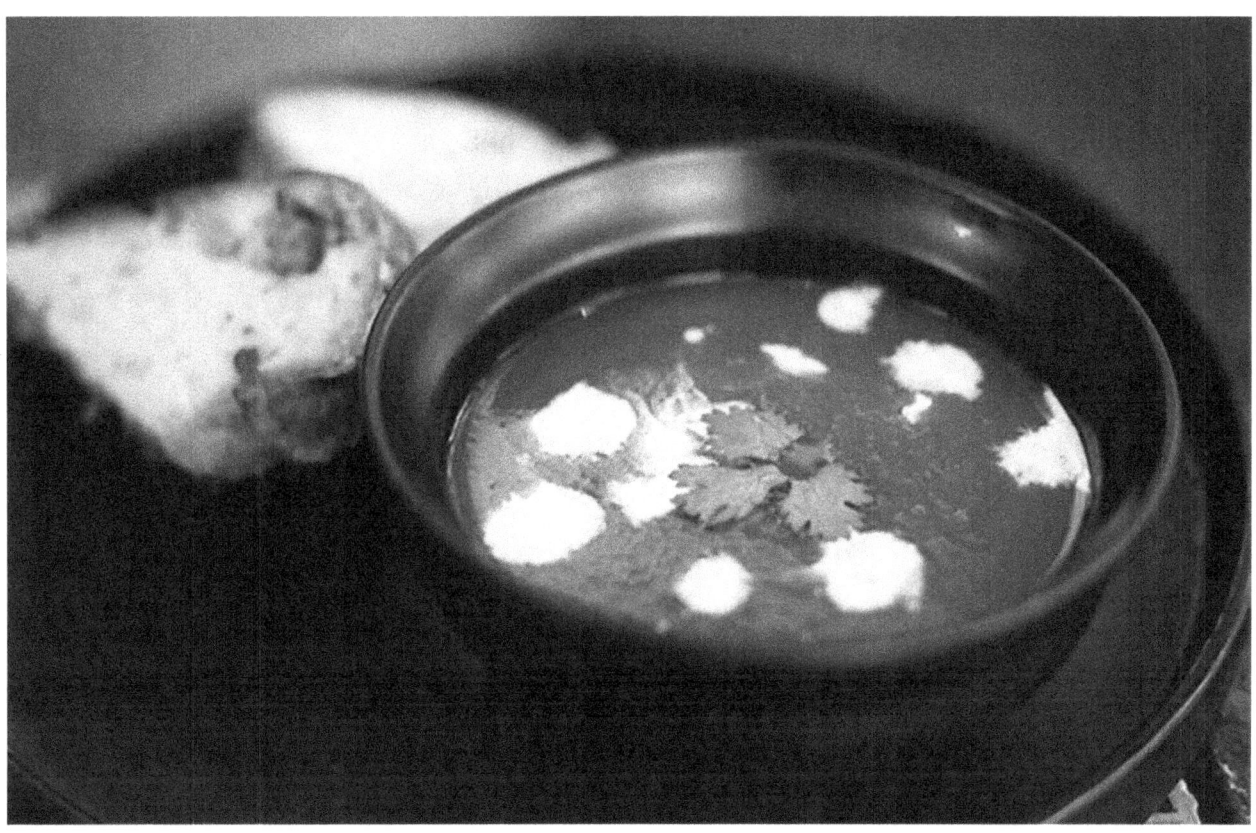

Ingredients

- ½ garlic clove, minced
- 1 small onion, chopped
- 1 ½ lbs fresh tomatoes, chopped
- 1 teaspoon dried parsley, crushed
- 1 tablespoon tomato sauce
- 1 teaspoon dried basil, crushed
- 1 ¼ cups vegetable broth
- 1 tablespoon sugar
- ½ tablespoon balsamic vinegar
- Freshly ground black pepper, to taste
- Cilantro and fresh cream (Garnish)

How to

1. Pour some oil into the inner pan of the instant pot and select the 'sauté" function.
2. Add the garlic and onions to the oil and cook for 3 minutes.
3. Hit 'cancel', then add the tomato sauce, the broth, herbs, tomatoes and black pepper.
4. Secure the lid and select the 'soup' function on your instant pot. Set the timer to cook for 10 minutes.
5. When you hear the beep, 'quick release' the steam and remove the lid.
6. Stir in the vinegar and sugar.
7. Garnish with fresh cream and cilantro, then serve hot.

Nutrition Values (Per Serving)

- Calories: 56
- Carbohydrate: 12g
- Protein: 2.4g
- Fat: 0.4g
- Sugar: 8.4g
- Sodium: 51mg

Delicious Potato and Corn Soup

(**Serves**: 4 / **Prep time:** 6 minutes / **Cooking time**: 12 minutes)

Ingredients

- 1 cup fresh corn kernels
- 1 tablespoon unsalted butter
- ½ medium onion, chopped
- 1 celery stalk, chopped
- 1 garlic clove, chopped
- 1 large russet potato, peeled and chopped
- 1 ½ carrots, peeled and chopped
- 1 tablespoon dried parsley, crushed
- 3 cups vegetable broth
- 1½ tablespoon corn starch
- Freshly ground black pepper, to taste
- ¼ cup water

How to

1. Pour the melted butter into the instant pot and press the 'sauté' key. Add the celery, onion, carrot and garlic to the pot, then cook for 3 minutes.
2. Now add the broth, potatoes, corns, black pepper and parsley to the pot, and secure the lid.
3. Select the 'manual' function, set to high pressure and the timer to 5 minutes.
4. After the beep, 'quick release' the steam and remove the lid.
5. Meanwhile, prepare the corn starch slurry by mixing it with some water.
6. Pour the corn starch slurry into the soup, stirring continuously.
7. Set the cooker to the 'sauté' function and cook for 3 minutes.
8. Serve hot

Nutrition Values (Per Serving)

- Calories: 168
- Carbohydrate: 30.5g
- Protein: 5.1g
- Fat: 3.5g
- Sugar: 3.9g
- Sodium: 282mg

Enticing Chicken and Kale Soup

(**Serves**: 8 / **Prep time:** 10 minutes / **Cooking time**: 10 minutes)

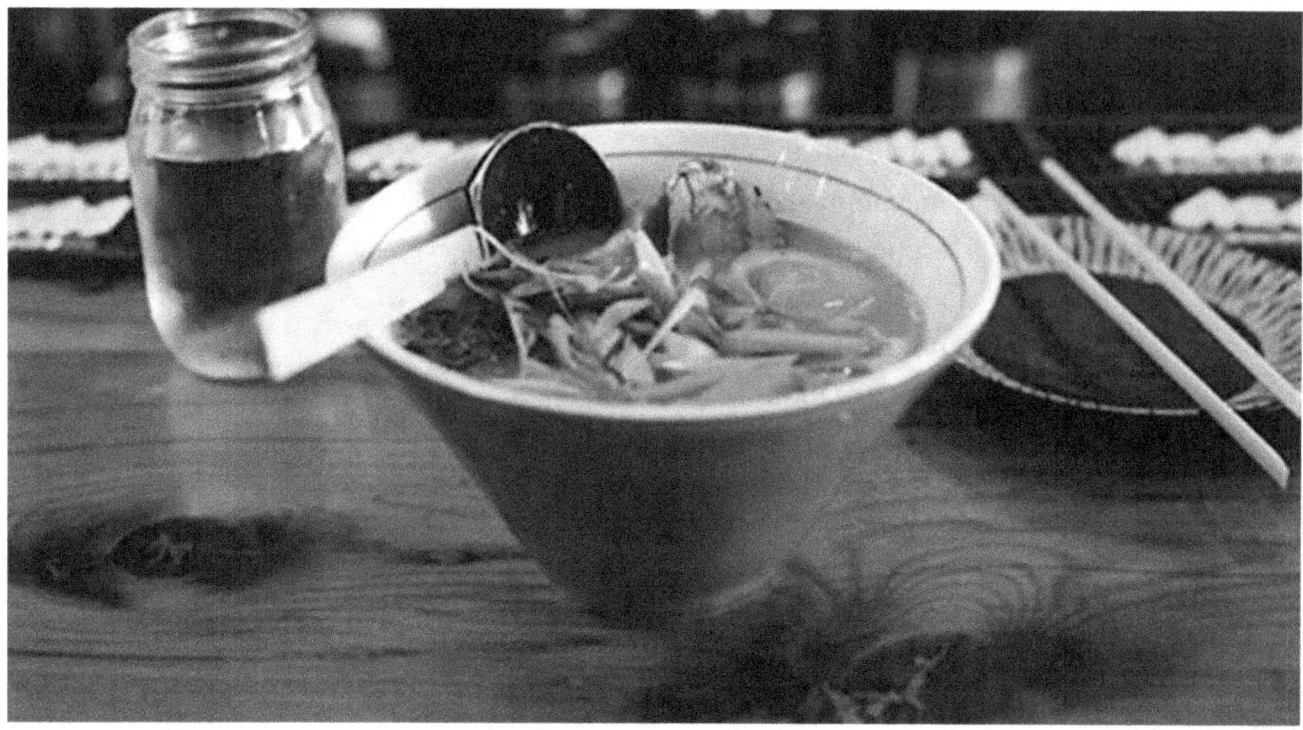

Ingredients

- 2 cups water
- 6 celery stalks, chopped
- 4 carrots, peeled and chopped
- 2 medium onions, chopped
- 4 bay leaves
- 2 tablespoons olive oil
- ½ teaspoon dried oregano, crushed
- Freshly ground black pepper to taste
- ½ teaspoon dried thyme, crushed
- 8 cups low-sodium chicken broth
- 2 lbs cooked chicken, shredded
- 4 cups fresh kale, trimmed and chopped
- 1 teaspoon Worcestershire sauce
- ¼ cup green onions, chopped

How to

1. Pour the oil into the instant pot and select the 'sauté' function.
2. Add the carrot, celery and onion to the oil and sauté for 5 minutes.
3. Now stir in the herbs, bay leaves and black pepper and cook for another minute.
4. Pour the water and broth into the pot and secure the lid.
5. Select the 'soup' function on the control panel and cook for 4 minutes.
6. When you hear the beep, 'quick release' the steam, then remove the lid.
7. Stir in the kale and chicken then cook on 'sauté' for 2 minutes.
8. Add Worcestershire sauce, then serve hot.

Nutrition Values (Per Serving)

- Calories: 261
- Carbohydrate: 11.2g
- Protein: 36.6g
- Fat: 7g
- Sugar: 3g
- Sodium: 198g

Green Bean Soup

(**Serves**: 3 / **Prep Time:** 10 minutes / **Cooking Time**: 30 minutes)

Ingredients

- ½ pound lean ground beef
- ½ tablespoon garlic, minced
- ½ tablespoon olive oil
- ½ medium onion, chopped
- 1 teaspoon dried thyme, crushed
- ½ teaspoon ground cumin
- 1½ cups fresh tomatoes, chopped finely
- ½ pound fresh green beans, trimmed and cut into 1-inch pieces
- 2 cups low-sodium beef broth
- Freshly ground black pepper, to taste
- ⅛ cup Parmesan cheese, freshly grated

How to

1. Select the 'sauté' function on your instant pot. Pour in the oil, add the beef, and cook for 5 minutes.
2. Add the thyme, cumin and garlic, then cook for 3 minutes.
3. Now stir in the beans, tomatoes and broth and secure the lid.
4. Set the 'manual' function to low pressure and cook for 20 minutes.
5. 'Quick release' the steam and remove the lid.
6. Drizzle some black pepper and Parmesan cheese on top.
7. Serve hot.

Nutrition Values (Per Serving)

- Calories: 226
- Carbohydrate: 11.5g
- Protein: 27.9g
- Fat: 7.7g
- Sugar: 4.2g
- Sodium: 371mg

Pork and Cabbage Soup

(**Serves**: 3 / **Prep Time:** 10 minutes / **Cooking Time**: 30 minutes)

Ingredients

- ½ tablespoon olive oil
- ½ lb ground pork
- ½ large onion, chopped
- 1 cup carrots, peeled and shredded
- ¼ head cabbage, chopped
- 2 cups chicken broth
- ½ cup coconut aminos*
- ½ teaspoon ground ginger
- Freshly ground black pepper, to taste

How to

1. Select the 'sauté' function on the instant pot, put the oil and pork in it and cook for 5 minutes.
2. Press 'cancel', add the remaining ingredients, and secure the lid.
3. Cook for 25 minutes at high pressure on the 'manual setting.
4. 'Quick release' the steam after the beep, then remove the lid.
5. Serve immediately.

Nutrition Values (Per Serving)

- Calories: 179
- Carbohydrate: 10.3g
- Protein: 22.5g
- Fat: 5.1g
- Sugar: 4.8g
- Sodium: 127mg

(**Note:** Coconut Aminos* - Coconut-based sauce satisfies, awesome tasting and healthy coconut sugar mixed with mineral-rich sea Salt-Aged to perfection)

Inviting Chicken and Mushroom Stew

(**Serves**: 3 / **Prep Time:** 10 minutes / **Cooking Time**: 15 minutes)

Ingredients

- ½ tablespoon olive oil
- ½ lb fresh cremini mushrooms, stemmed and quartered
- ½ small onion, chopped
- ½ tablespoon tomato paste
- 1½ garlic cloves, minced
- 4 (5-oz) skinless chicken thighs
- ½ cup green olives, pitted and halved
- 1 cup fresh cherry tomatoes
- ¼ cup low-sodium chicken broth
- Freshly ground black pepper to taste
- ¼ cup fresh parsley, chopped

How to

1. Place the oil, onion and mushrooms into the instant pot and cook on the 'sauté' function for 5 minutes.
2. Stir in the tomato paste, along with the garlic, and cook for another minute.
3. Add the broth, chicken, olives and tomatoes to the pot, then secure the lid.
4. Set the 'manual' function to high pressure for 10 minutes cooking time.
5. After the beep, 'Quick release' the steam and remove the lid.
6. Sprinkle some black pepper and parsley on top.
7. Serve immediately.

Nutrition Values (Per Serving)

- Calories: 423
- Carbohydrate: 7.8g
- Protein: 57.6g
- Fat: 16.7g
- Sugar: 3.7g
- Sodium: 202mg

Traditional Beef and Veggie Stew

(**Serves**: 4 / **Prep Time:** 10 minutes / **Cooking Time**: 40 minutes)

Ingredients

- 1½ tablespoons olive oil
- 1½ lb chuck roast, trimmed and cubed
- 1 cup homemade tomato sauce
- ½ teaspoon smoked paprika
- 1 cup low-sodium chicken broth
- 1 large onion, cut into bite-sized pieces
- ½ lb carrots, peeled and cut into bite-sized pieces
- ½ lb potatoes, peeled and cut into bite-sized pieces
- ½ garlic clove, minced
- ¼ cup fresh cilantro, chopped

How to

1. Put the oil and beef into the instant pot and cook on the 'sauté' function for 5 minutes.
2. Stir in the paprika, the broth and tomato paste, then secure the lid.
3. Cook on 'manual' settings high pressure for 15 minutes.
4. Once done, 'quick release' the steam pressure, then remove the lid.
5. Add all the vegetables and re-lock the lid. Cook for another 20 minutes at high pressure on 'manual' settings.
6. 'Quick release' the steam, remove the lid and add the cilantro.
7. Serve immediately.

Nutrition Values (Per Serving)

- Calories: 320
- Carbohydrate: 21.6g
- Protein: 26.9g
- Fat: 13.7g
- Sugar: 7.1g
- Sodium: 285mg

Tempting Mixed Veggie Stew

(**Serves**: 5 / **Prep Time:** 10 minutes / **Cooking Time**: 10 minutes)

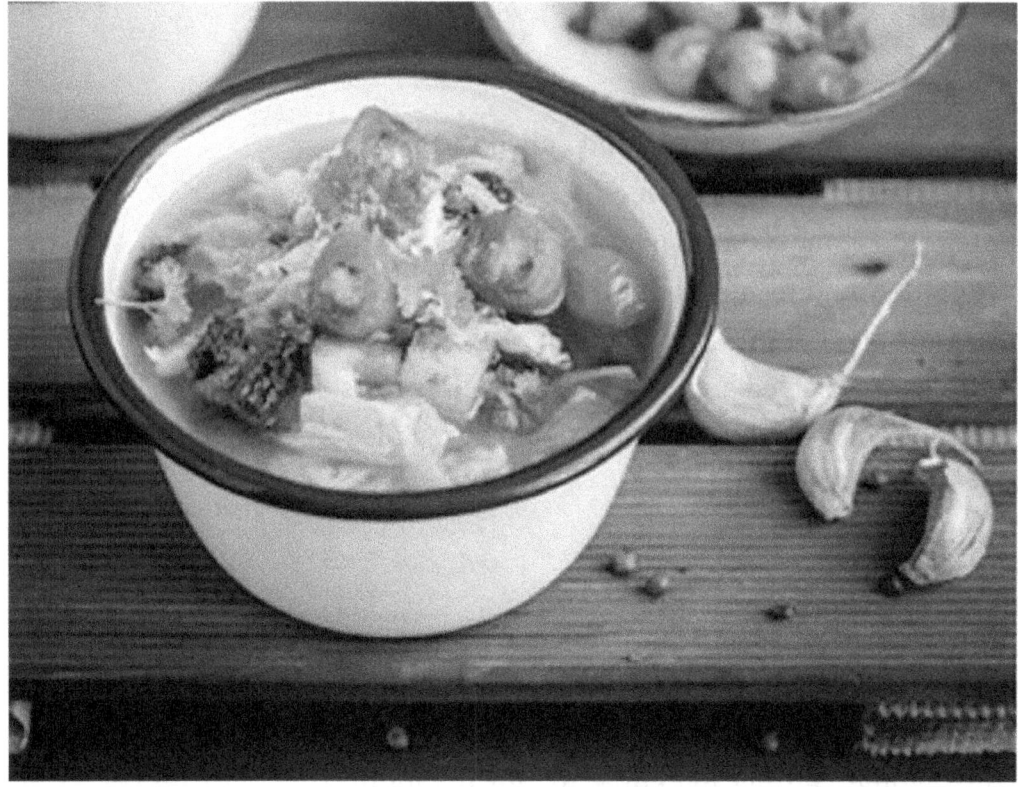

Ingredients

- 1 tablespoon olive oil
- ½ carrot, peeled and minced
- ½ celery stalk, minced
- ½ small onion, minced
- 1 garlic clove, minced
- ½ teaspoon dried sage, crushed
- ½ teaspoon dried rosemary, crushed
- 4 oz. fresh Portabella mushrooms, sliced
- 4 oz. fresh white mushrooms, sliced
- ¼ cup red wine
- 1 Yukon Gold potato, peeled and chopped
- ¾ cup fresh green beans, trimmed and chopped
- 1 cup tomatoes, chopped
- ½ cup tomato paste
- ½ tablespoon balsamic vinegar
- 1¼ cups water

- 1 tablespoon corn starch
- ⅛ cup water
- Salt and freshly ground black pepper to taste
- 2 oz. frozen peas

How to

1. Select the 'sauté' function on your instant pot and pour in the oil. Add the celery, carrot and onion. Cook for 3 minutes.
2. Add the herbs and garlic to the pot and cook for another minute.
3. Now add the mushrooms and sauté for 5 minutes. Stir in the wine and cook for 2 minutes.
4. Add the green beans, potatoes, carrots, tomato paste, water and vinegar, and secure the lid.
5. Set to high pressure in the 'manual' function for 15 minutes. When finished, 'quick release' the steam.
6. Combine the corn starch with water in a separate bowl to make a slurry.
7. Remove the lid of the cooker and add the corn starch slurry, the peas, onion, black pepper and salt.
8. Cook for 1 minute on the 'sauté' setting; transfer to a bowl and serve hot.

Nutrition Values (Per Serving)

- Calories: 197
- Carbohydrate: 36.9g
- Protein: 6.6g
- Fat: 3.2g
- Sugar: 12.6g
- Sodium: 224mg

Delectable Chicken Soup

(**Serves**: 4 / **Prep Time:** 20 minutes / **Cooking Time**: 25 minutes)

Ingredients

- 1½ pound grass-fed, boneless, skinless chicken thighs
- ½ (10-oz) can sugar-free diced tomatoes and green chillies
- ½ (14½-oz) can sugar-free diced tomatoes
- 5 oz. frozen mix veggies (yellow onion, celery, bell pepper)
- 4 cups homemade chicken broth
- 1 teaspoon chili powder
- ½ teaspoon garlic powder
- Salt and freshly ground black pepper to taste

How to

1. Put all the ingredients to the instant pot and secure the lid.
2. Select the 'soup' function on your cooker and set the timer to 25 minutes.
3. After the beep, use 'natural release' to vent the steam, then remove the lid.
4. Remove the chicken thighs and shred them using two forks.
5. Return the chicken to the pot and serve hot.

Nutrition Values (Per Serving)

- Calories: 805
- Carbohydrate: 2.5g
- Protein: 124.1g
- Fat: 34g
- Sugar: 1.4g
- Sodium: 1534mg

Beef with Beans Chili

(**Serves**: 8 / **Prep Time:** 10 minutes / **Cooking Time**: 20 minutes)

Ingredients

- 1 tablespoon olive oil
- 2 lbs ground beef
- 1 onion, chopped
- 1 green bell pepper, seeded and chopped
- 2 garlic cloves, minced
- 1 teaspoon dried oregano, crushed
- 3 tablespoons red chili powder
- 1 tablespoon ground cumin
- 3½ cups tomatoes, chopped finely
- 1½ cups cooked red kidney beans
- 1½ cups water
- ½ cup sour cream

How to

1. Place the oil and the beef in the instant pot and cook for 5 minutes on the 'sauté' function.
2. When cooked, transfer the beef to a plate.
3. Add all the vegetables and stir fry for 5 minutes.
4. Add the beef and all the remaining ingredients, except the sour cream, then secure the lid.
5. Cook on the 'manual' function for 10 minutes at high pressure.
6. 'Quick release' the steam and then remove the lid.
7. Serve with sour cream topping.

Nutrition Values (Per Serving)

- Calories: 769
- Carbohydrate: 96.4g
- Protein: 67.3g
- Fat: 14.6g
- Sugar: 13.4g
- Sodium: 150mg

Three Beans Mix Chili

(**Serves**: 4 / **Prep Time:** 5 minutes / **Cooking Time**: 20 minutes)

Ingredients

- 1 tablespoon olive oil
- 1 cup onion, chopped
- ½ green bell pepper, seeded and chopped
- ½ cup carrot, peeled and chopped
- 2 tablespoons celery stalk, chopped
- ½ tablespoon garlic, minced
- ¼ dried kidney beans, rinsed, soaked for 8 hours and drained
- ¼ cup dried pinto beans, rinsed, soaked for 8 hours and drained
- ¼ cup dried black beans, rinsed, soaked for 8 hours and drained
- 1 cup fresh tomatoes, chopped
- 1 cup homemade tomato paste
- 1 teaspoon dried oregano, crushed
- 1 tablespoon mild chili powder
- ½ teaspoon smoked paprika
- ½ teaspoons ground cumin
- ¼ teaspoon ground coriander
- 2 cups low-sodium vegetable broth

How to

1. Select the 'sauté' function on the instant pot, add the oil, bell pepper, celery, onion, carrot and garlic, and cook for 5 minutes.
2. Add the remaining ingredients to the pot then secure the lid.
3. Select the 'manual' function and set to high pressure. Cook for 15 minutes.
4. After the beep, use the 'natural release' function to vent the steam, then remove the lid.
5. Garnish with olives and scallion* then serve.

Nutrition Values (Per Serving)

- Calories: 282
- Carbohydrate: 50g
- Protein: 13g
- Fat: 4.7g
- Sugar: 12.8g
- Sodium: 213mg

(**Note:** Scallion* - Scallions are vegetables of various Allium onion species. Scallions have a milder taste than most onions.)

Nourishing Chicken Soup

(**Serves**: 3 / **Prep Time:** 15 minutes / **Cooking Time**: 12 minutes)

Ingredients

- 1 lb chicken breasts
- ½ teaspoon sea salt
- ½ onion, diced
- ½ tablespoon olive oil
- 2½ garlic cloves, minced
- ¼ cup organic chicken broth
- ½ teaspoon dried parsley
- ⅛ teaspoon black pepper
- ⅛ cup white wine
- ½ large lemon, juiced
- 2 teaspoons arrowroot flour

How to

1. Put the oil and onion in the instant pot and cook on the 'sauté' function until the onion turns golden brown.
2. Stir in all the remaining ingredients then switch the cooker to the 'poultry' function on its default settings.
3. When done, 'quick release' the steam and remove the lid.
4. Check if the consistency is thick enough. If not, add dissolved arrowroot flour to the soup.
5. Serve hot in a bowl.

Nutrition Values (Per Serving)

- Calories: 333
- Carbohydrate: 3.3g
- Protein: 44.7g
- Fat: 13.7g
- Sugar: 1.1g
- Sodium: 509mg

Full Meal Turkey Soup

(**Serves**: 3 / **Prep Time:** 15 minutes / **Cooking Time**: 30 minutes)

Ingredients

- ½ tablespoon olive oil
- ½ lb lean ground turkey
- ½ small yellow onion, chopped
- 1 cup carrots, peeled and shredded
- ¼ head cabbage, chopped
- 2 cups homemade chicken broth
- 2 teaspoons low-sodium soy sauce
- ½ teaspoon ground ginger
- Freshly ground black pepper to taste

How to

1. Place the oil and turkey in the instant pot and select the 'sauté' function to cook for 5 minutes.
2. Select 'cancel', then add the remaining ingredients. Cover and lock the lid.
3. Set the cooker to 'manual' and select high pressure for 25 minutes.
4. After the completion beep, 'quick release' the steam and then remove the lid.
5. Serve hot.

Nutrition Values (Per Serving)

- Calories: 190
- Carbohydrate: 9.2g
- Protein: 19.5g
- Fat: 8.7g
- Sugar: 4.9g
- Sodium: 798mg

Gourmet Mexican Beef Soup

(**Serves**: 4 / **Prep Time:** 15 minutes / **Cooking Time**: 15 minutes)

Ingredients

- ½ teaspoon olive oil
- 1 lb grass-fed, lean ground beef
- 10 oz. canned sugar-free diced tomatoes with green chilies
- 4 oz. cream cheese
- ¼ cup heavy cream
- 2 cups homemade beef broth
- 2 garlic cloves, minced
- 1 tablespoon chili powder
- 1 teaspoon ground cumin
- Salt and freshly ground black pepper to taste
- ¼ cup cheddar cheese, shredded

How to

1. Pour the oil into the instant pot and Select the 'sauté' function. Stir in the beef and cook for 10 minutes.
2. Add the remaining ingredients, except for the cheese, then secure the lid.
3. Select the 'soup' function and cook for 5 minutes. When done, vent the steam by using 'natural release'.
4. Remove the lid and serve hot with cheddar cheese on top.

Nutrition Values (Per Serving)

- Calories: 390
- Carbohydrate: 5.6g
- Protein: 29.5g
- Fat: 26.5g
- Sugar: 2.1g
- Sodium: 620mg

Nutrient Rich Beef Soup

(**Serves**: 3 / **Prep Time:** 15 minutes / **Cooking Time**: 33 minutes)

Ingredients

- ½ tablespoon olive oil
- ½ lb grass-fed, lean ground beef
- ½ small yellow onion, chopped
- ½ tablespoon garlic, minced
- 1 teaspoon dried thyme, crushed
- ½ teaspoon ground cumin
- 1½ cups fresh tomatoes, chopped finely
- ¼ lbs fresh green beans, trimmed and cut into 1-inch pieces
- 2¼ cups homemade beef broth
- Salt and freshly ground black pepper to taste
- ¼ cup Parmesan cheese, freshly grated

How to

1. Put the oil and beef into the instant pot and select the 'sauté' function. Cook for 5 minutes.
2. Now add the cumin, garlic, thyme and onion, and cook for another 3 minutes.
3. Add the broth, tomatoes and green beans, then secure the lid on the pot.
4. Switch the cooker to the 'manual' function at low pressure and cook for 25 minutes.
5. When it's cooked, 'quick release' the steam, then remove the lid.
6. Sprinkle some salt and black pepper on top, then garnish with Parmesan cheese.
7. Serve hot.

Nutrition Values (Per Serving)

- Calories: 227
- Carbohydrate: 8.4g
- Protein: 22.7g
- Fat: 10.8g
- Sugar: 3.4g
- Sodium: 1449mg

Earthy Bacon and Veggie Soup

(**Serves**: 3 / **Prep Time:** 15 minutes / **Cooking Time**: 20 minutes)

Ingredients

- ½ tablespoon olive oil
- ½ small yellow onion, chopped
- 1 garlic clove, minced
- ½ head cauliflower, chopped roughly
- ½ green bell pepper, seeded and chopped
- Freshly ground black pepper to taste
- 2 cups homemade chicken broth
- 1 cup Cheddar cheese, shredded
- ½ cup half-and-half cream*
- 3 cooked turkey bacon slices, chopped
- 2 dashes hot pepper sauce

How to

1. Add the oil with onion and garlic in the instant pot and "Sauté" for 3 minutes
2. Stir in the broth, salt, black pepper, cauliflower and bell pepper then secure the lid.
3. Select the 'soup'" function and cook for 15 minutes.
4. After the beep, 'quick release' the steam then remove the lid.
5. Stir in the remaining ingredients and cook on the 'sauté' function for 5 minutes.
6. Serve hot.

Nutrition Values (Per Serving)

- Calories: 293
- Carbohydrate: 18.1g
- Protein: 18.1g
- Fat: 21g
- Sugar: 3.3g
- Sodium: 894mg

(**Note:** Half-and-half cream* - Half-and-half, also known as half cream in the United Kingdom, is a simple blend of equal parts whole milk and light cream. It averages 10 to 12% fat, which is more than milk but less than light cream.)

Comforting Broccoli Soup

(**Serves**: 3 / **Prep Time:** 15 minutes / **Cooking Time**: 13 minutes)

Ingredients

- 1 tablespoon butter
- 1 medium carrot, peeled and chopped
- ½ small yellow onion, chopped
- 1 tablespoon almond flour
- ½ garlic clove, minced
- 1½ cups homemade vegetable broth
- 2½ cups broccoli florets
- ½ teaspoon dill weed
- ½ teaspoon smoked paprika
- Salt and freshly ground black pepper to taste
- 2 American cheese slices, cut into pieces
- ½ cup Colby Jack cheese, shredded
- ½ cup Pepper Jack cheese, shredded
- ¼ cup Parmesan cheese, shredded
- ½ cup half-and-half cream

How to

1. Select the 'sauté' function on the instant pot and add the oil, onion and carrot. Cook for 3 minutes.
2. Stir in the garlic and flour, then 'sauté' for another minute.
3. Pour in the broth and cook for one more minute, stirring continuously.
4. Add the broccoli and secure the lid. Cook on 'manual' settings, at high pressure for 8 minutes.
5. After the beep, 'quick release' the steam, then remove the lid.
6. Add the salt, paprika, black pepper, dill weed, and all the cheeses, and let it sit for 2 minutes until the cheeses melt completely.
7. Stir well to combine the ingredients, then serve hot

Nutrition Values (Per Serving)

- Calories: 525
- Carbohydrate: 59.8g
- Protein: 30.1g
- Fat: 19.3g
- Sugar: 17.3g
- Sodium: 897mg

Flavorsome Carrot Soup

(**Serves**: 2 / **Prep Time:** 15 minutes / **Cooking Time**: 12 minutes)

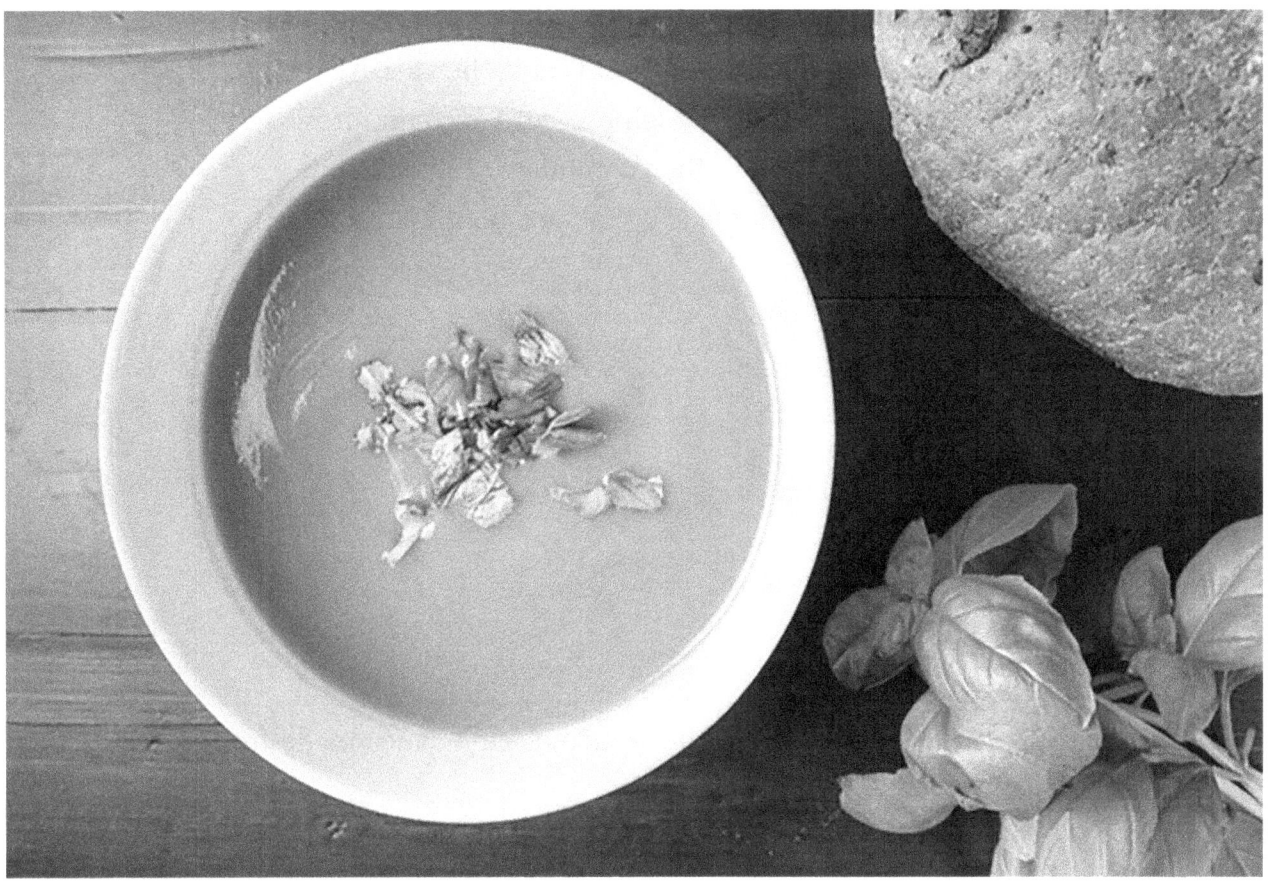

Ingredients

- 1 tablespoon olive oil
- ½ small yellow onion, chopped
- ½ garlic clove, minced
- ⅛ teaspoon dried parsley, crushed
- ⅛ teaspoon dried basil, crushed
- ½ lb carrots, peeled and chopped
- Salt and freshly ground black pepper to taste
- 1 (7-oz) can unsweetened coconut milk
- 1½ cups homemade chicken broth
- ½ tablespoon Sriracha*
- 1 tablespoon fresh cilantro, chopped

How to

1. Select the 'sauté' function on your instant pot, then add the oil, garlic and onion and cook for 3 minutes.
2. Add the salt, carrots and black pepper and cook for another 2 minutes.
3. Pour in the broth, Sriracha sauce and coconut milk, then secure the lid.
4. Set the cooker to 'manual' function at high pressure for 6 minutes.
5. Use 'natural release' for 10 minutes, then carefully remove the lid.
6. Use an immerse blender to blend the soup into a smooth puree.
7. Serve with fresh cilantro on top.

Nutrition Values (Per Serving)

- Calories: 376
- Carbohydrate: 20g
- Protein: 7.1g
- Fat: 31.7g
- Sugar: 10.2g
- Sodium: 693mg

(Note: Sriracha* - Sriracha is a type of hot sauce or chili sauce made from a paste of chili peppers, distilled vinegar, garlic, sugar, and salt.)

Scrumptious Veggie Soup

(**Serves**: 3 / **Prep Time:** 20 minutes / **Cooking Time**: 13 minutes)

Ingredients

- 1 teaspoon olive oil
- ½ small yellow onion, chopped
- ½ tablespoon garlic, minced
- ½ teaspoon dried thyme, crushed
- ½ lb fresh Baby Bella mushrooms, chopped
- 2 cups cauliflower, chopped
- 3 cups homemade vegetable broth
- ¼ cup Parmesan cheese, grated

How to

1. Put the oil, garlic and onion in the instant pot and select the 'sauté' function. Cook for 3 minutes.
2. Add the mushrooms and sauté for 5 minutes.
3. Pour in the broth and add the cauliflower to the mixture. Secure the lid.
4. Press the 'manual' key and adjust settings to high pressure. Cook for 5 minutes.
5. When done, use 'natural release' to vent the steam.
6. Remove the lid and blend the soup with an immerse blender.
7. Add Parmesan cheese and cook for 5 minutes on the 'sauté' function.
8. Serve hot.

Nutrition Values (Per Serving)

- Calories: 455
- Carbohydrate: 13.9g
- Protein: 44.3g
- Fat: 27.2g
- Sugar: 4.2g
- Sodium: 1892mg

Coconut Chicken Stew

(**Serves**: 4 / **Prep Time:** 15 minutes / **Cooking Time**: 25 minutes)

Ingredients

- 1½ tablespoons Worcestershire sauce
- 1 tablespoon fresh lime juice
- 1 tablespoon paprika
- ½ teaspoon ground cumin
- ½ teaspoon ground turmeric
- Salt and freshly ground black pepper to taste
- 2 grass-fed whole chicken legs (drumsticks and thighs separated into 8 pieces)
- ½ tablespoon coconut oil
- ½ cup yellow onion, sliced
- 1½ garlic cloves, minced
- 1 tablespoon homemade tomato puree
- 1 cup homemade chicken broth
- ¼ cup fresh parsley, chopped

How to

1. Prepare the marinade in a bowl by mixing all the spices, the Worcestershire sauce and the lime juice. Immerse the chicken in the marinade and mix well.
2. Place the chicken in the refrigerator for 1 hour to marinate.
3. Separate the chicken from the marinade and keep both to one side.
4. Select the 'sauté' function on your instant pot and add the oil and the chicken. Let it sauté for 3 minutes until each piece turns golden brown from both sides.
5. Remove the chicken and add the garlic and onion. Leave to cook for 3 minutes.
6. Now put chicken back in the pot and add the broth, tomato puree and marinade mixture.
7. Secure the lid and select 'manual' settings - 20 minutes on high pressure.
8. After the beep, use 'natural release' to vent the steam and carefully remove the lid.
9. Serve with fresh cilantro on top.

Nutrition Values (Per Serving)

- Calories: 131
- Carbohydrate: 7.7g
- Protein: 16.1g
- Fat: 3.9g
- Sugar: 3.6g
- Sodium: 293mg

Lamb Pepper Stew

(**Serves**: 3 / **Prep Time:** 20 minutes / **Cooking Time**: 25 minutes)

Ingredients

- ½ tablespoon olive oil
- ½ small yellow onion, chopped
- ½ celery stalk, chopped
- ½ tablespoon garlic, minced
- 1 lb grass-fed lamb shoulder, trimmed and cubed into 2-inch size
- 1 cup fresh tomatoes, chopped finely
- 1 tablespoon sugar-free tomato paste
- 1½ tablespoons fresh lemon juice
- ½ teaspoon dried oregano, crushed
- ½ teaspoon dried basil, crushed
- Salt and freshly ground black pepper to taste
- ¼ cup homemade chicken broth
- ½ large green bell pepper, seeded and cut into 8 slices
- ½ large red bell pepper, seeded and cut into 8 slices
- ¼ cup fresh parsley, minced

How to

1. Add the oil, onion and garlic to the instant pot and select 'sauté'. Cook for 2 minutes.
2. Now add all the remaining ingredients and secure the lid.
3. Select the 'manual' function and cook for 15 minutes on high pressure.
4. After the beep, use 'natural release' for 10 minutes, then vent any remaining steam by using 'quick release'.
5. Remove the lid and switch the cooker back to the 'sauté' mode.
6. Add the bell peppers and cook for 8 minutes stirring constantly.
7. Garnish with minced parsley and serve.

Nutrition Values (Per Serving)

- Calories: 252
- Carbohydrate: 5.3g
- Protein: 33.1g
- Fat: 10.4g
- Sugar: 3g
- Sodium: 142mg

3-Pepper Chicken Chili

(**Serves**: 4 / **Prep Time:** 25 minutes / **Cooking Time**: 15 minutes)

Ingredients

- 1 tablespoon olive oil
- 1½ lbs chicken thighs and drumsticks (bone-in, skin-on)
- ½ pound tomatillos, husks removed and quartered
- 1 Anaheim pepper, seeded and chopped
- 1 poblano pepper, seeded and chopped
- 1 serrano pepper, seeded and chopped
- ½ medium yellow onion, chopped
- 3 garlic cloves, peeled
- ¾ tablespoon ground cumin
- ½ tablespoon dried thyme
- Salt to taste
- ¼ cup fresh cilantro, chopped
- ¼ cup homemade chicken broth
- ½ tablespoon fish sauce
- 1 tablespoon fresh lime juice
- ¼ cup plain Greek yoghurt

How to

1. Pour the oil into the instant pot and select the 'sauté' function. Add the garlic, cumin, salt, thyme, tomatillos, chicken and peppers and stir-fry for 4 minutes.
2. Stir in the broth then cover with the lid. Press the 'manual' key and cook for 15 minutes at high pressure.
3. After the beep, use 'natural release' to vent the steam and remove the lid.
4. Transfer the chicken pieces to a bowl and remove all the skin and bones. Shred the remaining meat and keep it to one side.
5. Meanwhile, add the lime juice, fish sauce and cilantro to the instant pot and blend into a smooth puree using a hand blender.
6. Add the shredded chicken to the smooth puree.
7. Serve with yoghurt topping.

Nutrition Values (Per Serving)

- Calories: 490
- Carbohydrate: 9.6g
- Protein: 32.1g
- Fat: 36.7g
- Sugar: 2.5g
- Sodium: 354mg

Ground Turkey Chili

(**Serves**: 4 / **Prep Time:** 15 minutes / **Cooking Time**: 50 minutes)

Ingredients

- ½ tablespoon olive oil
- 1 small yellow onion, chopped
- 4 garlic cloves, minced
- 1½ lbs. lean ground turkey
- ¾ (15-oz) can sugar-free diced tomatoes with liquid
- 1 oz. sugar-free tomato paste
- ½ (4-oz) can green chilies with liquid
- 1 tablespoon Worcestershire sauce
- 2 tablespoons red chili powder
- 1 tablespoon ground cumin
- ½ tablespoon dried oregano, crushed
- Salt and freshly ground black pepper to taste
- 1 small avocado, peeled, pitted and sliced

How to

1. Select the 'sauté' function on your instant pot. Add the oil, onion and celery, and cook for 5 minutes.
2. Cook for 1 more minute after adding the garlic.
3. Add the turkey and let it cook for 9 minutes. Stir in all the remaining ingredients, except the avocado, then secure the lid.
4. Select the 'meat Stew' option on the cooker, and cook for the default time of 35 minutes.
5. When it's done, vent the steam using 'natural release', then remove the lid.
6. Serve with avocado slices on top.

Nutrition Values (Per Serving)

- Calories: 542
- Carbohydrate: 9.4g
- Protein: 67.6g
- Fat: 26.8g
- Sugar: 3.7g
- Sodium: 405mg

Pork and Beef Chili

(**Serves**: 4 / **Prep Time:** 15 minutes / **Cooking Time**: 40 minutes)

Ingredients

- ½ tablespoon olive oil
- ½ lb. grass-fed ground beef
- ½ lb. ground pork
- 1½ medium tomatillos, chopped
- ¼ small yellow onion, chopped
- 1 jalapeño pepper, chopped
- 1 garlic clove, minced
- ½ (6-oz) can sugar-free tomato sauce
- ½ tablespoon chili powder
- ½ tablespoon ground cumin
- Salt and freshly ground black pepper to taste
- 2 tablespoon water
- ¼ cup cheddar cheese, grated

How to

1. Add the oil to the instant pot and select the 'sauté' function. Place the pork and beef in the oil and sauté for 5 minutes.
2. Remove the excess grease and add the remaining ingredients, except the cheese.
3. Cook on 'manual" at high pressure for 35 minutes.
4. When done, vent the steam using 'natural release', then remove the lid.
5. Top with grated cheddar cheese and serve hot.

Nutrition Values (Per Serving)

- Calories: 270
- Carbohydrate: 6.9g
- Protein: 30.5g
- Fat: 12.7g
- Sugar: 1.6g
- Sodium: 183mg

Bacon Tomato Chili

(**Serves**: 8 / **Prep Time:** 15 minutes / **Cooking Time**: 45 minutes)

Ingredients

- 8 bacon slices, chopped
- 2 red bell peppers, seeded and chopped
- 1 small yellow onion, chopped
- 4 garlic cloves, minced
- 2 lbs. grass-fed, ground beef
- 3 tablespoons chili powder
- 2 tablespoon smoked paprika
- 4 teaspoons ground cumin
- Freshly ground black pepper, to taste
- 1 (28 oz.) can sugar-free, fire roasted tomatoes
- 4 oz. sugar-free tomato sauce
- ½ cup sour cream

How to

1. Place the bacon strips in the instant pot and cook on 'sauté' for 5 minutes until crispy.
2. Put the bacon on plate with a paper towel to soak away the fat.
3. Place the garlic, onion and bell pepper in the pot and 'sauté' for 5 minutes.
4. Now add the beef and spices and cook for another 5 minutes.
5. Stir in the tomato sauce, the tomatoes and crispy bacon, then secure the lid.
6. Select the 'bean/chili' function on your instant cooker and cook for 30 minutes using the default settings.
7. After the beep, use 'natural release' to vent the steam, and remove the lid.
8. Serve with sour cream on top.

Nutrition Values (Per Serving)

- Calories: 414
- Carbohydrate: 15.5g
- Protein: 33.5g
- Fat: 24.1g
- Sugar: 7.3g
- Sodium: 904mg

Spice Rich Beef Chili

(**Serves**: 3 / **Prep Time:** 15 minutes / **Cooking Time**: 27 minutes)

Ingredients

- ½ tablespoon avocado oil
- ¼ yellow onion, chopped
- ½ small red bell pepper, seeded and chopped
- Salt to taste
- 2 garlic cloves, minced
- 1 tablespoon sugar-free tomato paste
- 1 lb. grass-fed, lean ground beef
- 1½ tablespoons chili powder
- ½ tablespoon ground cumin
- ½ tablespoon dried oregano, crushed
- ½ (14½-oz) can sugar-free diced tomatoes, drained
- ¼ cup homemade chicken broth
- 1 tablespoon fresh lemon juice.
- ¼ cup cheddar cheese, shredded

How to

1. Pour the oil into the instant pot and heat it on the 'sauté' function. Add the bell pepper and the onion and cook for 3 minutes. Sprinkle on a pinch of salt while sautéing.
2. Add the tomato paste and garlic to the pot and cook for another minute.
3. Cook for 7 minutes after adding the beef.
4. Stir in the broth and tomatoes then switch the mode from 'sauté' to 'manual' and set to high pressure. Cook for 15 minutes.
5. After the beep, use 'natural release' to vent the steam then remove the lid carefully.
6. Drizzle some lemon juice and cheddar cheese on top.
7. Serve hot.

Nutrition Values (Per Serving)

- Calories: 357
- Carbohydrate: 9.8g
- Protein: 35.2g
- Fat: 17.9g
- Sugar: 4g
- Sodium: 312mg

Spinach Lentil Soup

(**Serves**: 2 / **Prep Time:** 5 minutes / **Cooking Time**: 20 minutes)

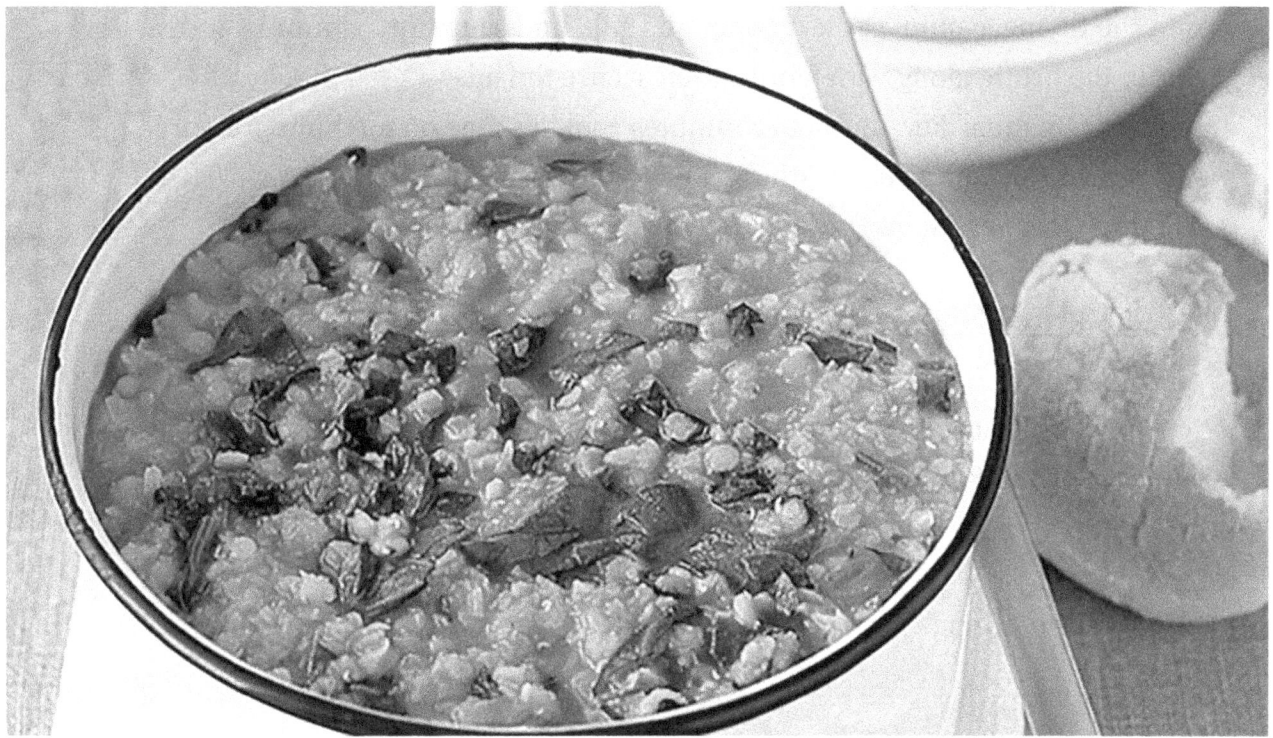

Ingredients

- 1 teaspoon olive oil
- ½ small yellow onion, diced
- 1 medium carrot, peeled and diced
- ½ medium stalk celery, diced
- 2 medium garlic cloves, minced
- 1 teaspoon ground cumin
- ½ teaspoon ground turmeric
- ½ teaspoon dried thyme
- Kosher salt to taste
- Freshly ground black pepper to taste
- ½ cup dry brown lentils, rinsed well in cold water
- 2 cups low-sodium vegetable broth
- 4 oz. (about 6 cups) baby spinach

How to

1. Select the 'sauté' function on the instant pot. Pour in the oil and add the onions, celery and carrots. Cook for 5 minutes.
2. Add the thyme, cumin, garlic, pepper and salt, and sauté for 1 minute.
3. Stir in the broth, along with lentils, then secure the lid.
4. Press the 'manual' key, and set 12 minutes cooking time on medium pressure.
5. After the beep, 'quick release' the steam, then remove the lid.
6. Add the spinach, salt and pepper to taste, then serve.

Nutrition Values (Per Serving)

- Calories: 190
- Carbohydrate: 30.5g
- Protein: 10.8g
- Fat: 3.5g
- Sugar: 4.2g
- Sodium: 461mg

Delightful Zuppa Toscana

(**Serves**: 2 / **Prep Time:** 10 minutes / **Cooking Time**: 10 minutes)

Ingredients

- 1 tablespoon olive oil
- ½ medium onion, diced
- ½ lb ground, mild Italian sausage
- 2 cloves garlic, minced
- 1½ large russet potatoes, unpeeled and sliced into 1/4-inch slices.
- 3 cups (1½ quarts) chicken broth
- 2 tablespoons water
- 1 cup fresh kale, chiffonade
- ½ cup heavy cream

How to

1. Add the oil and onion to the instant pot and cook on the 'sauté' function for 3 minutes.
2. Add the Italian sausage and cook until it turns brown.
3. Stir in the garlic and cook for 1 minute.
4. Add the water, broth and potato slices and seal the lid.
5. Cook on 'manual' setting for 5 minutes at high pressure.
6. After 10 minutes, use 'natural release', and then 'quick release' to vent all the steam.
7. Remove the lid and stir in the kale and cream. Serve hot

Nutrition Values (Per Serving)

- Calories: 784
- Carbohydrate: 54.8g
- Protein: 34g
- Fat: 46.5g
- Sugar: 7.5g
- Sodium: 2149mg

Special Minestrone Soup

(**Serves**: 4 / **Prep Time:** 12 minutes / **Cooking Time**: 6 minutes)

Ingredients

- 2 tablespoons olive oil
- 2 stalks celery, diced
- 1 large onion, diced
- 1 large carrot, diced
- 3 cloves garlic, minced
- 1 teaspoon dried oregano
- 1 teaspoon dried basil
- Sea salt and pepper to taste
- 1 (28 oz.) can San Marzano tomatoes
- 1 (15 oz.) can white or cannellini beans
- 4 cups bone broth or vegetable broth
- 1 bay leaf
- ½ cup fresh spinach
- 1 cup gluten-free elbow pasta
- 1/3 cup finely grated parmesan cheese
- 2 tablespoons fresh pesto

How to

1. Switch the instant pot to 'sauté' mode and add the oil, onion, garlic, celery and carrot. Cook for 3 minutes.
2. Drizzle the salt, pepper, oregano and basil into the mix to add more flavour.
3. Add the broth, spinach, pasta, tomatoes and bay leaf to the pot and select 'manual' settings. Cook for 6 minutes at high pressure.
4. Let it sit for 2 minutes after the beep, then 'quick release' the steam. Remove the lid carefully.
5. Stir in the white kidney beans.
6. Serve with a grating of parmesan cheese and pesto on top.

Nutrition Values (Per Serving)

- Calories: 629
- Carbohydrate: 96.9g
- Protein: 37.3g
- Fat: 12.6g
- Sugar: 11.2g
- Sodium: 876mg

Super Easy Chicken Tortilla Soup

(**Serves**: 4 / **Prep Time:** 10 minutes / **Cooking Time**: 20 minutes)

Ingredients

- 2½ cups chicken broth
- ½ (14.5 oz.) can tomatoes, undrained, diced
- 1 small onion, diced
- 2 garlic cloves, finely minced
- 1 teaspoon chili powder
- 1 teaspoon cumin
- ½ teaspoon paprika
- ½ teaspoon coriander (ground)
- Salt and pepper to taste
- 1 lb boneless, skinless chicken breast
- 14.5 oz. (½ can) black beans, drained and rinsed
- 1 cup frozen corn kernels
- ½ tablespoon lime juice
- 2 tablespoons cilantro, chopped
- Tortilla chips

How to

1. Pour the chicken broth into the instant pot, add the tomatoes and garlic, then the chicken breasts.
2. Sprinkle all the spices into the pot and add the corn and the beans.
3. Seal the lid and cook on the 'manual' setting at high pressure for 5 minutes.
4. 'natural release' the steam when the timer goes off. Remove the lid.
5. Remove the chicken and shred it in a bowl using two forks.
6. Put the chicken back in the pot and add the lime juice.
7. Garnish with cilantro and serve with tortilla chips.

Nutrition Values (Per Serving)

- Calories: 625
- Carbohydrate: 76.6g
- Protein: 57.2g
- Fat: 10.8g
- Sugar: 5.4g
- Sodium: 590mg

Japanese Ramen Soup

(**Serves**: 4 / **Prep Time:** 10 minutes / **Cooking Time**: 90 minutes)

Ingredients

- 1½ lbs. pork spareribs, cut into 2" pieces
- ¾ lb chicken wings
- 1 tablespoon cooking oil
- 1 large onion, peeled, thick sliced
- 1½ cloves garlic, smashed
- 1 teaspoon ginger, grated
- Soy sauce or salt to taste
- 1 cup boiled egg noodles.
- ¼ cup green onion, chopped.
- 1 boiled egg (cut in half)

How to

1. Pour the water into a large pot. Add the pork spareribs and chicken wings. Boil the mixture for 8 minutes, then remove the wing and spareribs. Dispose of the remaining water.
2. Now set the instant pot on the 'sauté' function and add the onion and oil. Cook for 5 minutes
3. When the onion turns brown, add the garlic, ginger, wings and ribs. Fill the inner pot with water up to the 'MAX' limit. Secure the lid.
4. Select the 'manual' function on the instant pot, and cook for 90 minutes at high pressure.
5. After the beep, 'natural release' the steam, then remove the lid.
6. Strain the soup, discard all the solids and skim off the surface fats.
7. Serve with boiled noodles, chopped green onions and boiled egg on top.

Nutrition Values (Per Serving)

- Calories: 662
- Carbohydrate: 14.8g
- Protein: 75.5g
- Fat: 31.8g
- Sugar: 2g
- Sodium: 191mg

Barley Soup

(**Serves**: 6 / **Prep Time:** 10 minutes / **Cooking Time**: 1 hr 30 min)

Ingredients

- 1½ lb stew meat
- Salt and pepper to taste
- 2 tablespoons oil
- 10 baby Bella mushrooms, quartered
- 1 cup onion, chopped
- 1 cup carrots, chopped
- 4 celery stalks, chopped
- 6 cloves garlic, minced
- 6 cups low sodium beef broth
- 1 cup water
- 2 bay leaves
- ½ teaspoon dried thyme
- 1 large potato, shredded
- 2/3 cup pearl barley, rinsed

How to

1. Put the oil and the stew meat in the instant pot and 'sauté' until all the meat turns golden brown on both sides. Sprinkle in the salt and pepper for seasoning.
2. When cooked, remove the beef and add the mushrooms to the oil. Cook for 2 minutes, then transfer them on to a plate.
3. Put the onion, carrot and celery into the pot and cook for 5 minutes, stirring constantly. Add the garlic and cook for another minute.
4. Now put the beef and mushrooms back in the pot and add the thyme, bay leaves, water and broth, and secure the lid.
5. Cook the mixture on the 'manual' function at high pressure for 16 minutes.
6. Use 'natural release' to vent the steam and remove the lid.
7. Stir in the potatoes and barley, then cover with the lid.
8. Cook on 'slow cook' for 1 hour, then press 'cancel'.
9. Remove the lid and serve hot.

Nutrition Values (Per Serving)

- Calories: 518
- Carbohydrate: 35.5g
- Protein: 44.9g
- Fat: 21.2g
- Sugar: 3.8g
- Sodium: 875mg

Coconut Celery Soup

(**Serves**: 8 / **Prep Time:** 10 minutes / **Cooking Time**: 30 minutes)

Ingredients

- 2 bunches celery, diced
- 2 sweet yellow onions, diced
- 2 cups coconut milk
- 4 cups chicken broth
- 1 teaspoon dill
- 2 pinches of sea salt

How to

1. Put all the ingredients into the instant pot.
2. Secure the lid and set the cooker on the 'soup' function for 30 minutes.
3. After the beep, use 'natural release' to vent the steam, then remove the lid.
4. Use an immerse blender to blend the soup into a smooth mixture.
5. Serve hot.

Nutrition Values (Per Serving)

- Calories: 169
- Carbohydrate: 5.4g
- Protein: 4.2g
- Fat: 15g
- Sugar: 3.9g
- Sodium: 419mg

Cauliflower Butternut Soup

(**Serves**: 3 / **Prep Time:** 05 minutes / **Cooking Time**: 25 minutes)

Ingredients

- ½ medium onion, diced
- 2 teaspoons oil
- 1 garlic clove, minced
- ½ lb frozen cauliflower
- ½ lb frozen, cubed, butternut squash
- 1 cup vegetable broth
- ½ teaspoon paprika
- ¼ teaspoon dried thyme
- 2 pinches of sea salt
- ½ cup milk

How to

1. Put the oil and garlic into the instant pot and select the 'sauté' function. Cook for 2 minutes.
2. Add the broth, cauliflower, butternut and all the spices and secure the lid.
3. Cook under 'manual' settings at high pressure for 5 minutes.
4. After the beep, 'quick release' the steam and remove the lid.
5. Add the milk to the soup and blend well using an immerse blender.
6. Serve hot.

Nutrition Values (Per Serving)

- Calories: 125
- Carbohydrate: 15.4g
- Protein: 4.7g
- Fat: 6g
- Sugar: 4.4g
- Sodium: 445mg

Instant Lasagne Soup

(**Serves**: 4 / **Prep Time:** 10 minutes / **Cooking Time**: 9 minutes)

Ingredients

- 2 tablespoons olive oil
- 1 medium onion, chopped
- ½ green pepper, chopped
- 2 carrots, chopped
- 1 medium zucchini, chopped
- 2 cups ground meat
- 1 large can diced tomatoes
- 4 cups vegetable stock
- 2 cups water
- ½ box of lasagne noodles (small pieces)
- ½ teaspoon onion powder
- 1 teaspoon black pepper
- 1 teaspoon oregano
- Sea salt to taste

How to

1. Put the oil, the green pepper, onion and carrots, into the instant pot and select the 'sauté' function. Cook for 5 minutes.
2. Stir in the ground meat, zucchini and all the spices, and cook for 3 minutes
3. Add the broth, tomatoes, water and lasagne noodles to the cooker, and secure the lid.
4. Cook under 'manual' settings, at high pressure, for 4 minutes.
5. After the beep, 'quick release' the steam and remove the lid.
6. Serve hot.

Nutrition Values (Per Serving)

- Calories: 231
- Carbohydrate: 19.1g
- Protein: 15.8g
- Fat: 10.7g
- Sugar: 6g
- Sodium: 180mg

Italian Chicken Soup

(**Serves**: 6 / **Prep Time:** 10 minutes / **Cooking Time**: 15 minutes)

Ingredients

- 1 (3-4 lb) whole chicken
- 1 cup large cut up carrots
- 1 head of escarole
- 1 (28 oz.) can of diced tomatoes
- 32 oz. chicken Broth
- 10 meat balls, cut in quarters
- 2 celery stalks chopped
- ½ lb egg noodles

How to

1. Fill the instant pot with water up to the 'Max' limit, and put the whole chicken in.
2. Secure the lid and select 'poultry' settings. Set timer for 20 minutes.
3. After the beep, 'natural release' the steam and remove the lid.
4. Strain the chicken. Pull all the meat from the bones, shred it and keep it aside.
5. Now put the tomatoes, broth, celery and meatballs into the pot and secure the lid.
6. Cook on the 'soup' function for 10 minutes, then 'natural release' the steam after you hear the beep.
7. Remove the lid and stir in the shredded chicken, the egg noodles and escarole. Secure the lid again.
8. Cook for 2 minutes, on the 'soup' function then 'quick release' the steam.
9. Remove the lid and serve hot.

Nutrition Values (Per Serving)

- Calories: 814
- Carbohydrate: 25.3g
- Protein: 87.8g
- Fat: 38.9g
- Sugar: 5.9g
- Sodium: 1708mg

Chinese Congee

(**Serves**: 6 / **Prep Time:** 5 minutes / **Cooking Time**: 20minutes)

Ingredients

- 1 lb ground chicken
- 6 cups chicken broth
- ½ tablespoon salt
- 1½ cups short grain rice, rinsed until water is clear
- 1 tablespoon grated fresh ginger
- 4 cups cabbage, shredded
- Green onions to garnish

How to

1. Put all the ingredients, except the cabbage and green onions, in the instant pot.
2. Select the 'porridge' function and cook on the default time and settings.
3. After the beep, 'quick release' the steam and remove the lid.
4. Stir in the shredded cabbage and cover with the lid.
5. Serve after 10 minutes with chopped green onions on top.

Nutrition Values (Per Serving)

- Calories: 237
- Carbohydrate: 13.2g
- Protein: 28.1g
- Fat: 7.1g
- Sugar: 2.2g
- Sodium: 1418mg

Ham and White Bean Soup

(**Serves**: 4 / **Prep Time:** 10 minutes / **Cooking Time**: 15 minutes)

Ingredients

- ½ lb Great Northern beans, soaked
- ½ tablespoon olive oil
- ½ medium carrot, chopped
- ½ medium onion, chopped
- 1½ cloves garlic, minced
- ½ medium tomato, peeled and chopped
- ½ lb ham, cubed
- 2 cups vegetable stock
- 1 cup water
- 1 teaspoon salt
- ½ teaspoon freshly ground black pepper
- ½ teaspoon dried mint
- ½ teaspoon thyme
- ½ teaspoon paprika

How to

1. Put the and all the vegetables in the instant pot. Stir fry the veggies for 5 minutes on the 'sauté' function.
2. Add the remaining ingredients to the pot and secure the lid.
3. Use the 'manual' function to cook for 15 minutes at high pressure.
4. After the beep, 'natural release' and 'quick release' to vent all the steam.
5. Remove the lid and serve hot.

Nutrition Values (Per Serving)

- Calories: 295
- Carbohydrate: 42g
- Protein: 23.4g
- Fat: 4g
- Sugar: 5.7g
- Sodium: 1252mg

Cheesy Leek Soup

(**Serves**: 4 / **Prep Time:** 15 minutes / **Cooking Time**: 10 minutes)

Ingredients

- 1 tablespoon unsalted butter
- 1½ leeks, cleaned and sliced
- ½ teaspoon kosher salt
- 2 garlic cloves, crushed
- 2 sprigs fresh thyme
- 1/3 teaspoon dried oregano
- 1 bay leaf
- ½ cup white wine
- 2½ cups vegetable broth
- 2 cups medium gold potatoes, peeled and diced
- ¾ cups cream
- ¼ cup grated cheddar cheese

How to

1. 'Sauté' the leeks with melted butter in the instant pot for 1 minute, then add the garlic to cook for 30 seconds.
2. Add all the remaining ingredients, except the cream, and secure the lid.
3. Select the 'manual' function on the instant pot and cook for 10 minutes at high pressure.
4. After the beep, 'quick release' the steam and remove the lid.
5. Stir the cream into the soup and remove the bay leaf.
6. Serve hot.

Nutrition Values (Per Serving)

- Calories: 878
- Carbohydrate: 94.2g
- Protein: 30.4g
- Fat: 35.3g
- Sugar: 14.1g
- Sodium: 3455mg

Spicy Pork Vindaloo

(**Serves**: 6 / **Prep Time:** 10 minutes / **Cooking Time**: 25 minutes)

Ingredients

- 3 lbs boneless pork shoulder, cubed
- 1 teaspoon sea salt
- ¼ cup olive oil
- 1 large white onion, peeled and finely chopped
- 4 cloves garlic, peeled and minced
- 1-piece fresh ginger, peeled and grated
- 2 tablespoons vindaloo seasoning
- 1 teaspoon hot paprika
- ½ teaspoon ground turmeric
- 3 tablespoons all-purpose flour
- 1/3 cup Champagne vinegar
- 1 (14½ oz.) can diced tomatoes in juice, undrained
- 1 cup chicken broth

How to

1. Pour all the oil into the instant pot and stir-fry the pork meat on the 'sauté' function for 7 minutes until brown.
2. Remove the meat and place it to one side. Add the onion, garlic and ginger to the oil and stir-fry for 5 minutes.
3. Add the remaining ingredients to the pot, including the pork meat, and secure the lid.
4. Cook on 'manual' setting at high pressure for 25 minutes.
5. After the beep, 'quick release' the steam and remove the lid.
6. Skim the surface fats and serve hot.

Nutrition Values (Per Serving)

- Calories: 518
- Carbohydrate: 25g
- Protein: 65.4g
- Fat: 17.4g
- Sugar: 1.4g
- Sodium: 923mg

Salsa Chicken Soup

(**Serves**: 4 / **Prep Time:** 10 minutes / **Cooking Time**: 11 minutes)

Ingredients

- 1 tablespoon olive oil
- 1 onion, diced
- 2 chicken breasts
- 4 cups chicken broth
- 2 cans diced tomatoes
- ½ teaspoon ground cumin
- ½ teaspoon kosher salt
- ¼ teaspoon chili powder
- 1 cup salsa
- 2 cups shredded cheese
- 1 cup milk

How to

1. Put the oil and onions into the instant pot and 'sauté' for 3 minutes.
2. Push the onions to one side and place the chicken breasts in the pot. Let them cook for 3 minutes on each side
3. Add the remaining ingredients, except the salsa, and secure the lid.
4. Select 'manual' settings and cook at high pressure for 8 minutes.
5. After the beep, 'quick release' the steam and remove the lid.
6. Stir in the salsa and serve hot.

Nutrition Values (Per Serving)

- Calories: 512
- Carbohydrate: 15g
- Protein: 44.2g
- Fat: 30.7g
- Sugar: 9.3g
- Sodium: 1894mg

Cheese Potato Soup

(**Serves**: 4 / **Prep Time:** 10 minutes / **Cooking Time**: 15 Min)

Ingredients

- 1 tablespoon butter
- ¼ cup chopped onion
- 3 cups potatoes, peeled and cubed
- 1 (14 oz.) can chicken broth
- ½ teaspoon salt
- ¼ teaspoon black pepper
- 1 tablespoon dried parsley
- 1 tablespoon corn starch
- 1 tablespoon water
- 1½ oz. cream cheese, cut into cubes
- ½ cup shredded cheddar cheese
- 1 cup half and half
- ½ cup frozen corn
- 3 slices crisply cooked bacon, crumbled

How to

1. Put the butter and onion in the instant pot and cook for 5 minutes on the 'sauté' function.
2. Add half the can of chicken broth, pepper, salt and parsley to the onions.
3. Place the steamer trivet in the pot and arrange the diced potatoes on it.
4. Secure the lid and select the 'manual' function. Cook for 4 minutes at high pressure.
5. After the beep, 'quick release' the steam and remove the lid.
6. Remove the steamer trivet and the potatoes.
7. Dissolve the corn starch in water in a small bowl and add this slurry to the instant pot. Select 'sauté' to cook.
8. Add the remaining ingredients, including the potatoes, and cook for 5 minutes.
9. Serve hot.

Nutrition Values (Per Serving)

- Calories: 338
- Carbohydrate: 32.5g
- Protein: 11.5g
- Fat: 192g
- Sugar: 2.3g
- Sodium: 788mg

Borscht Beet Soup

(**Serves**: 8 / **Prep Time:** 15 minutes / **Cooking Time**: 15 minutes)

Ingredients

- 2 medium white onions, chopped
- 2 teaspoons salt
- 4 tablespoons olive oil
- 4 large white potatoes, peeled and diced
- 2 large carrots, grated
- 4 medium beets
- ½ medium white cabbage, thinly sliced
- 8 medium cloves of garlic, diced
- ½ cup dried porcini mushrooms
- 4 tablespoons apple cider vinegar
- 3 tablespoons tomato paste
- 2 cups beef stock
- 2 cups vegetable stock
- 1 teaspoon pepper
- 10 cups water
- Fresh parsley and sour cream (garnish)

How to

1. Put the oil and onion in the instant pot and cook for 3 minutes on the 'sauté' function.
2. Add the carrots, beets, potatoes and cabbage, and cook for 1 minute.
3. Stir in the rest of the ingredients and secure the lid.
4. Select the 'manual' function and cook for 10 minutes at high pressure.
5. After the beep, 'natural release' the steam, then remove the lid.
6. Serve hot with parsley and cream on top.

Nutrition Values (Per Serving)

- Calories: 250
- Carbohydrate: 46g
- Protein: 7.5g
- Fat: 7.6g
- Sugar: 10.6g
- Sodium: 876mg

Creamy Buffalo Chicken Soup

(**Serves**: 4 / **Prep Time:** 5 minutes / **Cooking Time**: 10 minutes)

Ingredients

- 4 boneless, skinless chicken breasts
- 6 cups chicken bone broth
- 1 cup diced celery
- ½ cup diced onion
- 2 cloves garlic, chopped
- 2 tablespoons ranch dressing mix
- 2 tablespoons butter
- ¾ cup hot sauce
- 2 cups cheddar cheese, shredded
- 2 cups heavy cream

How to

1. Put all the ingredients, except the cheese and cream, into the instant pot.
2. Secure the lid and select the 'manual' function. Cook for 10 minutes on high pressure.
3. After the beep, 'quick release' the steam and remove the lid.
4. Stir in the cheese and cream.
5. Serve hot.

Nutrition Values (Per Serving)

- Calories: 840
- Carbohydrate: 7.5g
- Protein: 65.6g
- Fat: 59.8g
- Sugar: 3.1g
- Sodium: 2890mg

Chicken Spinach Corn Soup

(**Serves**: 6 / **Prep Time:** 10 minutes / **Cooking Time**: 10 Min)

Ingredients

- 1 tablespoon olive oil
- 2 medium chicken breasts, thinly sliced
- 3 scallions, chopped
- 1 large white potato, peeled and diced
- 1 tablespoon ginger, grated
- 3 cups frozen corn kernels
- 4 cups chicken stock
- 1 tablespoon fish sauce
- 2 tablespoons light soy sauce
- 2 large cloves of garlic, diced
- ⅓ teaspoon white pepper
- 1 teaspoon salt
- 1 tablespoon arrowroot powder
- 3-4 handfuls of baby spinach leaves
- 2 eggs
- Juice of ½ lemon

How to

1. Put the oil, green onions, chicken, potato and ginger, into the instant pot and stir fry on the 'sauté' function for 5 minutes.
2. Place the corn kernels and 1 cup chicken broth into a blender. Blend well to form a smooth puree.
3. Now put the remaining ingredients and corn mixture into the cooker and secure the lid.
4. Cook for 5 minutes at high pressure on 'manual' function.
5. After the beep, 'natural release' the steam and remove the lid.
6. Switch the cooker to the 'sauté' mode.
7. Crack the eggs into a small bowl and whisk them well. Pour the egg mix into the soup, stirring constantly.
8. Dissolve the arrowroot powder in water and stir it into the soup.
9. Cook for 1 minute then serve hot.

Nutrition Values (Per Serving)

- Calories: 246
- Carbohydrate: 29.7g
- Protein: 20.7g
- Fat: 8.5g
- Sugar: 6.7g
- Sodium: 2767mg

BEEF, LAMB AND PORK

Beef Mushroom Stroganoff

(**Serves**: 6 / **Prep time:** 5 minutes / **Cooking time**: 35 minutes)

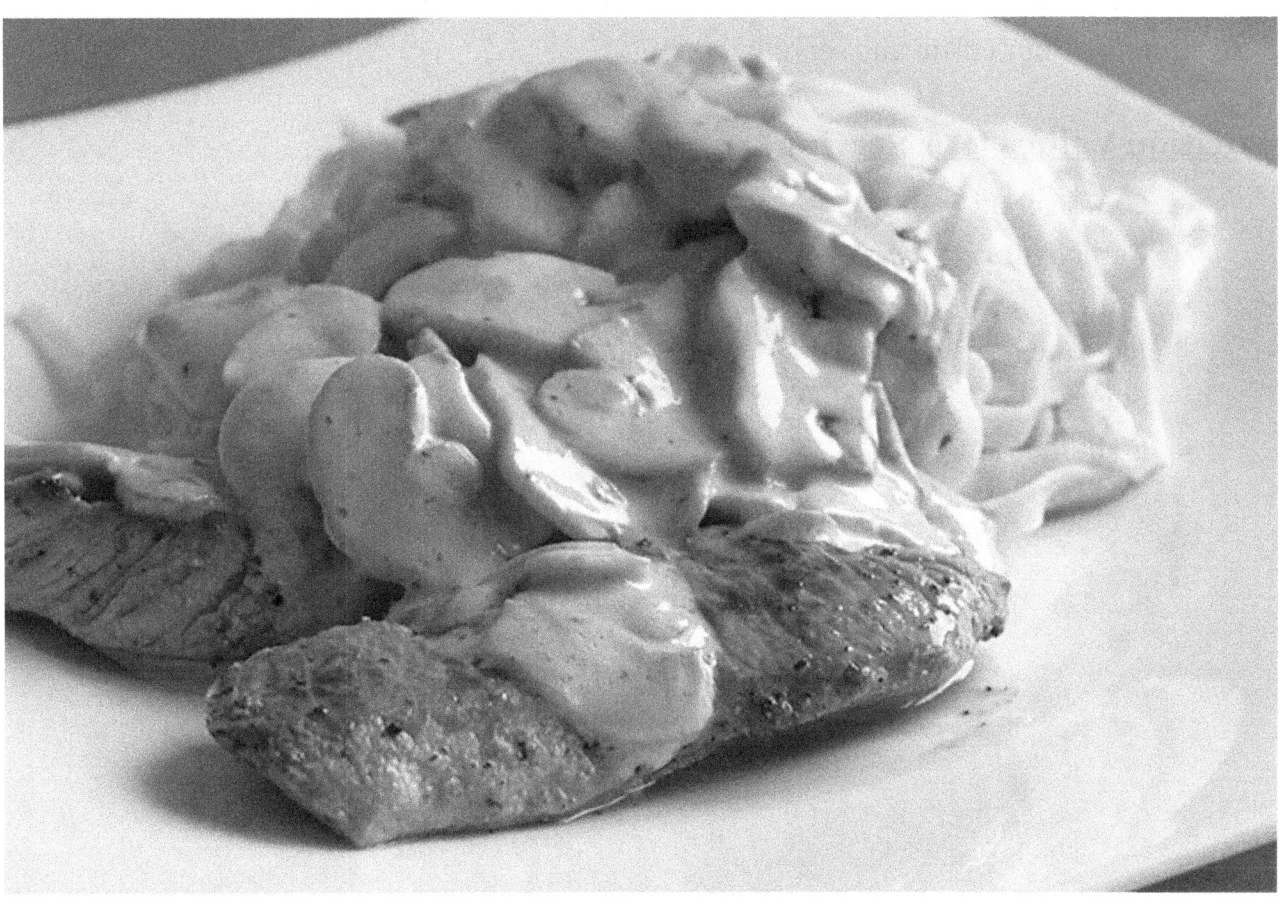

Ingredients

- 1½ lbs beef stew meat
- 1½ tablespoons oil
- 1½ tablespoons garlic
- ¾ cup diced onions
- 1½ teaspoons salt
- 2 cups mushroom, chopped
- 1 cup water
- 1½ teaspoons black pepper
- ¾ cup sour cream

How to

1. Select the 'sauté' function on the instant pot.
2. Add the oil. the onions and garlic. Cook for 3 minutes.
3. Add the remaining ingredients, except the sour cream.
4. Secure the lid and set the cooker on 'manual' for 20 minutes at high pressure.
5. After the beep, 'natural release' the steam and remove the lid after 20 minutes.
6. Stir in the sour cream and serve.

Nutrition Values (Per Serving)

- Calories: 317
- Carbohydrate: 4.4g
- Protein: 36.4g
- Fat: 16.6g
- Sugar: 1.1g
- Sodium: 675mg

Eastern Lamb Stew

(**Serves**: 8 / **Prep time**: 15 minutes / **Cooking time**: 1 hour 20 minutes)

Ingredients

- 4 tablespoons olive oil
- 1 (½ -1¾) lb lamb stew meat
- 2 onions, diced
- 8 garlic cloves, chopped
- 2 teaspoons salt
- 2 teaspoons pepper
- 2 teaspoons cumin
- 2 teaspoons coriander
- 2 teaspoons turmeric,
- 2 teaspoons cinnamon
- 1 teaspoon chilli flakes
- 4 tablespoons tomato paste
- ½ cup apple cider vinegar
- 4 tablespoons honey or brown sugar
- 2½ cups chicken broth
- 2 (15 oz.) cans chickpeas, rinsed and drained
- ½ cup raisins, chopped

How to

1. Select the 'sauté' function on the instant pot.
2. Add the oil, garlic and all the spices. Sauté for 4 minutes.
3. Stir in all the remaining ingredients and secure the lid.
4. Switch the cooker to the 'meat stew' mode for 1 hour 15 minutes.
5. After the beep, 'natural release' the steam and remove the lid.
6. Stir the stew and serve with fresh cilantro on top.

Nutrition Values (Per Serving)

- Calories: 1010
- Carbohydrate: 87.2g
- Protein: 65.4g
- Fat: 44.2g
- Sugar: 27.9g
- Sodium: 1018mg

Garlic Beef Sirloin

(**Serves**: 8 / **Prep time:** 10 minutes / **Cooking time**: 50 minutes)

Ingredients

- 6 lbs beef top sirloin steak
- 4 teaspoons garlic powder
- 8 cloves garlic, minced
- 1 cup butter
- Salt and pepper to taste

How to

1. Select the 'sauté' function on the instant pot.
2. Pour in the oil and add the sirloin steaks. Cook for 5 minutes. Let the meat brown on each side.
3. Stir in all the remaining ingredients and secure the lid.
4. Switch the cooker to the 'meat stew' mode and cook for 30 minutes.
5. After the beep, 'natural release' the steam and remove the lid.
6. Serve hot.

Nutrition Values (Per Serving)

- Calories: 865
- Carbohydrate: 2g
- Protein: 103.9g
- Fat: 44.3g
- Sugar: 0.4g
- Sodium: 368g

Lamb Meat Balls

(**Serves**: 3 / **Prep Time:** 10 minutes / **Cooking Time**: 40 minutes)

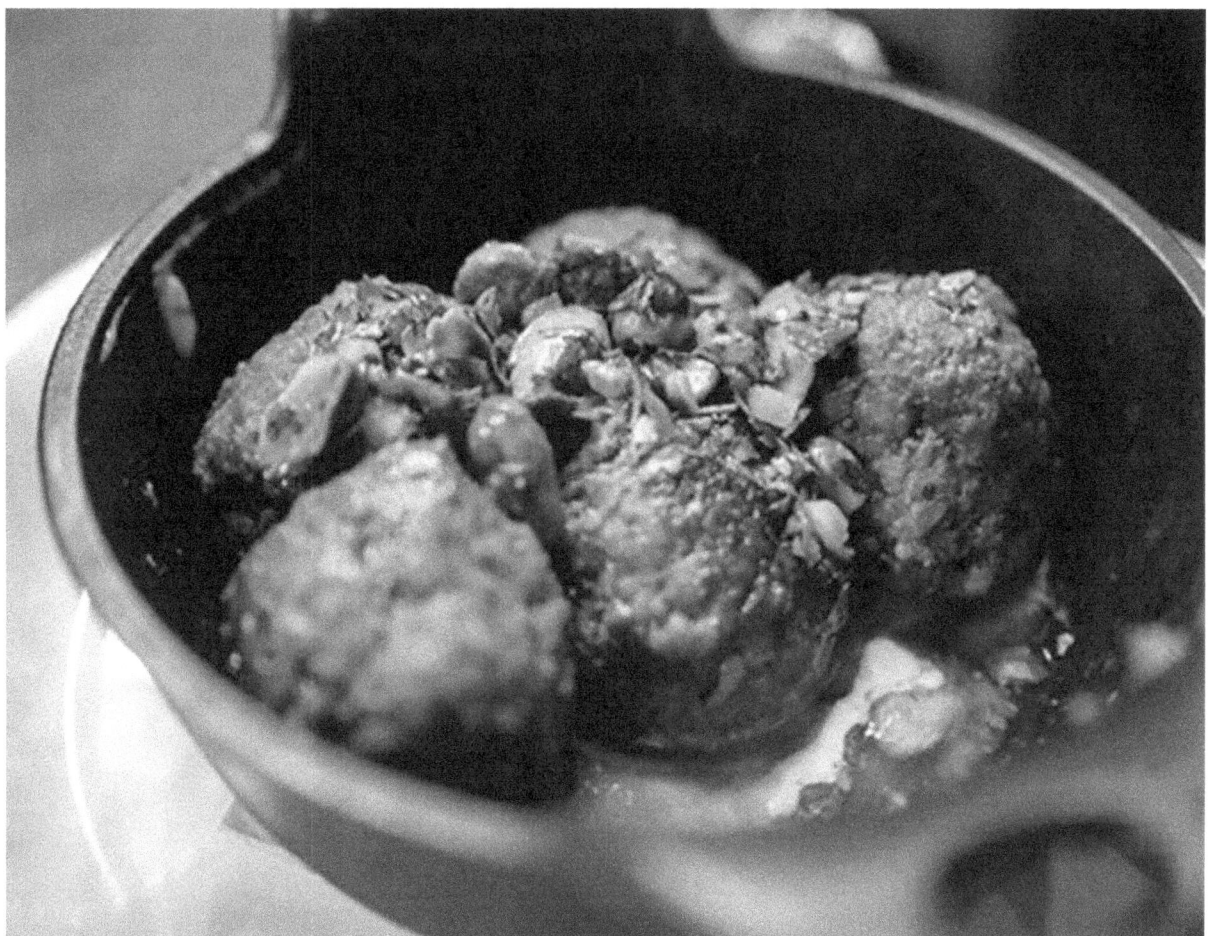

Ingredients

- ¾ lbs ground lamb meat
- Salt and freshly ground black pepper, to taste
- 2 small tomatoes, chopped roughly
- ½ small yellow onion, chopped roughly
- ½ cup sugar-free tomato sauce
- ¼ teaspoon red pepper flakes, crushed
- 2 garlic cloves, peeled
- 5 mini bell peppers, seeded and halved
- ½ tablespoon olive oil
- 1 teaspoon adobo seasoning

How to

1. In a bowl, combine the lamb meat with the adobo seasoning, black pepper and salt. 2. Prepare small meatballs out of this mixture.
3. Set the cooker to the 'sauté' mode and add oil to it.
4. Add the meatballs to the hot oil and cook until they turn golden brown.
5. Transfer the meatballs to a separate bowl.
6. Add all the remaining ingredients to the pot and secure the lid.
7. Switch the cooker to the 'meat stew' mode and cook for 35 minutes.
8. After the beep, 'natural release the steam and remove the lid.
9. Use an immerse blender to blend the vegetable mix.
10. Stir in the meatballs, garnish with herbs, and serve hot.

Nutrition Values (Per Serving)

- Calories: 445
- Carbohydrate: 24.3g
- Protein: 32g
- Fat: 25.5g
- Sugar: 15.7g
- Sodium: 430mg

Traditional Country Steak

(**Serves**: 8 / **Prep Time:** 10 minutes / **Cooking Time**: 40 minutes)

Ingredients

- 4 lbs beef round steak
- 2 tablespoons vegetable oil
- 4 teaspoons Worcestershire sauce
- 6 garlic cloves
- 1 cup all-purpose flour
- 1 teaspoon salt
- 1 teaspoon black pepper
- 1 cup ketchup
- 1 cup diced onions

How to

1. Add the steaks and flour to a bowl and dredge the steaks through to cover both sides with flour.
2. Set the instant pot on the 'sauté' function and add oil to it.
3. Add the steaks in batches and cook well to turn them brown on both sides.
4. Add the remaining ingredients and secure the lid.
5. Cook on the 'manual' function for 30 minutes at high pressure.
6. 'Natural release' the steam, then remove the lid.
7. Serve immediately.

Nutrition Values (Per Serving)

- Calories: 616
- Carbohydrate: 22.2g
- Protein: 74.3g
- Fat: 23.8g
- Sugar: 8g
- Sodium: 792mg

3 Peppers Lamb

(**Serves**: 10 / **Prep Time:** 10 minutes / **Cooking Time**: 35 minutes)

Ingredients

- 2 lbs grass-fed, boneless beef, trimmed
- 4 cups tomatoes, chopped finely
- 6 garlic cloves, minced
- 2 cups water
- 2 tablespoons olive oil
- Salt and black pepper to taste
- 2 teaspoons dried rosemary, crushed
- 2 large green bell peppers, seeded and sliced
- 2 large yellow bell peppers, seeded and sliced
- 2 large red bell peppers, seeded and sliced
- 3 cups sugar-free tomato sauce

How to

1. Turn the instant pot to the 'sauté' function and add oil to it.
2. Stir in the lamb meat along with salt and pepper. Cook for 5 minutes.
3. Dish the meat out onto a plate.
4. Add the water, salt, garlic, rosemary and black pepper.
5. Stir in all the peppers and return the meat to the pot.
6. Secure the lid and set it to the 'manual' function for 25 minutes at high pressure.
7. 'Quick release' the steam and remove the lid. Serve hot.

Nutrition Values (Per Serving)

- Calories: 224
- Carbohydrate: 10.1g
- Protein: 26g
- Fat: 9.2g
- Sugar: 6.6g
- Sodium: 451mg

Healthy Prime Rib

(**Serves**: 7 / **Prep Time:** 5 minutes / **Cooking Time**: 46 minutes)

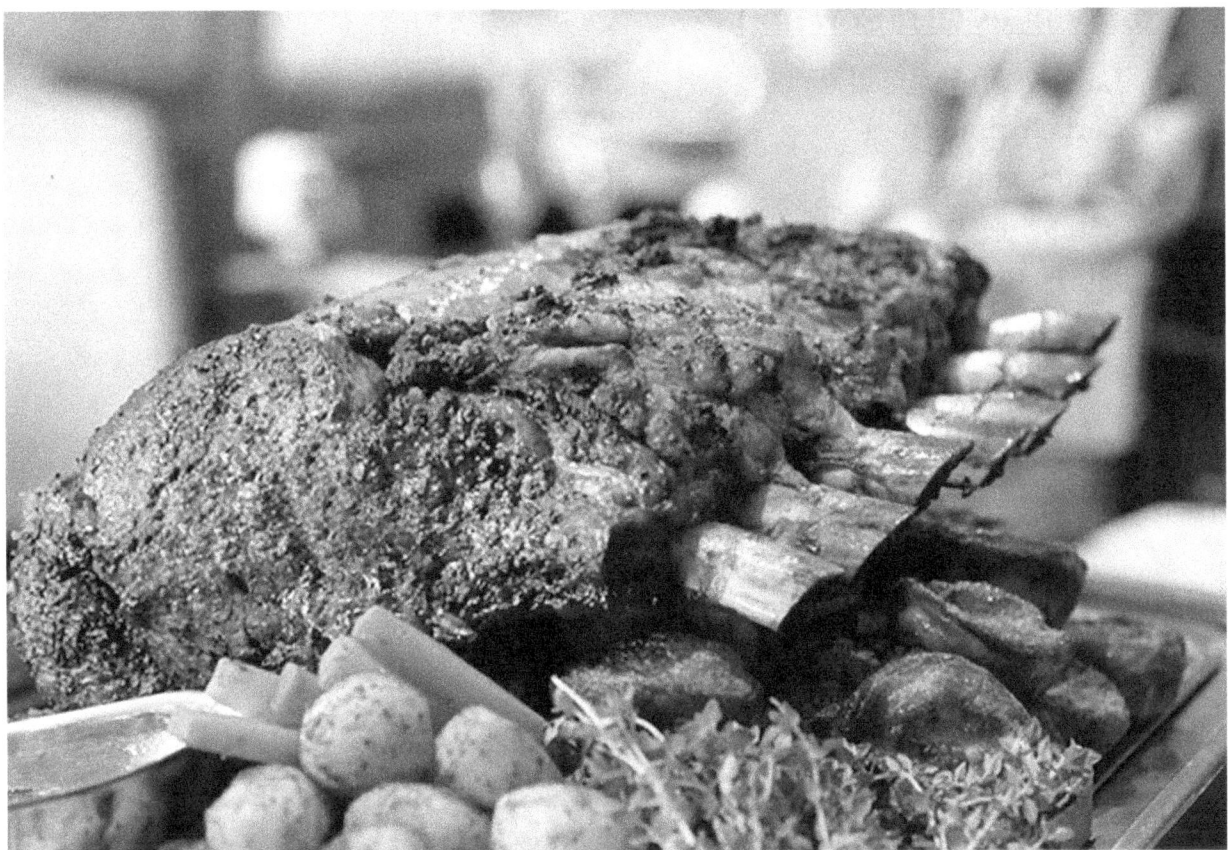

Ingredients

- ½ (5 lbs) prime rib roast
- 1 tablespoon olive oil
- 1 teaspoon ground black pepper
- 1 teaspoon salt
- 5 cloves garlic, minced
- 1 teaspoon dried thyme

How to

1. In a large bowl, combine the oil, salt, thyme and pepper.
2. Add the beef to the mix and marinate for 5 minutes.
3. Pour water into the pot and place in the streamer trivet.
4. Place the marinated prime rib roast over the trivet and secure the lid.
5. Select the 'meat stew' option and cook for 25 minutes at high pressure.
6. 'Quick release' the steam and remove the lid.
7. Meanwhile, set the oven to 475º F.

8. Bake the ribs in the oven for 15 minutes.
9. Serve hot.

Nutrition Values (Per Serving)
- Calories: 1164
- Carbohydrate: 6.7g
- Protein: 80.2g
- Fat: 87.9g
- Sugar: 0g
- Sodium: 3020mg

Bacon Lamb Chili

(**Serves**: 8 / **Prep Time:** 10 minutes / **Cooking Time**: 50 minutes)

Ingredients

- 2 lbs grass-fed ground lamb
- 8 bacon slices, chopped
- 1 small onion, chopped
- 3 tablespoons chilli powder
- 2 tablespoons smoked paprika
- 4 teaspoons ground cumin
- 2 red bell peppers, seeded and chopped
- Freshly ground black pepper to taste
- 4 garlic cloves, minced

How to

1. Set the instant pot to 'sauté' mode and place the bacon inside.
2. Sauté the bacon for 5 minutes, then transfer onto a paper towel on a plate.
3. Now add the garlic, onion and bell peppers to the pot and cook for 5 minutes.
4. Add the lamb, the spices and cooked bacon to the pot and secure the lid.
5. Use the 'bean/Chili' function to cook for 30 minutes.
6. 'Natural release' the steam then, remove the lid.
7. Serve hot.

Nutrition Values (Per Serving)

- Calories: 427
- Carbohydrate: 6.8g
- Protein: 27.4g
- Fat: 23g
- Sugar: 2.3g
- Sodium: 536mg

Super Easy Hot Dogs

(**Serves**: 3 / **Prep Time:** 5 minutes / **Cooking Time**: 3 minutes)

Ingredients

- 3 beef sausages, cured, cooked and smoked
- ½ tablespoon cider vinegar
- ½ quart fresh water
- ¼ teaspoon ground cumin
- 3 whole grain white buns

How to

1. Pour the water into the instant pot and add the cumin and vinegar.
2. Add the sausages and secure the lid.
3. Cook on the 'manual' setting for 3 minutes at low pressure.
4. 'Natural release' the steam and remove the lid
5. Place the sausages in the white buns and serve with the tomato sauce.

Nutrition Values (Per Serving)

- Calories: 298
- Carbohydrate: 37.8g
- Protein: 10.8g
- Fat: 11.3g
- Sugar: 4g
- Sodium: 563mg

Sauce Glazed Lamb Chops

(**Serves**: 2 / **Prep Time:** 5 minutes / **Cooking Time**: 30 minutes)

Ingredients

- 1 lb lamb loin chops
- 1 garlic clove, crushed
- ½ cup bone broth
- ¾ teaspoon dried rosemary, crushed
- 1 tablespoon arrowroot starch
- 1½ tablespoons butter
- ½ small onion, sliced
- ¾ cup sugar-free, diced tomatoes
- 1 cup carrots, peeled and sliced
- Salt and black pepper **to taste**
- ½ tablespoon cold water

How to

1. Add butter to the instant pot and heat it on the 'sauté' function.
2. Place the lamb chops in the pot and cook for 3 minutes each side.
3. Take the chops out of the pot and place them on a plate.
4. Put the onion and garlic into the pot and cook for 3 minutes.
5. Add the remaining ingredients and secure the lid.
6. Cook on the 'manual' setting for 15 minutes at high pressure.
7. 'Quick release' the steam and remove the lid.
8. Meanwhile, dissolve the arrowroot flour in some water and add the slurry to the pot.
9. Cook for 5 minutes then pour this sauce over the fried chops.
10. Serve hot.

Nutrition Values (Per Serving)

- Calories: 579
- Carbohydrate: 14g
- Protein: 70.1g
- Fat: 25.5g
- Sugar: 5.3g
- Sodium: 314mg

Turmeric Beef Steaks

(**Serves**: 3 / **Prep Time:** 5 minutes / **Cooking Time**: 35 minutes)

Ingredients

- ½ lb beef steak pieces
- 1 tablespoon salt
- ½ cup yoghurt
- 1½ tablespoons oil
- 1 tablespoon turmeric powder
- 1 tablespoon red chili powder
- 1 tablespoon coriander powder
- 1 tablespoon lemon juice
- 1 tablespoon cumin powder
- 1 tablespoon vinegar

How to

1. In a bowl, combine the red chili powder with the cumin powder, salt, coriander powder, vinegar, oil, lemon juice, and turmeric powder.
2. Place the beef pieces in the marinade, mix well and refrigerate overnight.
3. Pour a cup of water into the instant pot and place a steamer trivet inside.
4. Arrange the beef pieces in a single layer over the trivet and secure the lid.
5. Cook for 30 minutes on the 'meat stew' setting at high pressure.
6. 'Natural release' the steam and remove the lid.
7. Serve hot with boiled white rice.

Nutrition Values (Per Serving)

- Calories: 255
- Carbohydrate: 6.8g
- Protein: 26.6g
- Fat: 13.1g
- Sugar: 3.3g
- Sodium: 2435mg

Full Meal Lamb Shanks

(**Serves**: 3 / **Prep Time:** 15 minutes / **Cooking Time**: 45 minutes)

Ingredients

- 1½ lbs grass-fed lamb shanks, trimmed
- 1 tablespoon olive oil
- ¾ cup bone broth
- ½ teaspoon dried rosemary, crushed
- 1 tablespoon melted butter
- 7 whole garlic cloves, peeled
- Salt and black pepper to taste
- ¾ tablespoon sugar-free tomato paste
- 1¼ tablespoons fresh lemon juice

How to

1. Turn the instant pot to the 'sauté' setting, and add the oil to the insert.
2. Place the shanks in the pot and sprinkle salt and pepper over them.
3. Cook each side for 3 minutes, then add the garlic cloves.
4. Stir-fry for 2 minutes, then add all the remaining ingredients.
5. Secure the lid and select the 'manual' function and cook at high pressure for 30 minutes.
6. 'Natural release' the steam for 10 minutes, then remove the lid.
7. Transfer the lamb to a platter.
8. Pour the melted butter and lemon juice on top and serve.

Nutrition Values (Per Serving)

- Calories: 533
- Carbohydrate: 1.2g
- Protein: 69.1g
- Fat: 23.7g
- Sugar: 0.6g
- Sodium: 382mg

Cheesy Beef Meatballs

(**Serves**: 3 / **Prep Time:** 15 minutes / **Cooking Time**: 15 minutes)

Ingredients

- 1 lb ground beef
- 1 tablespoon Parmesan cheese, grated
- ½ teaspoon dried oregano
- ½ tablespoon olive oil
- ½ egg
- ½ tablespoon flaxseed meal
- Salt and ground black pepper to taste
- ½ (14 oz) can tomato sauce

How to

1. In a bowl, combine he Parmesan cheese with the ground beef, oregano, egg, salt, pepper and flaxseed.
2. Use this mixture to make small meatballs of 1-inch diameter.
3. Add the oil to the instant pot and select the 'sauté' function.
4. Put the meatballs into the oil and sauté until they turn brown.
5. Stir in the tomato sauce and water, then secure the lid.
6. Cook on 'manual' setting for 6 minutes at high pressure.
7. 'Natural release' the steam for 5 minutes, then remove the lid.
8. Serve warm.

Nutrition Values (Per Serving)

- Calories: 358
- Carbohydrate: 3.1g
- Protein: 50.6g
- Fat: 15g
- Sugar: 1.8g
- Sodium: 411mg

Coconut Lamb Curry

(**Serves**: 4 / **Prep Time:** 15 minutes / **Cooking Time**: 50 minutes)

Ingredients

- 1 lb grass-fed lamb shoulder, cut into bite-sized pieces
- 1 tablespoon curry powder, divided
- ¼ cup unsweetened coconut milk
- 2 tablespoons coconut cream
- 1 tablespoon coconut oil
- 1 medium yellow onion, chopped
- ½ cup chicken broth
- 1 tablespoon fresh lemon juice
- Salt and black pepper to taste
- 2 tablespoons fresh basil, chopped

How to

1. Combine the coconut cream, milk and curry powder in a bowl and then add the lamb. Allow to marinate for 20 minutes.
2. Heat the oil and butter in the instant pot on 'sauté' function.
3. Stir in the onion and garlic and cook for 4 minutes.
4. Add the curry powder to the pot and cook for a minute.
5. Now put the lamb into the pot, keeping the marinade to one side.
6. Stir in the chicken broth, the pepper, salt and lemon juice, then secure the lid.
7. Cook on 'manual' setting at high pressure for 20 minutes.
8. 'Quick release' the steam, remove the lid, and add the cream marinade to the lamb.
9. Cook for 5 minutes on 'sauté' mode.
10. Serve with fresh basil on top.

Nutrition Values (Per Serving)

- Calories: 340
- Carbohydrate: 7.1g
- Protein: 29.5g
- Fat: 21.3g
- Sugar: 4.3g
- Sodium: 179mg

Japanese Beef Bowl

(**Serves**: 4 / **Prep Time:** 15 minutes / **Cooking Time**: 20 minutes)

Ingredients

- 1 lb beef ribeye steak, thinly sliced
- 2 large white onions
- 1 cup water
- 2 tablespoons brown sugar
- 2 tablespoons sake
- 2 teaspoons vegetable oil
- 4 tablespoons soy sauce
- 2 tablespoons mirin

How to

1. Put the oil and onions into the instant pot and cook until brown.
2. Stir in the soy sauce, the mirin, sake, water and brown sugar.
3. Add the beef steaks to the instant pot and secure the lid.
4. Cook on 'manual' function for 15 minutes at high pressure.
5. 'Quick release' the steam and remove the lid.
6. Serve hot.

Nutrition Values (Per Serving)

- Calories: 316
- Carbohydrate: 16.9g
- Protein: 22.7g
- Fat: 16.3g
- Sugar: 9.8g
- Sodium: 1274mg

Mouth Watering Lamb Stew

(**Serves**: 3 / **Prep Time:** 15 minutes / **Cooking Time**: 45 minutes)

Ingredients

- 1 lb grass-fed lamb shoulder, trimmed and cut into 2-inch cubes
- ¾ tablespoon olive oil
- 1 celery stalk, chopped
- 1 cup fresh tomatoes, chopped finely
- 1½ tablespoon fresh lemon juice
- ½ teaspoon salt
- ½ teaspoon black pepper
- ½ large green bell pepper, cut into 8 slices
- ½ large red bell pepper, cut into 8 slices
- ½ cup bone broth
- ½ small onion, chopped
- ½ tablespoon garlic, minced
- ½ teaspoon dried oregano, crushed
- ½ teaspoon dried basil, crushed

How to

1. Turn the instant pot to the 'sauté' function and heat the oil.
2. Add the garlic and onion and cook for 2 minutes.
3. Stir in all the remaining ingredients except the bell peppers.
4. Secure the lid and cook for 15 minutes on 'manual' function at high pressure.
5. 'Natural release' the steam for 10 minutes, then remove the lid.
6. Stir in the bell peppers and 'sauté' for 8 minutes.
7. Serve hot.

Nutrition Values (Per Serving)

- Calories: 381
- Carbohydrate: 6.3g
- Protein: 39.1g
- Fat: 21.5g
- Sugar: 3.5g
- Sodium: 628mg

Beef & Bacon Casserole

(**Serves**: 4 / **Prep Time:** 15 minutes / **Cooking Time**: 35 minutes)

Ingredients

- 1 lb ground beef
- ¼ teaspoon onion powder
- 4 eggs
- ½ cup heavy cream
- ¼ teaspoon ground pepper
- 1½ garlic cloves
- ½ lb bacon, cooked and chopped
- 3 oz. tomato paste
- ¼ teaspoon salt
- 6 oz. cheddar cheese, grated

How to

1. Put the beef, bacon, garlic and onion powder into the instant pot and 'sauté' for 5 minutes.
2. Combine the cream, eggs, salt, tomato paste and cheddar cheese, in a bowl.
3. Pour this mixture over the beef and bacon. Secure the lid.
4. Cook on 'the manual' function for 25 minutes at high pressure.
5. 'Natural release the steam for 5 minutes, then remove the lid.
6. Serve hot.

Nutrition Values (Per Serving)

- Calories: 823
- Carbohydrate: 6.7g
- Protein: 72.9g
- Fat: 54.9g
- Sugar: 3.2g
- Sodium: 1884mg

Lamb and Zucchini Curry

(**Serves**: 3 / **Prep Time:** 15 minutes / **Cooking Time**: 50 minutes)

Ingredients

- 1 lb cubed lamb stew meat
- 1 tablespoon fresh ginger, grated
- ½ teaspoon lime juice
- ¼ teaspoon black pepper
- ¾ cup diced tomatoes
- ½ teaspoon turmeric powder
- 1½ medium carrots, sliced
- 2 garlic cloves, minced
- ½ cup coconut milk
- ¼ teaspoon salt
- 1 tablespoon olive oil
- ½ medium onion, diced
- ½ medium zucchini, diced

How to

1. Combine the garlic, ginger, salt, pepper, coconut milk and lime juice in a bowl and add meat to marinate for 30 minutes.
2. Put the oil and meat, along with the marinade, tomatoes, carrots, turmeric powder and onions, into the instant pot.
3. Secure the lid and cook for 20 minutes on 'manual' function at high pressure.
4. 'Natural release' for 15 minutes, then remove the lid.
5. Add the zucchini to the curry and let it simmer for 5 minutes.
6. Serve hot.

Nutrition Values (Per Serving)

- Calories: 255
- Carbohydrate: 12.7g
- Protein: 9,5g
- Fat: 19.6g
- Sugar: 5.6g
- Sodium: 255mg

Beef Potato Tots

(**Serves**: 4 / **Prep Time:** 10 minutes / **Cooking Time**: 35 minutes)

Ingredients

- ¾ lbs lean ground beef
- 16 oz. frozen potato rounds, tater tots
- ¼ onion, chopped
- 8 oz. cream of chicken soup
- 2 tablespoons oil

How to

1. Heat the oil in the instant pot on 'sauté' mode.
2. Stir in the beef and onion. Sauté for 5 minutes.
3. Add the cream of chicken soup and place the potato tater tots on top.
4. Secure the lid and cook for 25 minutes at medium pressure on the 'manual' setting.
5. 'Natural release for 5 minutes, then remove the lid.
6. Serve warm.

Nutrition Values (Per Serving)

- Calories: 1100
- Carbohydrate: 92.7g
- Protein: 35.2g
- Fat: 63.4g
- Sugar: 0.6g
- Sodium: 1552mg

Juicy Lamb Leg

(**Serves**: 6 / **Prep Time:** 15 minutes / **Cooking Time**: 60 minutes)

Ingredients

- 2 lbs leg of lamb
- 1 teaspoon fine sea salt
- 2½ tablespoons olive oil
- 6 sprigs thyme
- 1½ cups bone broth
- 6 garlic cloves, minced
- 1½ teaspoons black pepper
- 1½ small onions
- ¾ cup orange juice

How to

1. Add the salt, pepper and garlic to the lamb and marinate.
2. Heat the oil in the instant pot using the 'sauté' function, then add the onions.
3. Cook for 4 minutes then remove the onions from the pot.
4. put the marinated lamb in the pot and cook for 3 minutes on each side.
5. Stir in the broth, the onion, orange juice and thyme. Secure the lid.
6. Select 'meat stew' mode and cook for 40 minutes.
7. 'Natural release' the steam for 10 minutes, then remove the lid.
8. Serve hot.

Nutrition Values (Per Serving)

- Calories: 380
- Carbohydrate: 6.3g
- Protein: 48.1g
- Fat: 17g
- Sugar: 3.4g
- Sodium: 466mg

Mexican Butter Beef

(**Serves**: 3 / **Prep Time:** 20 minutes / **Cooking Time**: 35 minutes)

Ingredients

- 1 lb boneless beef
- ¾ teaspoon salt
- ½ teaspoon black pepper
- ½ medium onion, thinly sliced
- 3 garlic cloves, minced
- ¼ cup bone broth
- ½ tablespoon chili powder
- 1 tablespoon butter
- ½ tablespoon tomato paste
- ¼ teaspoon red boat fish sauce

How to

1. Add the chili powder and salt to the beef in a bowl. Mix well.
2. Heat the butter in the instant pot on the 'sauté' function.
3. Sauté the onion for 4 minutes, then add the tomato paste and garlic.
4. Add the fish sauce, beef and broth to the cooker and lock the lid.
5. Select the 'meat stew' function and cook for 30 minutes at high pressure.
6. 'Natural release' the steam for 15 minutes, then remove the lid.
7. Sprinkle some salt and pepper on top, then serve.

Nutrition Values (Per Serving)

- Calories: 649
- Carbohydrate: 4.1g
- Protein: 23.9g
- Fat: 59g
- Sugar: 1.2g
- Sodium: 753mg

Greek Style Lamb

(**Serves**: 2 / **Prep Time:** 25 minutes / **Cooking Time**: 45 minutes)

Ingredients

- 1 lb lamb meat, ground
- 4 garlic cloves
- 1 teaspoon rosemary
- ¾ teaspoon salt
- ¼ teaspoon black pepper
- ½ small onion, chopped
- 1 teaspoon dried oregano
- 1 teaspoon ground marjoram
- ¾ cup water

How to

1. Chop the garlic, onions, rosemary and marjoram in a food processor.
2. Add the ground beef and the salt and pepper to the mixture and combine well.
3. Compress the beef mixture to make a compact 'loaf'.
4. Cover it tightly with tin foil and make some holes in it.
5. Pour water into the instant pot and place the trivet inside.
6. Place the loaf pan over the trivet and secure the lid.
7. Cook on 'manual' at high pressure for 15 minutes.
8. 'Quick release' the steam, then remove the lid.
9. Serve warm.

Nutrition Values (Per Serving)

- Calories: 664
- Carbohydrate: 4.8g
- Protein: 56.9g
- Fat: 44.8g
- Sugar: 0.8g
- Sodium: 1061mg

Beef Broccoli Stew

(**Serves**: 3 / **Prep Time:** 15 minutes / **Cooking Time**: 55 minutes)

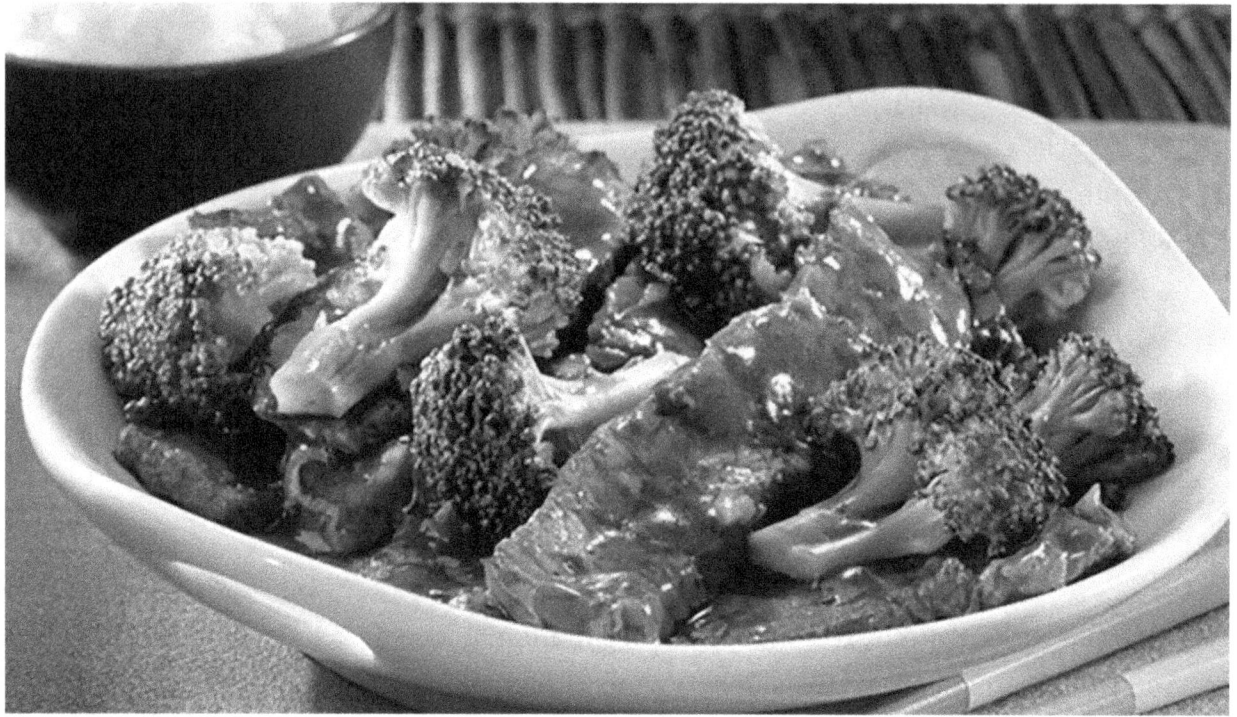

Ingredients

- 1¼ lbs beef stew chunks
- 1 zucchini, chopped
- 1 tablespoon curry powder
- ½ teaspoon salt
- ½ lb broccoli florets
- ¼ cup chicken broth
- ½ tablespoon garlic powder
- ½ cup coconut milk

How to

1. Place all the ingredients, except the coconut milk, into the instant pot.
2. Secure the lid and turn on the 'manual' function.
3. Cook for 45 minutes at high pressure.
4. 'Natural release' the steam and remove the lid.
5. Stir in the coconut milk and let it simmer for 2 minutes.
6. Serve immediately.

Nutrition Values (Per Serving)

- Calories: 227
- Carbohydrate: 24.4g
- Protein: 12.3g
- Fat: 16.2g
- Sugar: 5.9g
- Sodium: 1297mg

Beef and Pork Gumbo

(**Serves**: 3 / **Prep Time:** 15 minutes / **Cooking Time**: 4 hours 25 minutes)

Ingredients

- ¼ tablespoon olive oil
- ¼ lbs. grass-fed ground beef
- ¼ lbs. ground pork
- 1 medium tomatillo, chopped
- ⅛ small yellow onion, chopped
- ½ jalapeño pepper, chopped
- ½ garlic clove, minced
- ¼ (6oz) can sugar-free tomato sauce
- ¼ tablespoon chili powder
- ¼ tablespoon ground cumin
- Salt and freshly ground black pepper to taste
- 1 tablespoon water
- 2 tablespoons cheddar cheese, shredded

How to

1. Put the oil and all the ingredients into the instant pot.
2. Stir well and secure the lid.
3. Set the cooker to 'slow cook' at high heat for 4 hours.
4. 'Natural release' the steam and remove the lid.
5. Serve hot.

Nutrition Values (Per Serving)

- Calories: 181
- Carbohydrate: 4.8g
- Protein: 20.4g
- Fat: 8.5g
- Sugar: 1g
- Sodium: 122mg

Wine Glazed Short Ribs

(**Serves**: 2 / **Prep Time:** 15 minutes / **Cooking Time**: 60 minutes)

Ingredients

- 1 lb boneless beef short ribs
- 1 tablespoon curry powder
- 1 cup water
- 1 tablespoon white wine
- ½ large onion, diced
- 1½ tablespoons tamari sauce
- ½ tablespoon salt

How to

1. Put all the ingredients into the instant pot.
2. Cover with the lid and select the 'slow Cook' function. Cook for 1 hour.
3. Remove the lid.
4. Serve hot.

Nutrition Values (Per Serving)

- Calories: 482
- Carbohydrate: 8.3g
- Protein: 74.8g
- Fat: 14.7g
- Sugar: 2.6g
- Sodium: 570mg

Spicy Minced Meat

(**Serves**: 2 / **Prep Time:** 15 minutes / **Cooking Time**: 25 minutes)

Ingredients

- ½ lb ground lamb meat
- ½ cup onion, chopped
- ½ tablespoon garlic
- ½ tablespoon minced ginger
- ¼ teaspoon turmeric
- ¼ teaspoon ground coriander
- ½ teaspoon salt
- ¼ teaspoon cumin
- ¼ teaspoon cayenne pepper

How to

1. Set the instant pot to 'sauté' mode.
2. Add the onions, garlic and ginger, and sauté for 5 minutes.
3. Add the remaining ingredients to the pot and secure the lid.
4. Cook on the 'manual' function for 15 minutes at high pressure.
5. After the beep, 'natural release' the steam for 15 minutes.
6. Remove the lid and serve immediately.

Nutrition Values (Per Serving)

- Calories: 343
- Carbohydrate: 4.8g
- Protein: 28.7g
- Fat: 22.5g
- Sugar: 1.3g
- Sodium: 676mg

Beef Pot Roast

(**Serves**: 6 / **Prep Time:** 5 minutes / **Cooking Time**: 2 hours 20 minutes)

Ingredients

- 2½ lbs beef roast
- 1 teaspoon garlic powder
- 1 tablespoon avocado oil
- 1 teaspoon salt
- ½ teaspoon black pepper

How to

1. Select the 'sauté' function on the instant pot.
2. Combine the salt, pepper and garlic powder and stir to form an even mix. Now coat the beef roast evenly with the mix.
3. Place the beef in the pot, add the oil and cover with the lid.
4. Cook for 10 minutes then flip the roast on to the other side.
5. Cover with the lid again and cook for a further 10 minutes.
6. Lock the lid and select the 'meat stew' option. Set to cook for 85 minutes.
7. 'Natural release' the steam for 30 minutes, then remove the lid.
8. Serve warm.

Nutrition Values (Per Serving)

- Calories: 356
- Carbohydrate: 0.6g
- Protein: 57.5g
- Fat: 12.1g
- Sugar: 0.1g
- Sodium: 512mg

Potato Lamb Roast

(Serves: 2 / **Prep Time:** 10 minutes / **Cooking Time**: 1 hour 30 minutes)

Ingredients

- 2 lbs lamb roasted
- 1 cup onion soup
- ¼ cup carrots
- ¼ cup potatoes
- 1 cup beef broth

How to

1. Place the lamb roast in the instant pot and add the remaining ingredients.
2. Set the timer for 70 minutes at high pressure on 'manual' mode.
3. 'Natural release' the steam for 15 minutes, then remove the lid.
4. Serve warm.

Nutrition Values (Per Serving)

- Calories: 1066
- Carbohydrate: 13g
- Protein: 120g
- Fat: 56.7g
- Sugar: 4.6g
- Sodium: 1450mg

Beef Carne Asada

(**Serves**: 6 / **Prep Time:** 10 minutes / **Cooking Time**: 2 hours 15 minutes)

Ingredients

- 2 lbs beef stew meat
- ¾ tablespoon chili powder
- 2 tablespoon salt
- 1½ tablespoons olive oil
- ½ cup beef bone broth
- ½ large onion, sliced
- ¾ tablespoon cumin
- 1 tablespoon lemon juice
- 1½ oz. tomato paste

How to

1. Season the stew meat with salt, cumin and chili powder.
2. Select the 'sauté' function on your instant pot to heat the oil.
3. Place the beef in the pot and secure the lid.
4. Cook on 'manual' function for 35 minutes at high pressure.
5. 'Natural release' the steam and remove the lid.
6. Add the remaining ingredients and let it sit for 5 minutes.
7. Serve warm.

Nutrition Values (Per Serving)

- Calories: 408
- Carbohydrate: 13.4g
- Protein: 58.6g
- Fat: 15.3g
- Sugar: 3.5g
- Sodium: 2556mg

Lamb Chop Irish Stew

(**Serves**: 8 / **Prep Time:** 10 minutes / **Cooking Time:** 30 minutes)

Ingredients

- 8 lamb shoulder chops, cubed
- 8 large onions, sliced into thin rounds
- 4 cups water
- 4 tablespoons olive oil
- 9 large carrots, chunked
- 4 sprigs thyme
- 2 teaspoons salt
- 2 teaspoons black pepper

How to

1. Select 'sauté' on the instant pot and heat the oil in it.
2. Add the lamb chops and cook until they turn brown.
3. Transfer the chops to a plate.
4. Pour water into the pot and add the thyme.
5. Put the chops back into the pot and arrange the vegetables over them.
6. Sprinkle with salt and secure the lid.
7. Cook for 15 minutes on 'manual' at high pressure.
8. 'Natural release' the steam, then remove the lid.
9. Serve warm.

Nutrition Values (Per Serving)

- Calories: 325
- Carbohydrate: 22.5g
- Protein: 24.4g
- Fat: 16.2g
- Sugar: 10.3g
- Sodium: 727mg

Pork Lettuce Wraps

(**Serves**: 6 / **Prep Time:** 10 minutes / **Cooking Time**: 55 minutes)

Ingredients

- 3 lbs bone-in pork shoulder
- ¾ teaspoon ground cumin
- 1¼ pinches cayenne
- ½ teaspoon black pepper
- ½ teaspoon dried oregano
- ¾ teaspoon garlic powder
- ¾ teaspoon sea salt
- 1¼ tablespoon olive oil
- 1¼ onions, chopped
- 1¼ oranges, juiced
- 6 lettuce leaves

How to

1. Put all the ingredients in with the pork and mix well. Refrigerate overnight.
2. Heat the oil in the instant pot using the 'sauté' function.
3. Put the marinated pork into the oil and sear for 10 minutes.
4. Pour in 2 cups of water and secure the lid.
5. Select the 'manual' function and cook for 45 minutes at medium pressure.
6. Release the pressure for 10 minutes using 'Natural release'.
7. Serve the cooked pork on lettuce leaves.

Nutrition Values (Per Serving)

- Calories: 514
- Carbohydrate: 7.6g
- Protein: 39.2g
- Fat: 35.5g
- Sugar: 5.7g
- Sodium: 781mg

Picante Lamb Chops

(**Serves**: 6 / **Prep Time:** 10 minutes / **Cooking Time**: 50 minutes)

Ingredients

- 6 lamb chops, bone-in
- 1¼ apples, peeled and pieced
- 1¼ cup Picante sauce
- 3 tablespoons olive oil
- 3 tablespoons all-purpose flour
- 3 tablespoons brown sugar, packed

How to

1. Dredge the mutton chops through a bowl of flour.
2. Mix the apple slices, picante sauce and brown sugar in a bowl.
3. Pour the oil into the instant pot and select 'sauté'.
4. Add the flour covered chops to the oil and sear for 5 minutes.
5. Secure the lid and select the 'meat stew" function. Cook for 35 minutes at high pressure.
6. 'Natural release' the steam for 10 minutes, then remove the lid.
7. Serve warm.

Nutrition Values (Per Serving)

- Calories: 449
- Carbohydrate: 16.3g
- Protein: 20.1g
- Fat: 33.3g
- Sugar: 10.7g
- Sodium: 316mg

Pork with Calabacita Squash

(**Serves**: 3 / **Prep Time:** 10 minutes / **Cooking Time**: 1 hour 45 minutes)

Ingredients

- ½ pork tenderloin
- ½ tablespoon ground cumin
- 1 teaspoon salt
- ½ tablespoon chili powder
- ½ tablespoon garlic powder
- ½ tablespoon butter
- 3 calabacita squashes, seeds removed

How to

1. Season the pork with half the cumin, garlic powder, salt and chili powder.
2. Switch the instant pot to 'sauté' mode and add butter to heat.
3. Place the seasoned pork in the pot and cook it for 4 minutes per side.
4. Pour in 4 cups of water and secure the lid.
5. Select 'meat stew' option and cook for 1 hour.
6. 'Natural release' the steam for 30 minutes, and remove the lid.
7. Stuff the calabacita squashes with the pork mixture.
8. Serve hot.

Nutrition Values (Per Serving)

- Calories: 146
- Carbohydrate: 11.5g
- Protein: 16.7g
- Fat: 4.3g
- Sugar: 3.9g
- Sodium: 1408mg

Instant Pork Thai Curry

(**Serves**: 2 / **Prep Time:** 5 minutes / **Cooking Time**: 35 minutes)

Ingredients

- ½ lbs pork meat, boneless
- ½ cup coconut milk, canned
- 1 tablespoon Thai curry paste
- ¼ cup water

How to

1. Prepare the Thai curry sauce by mixing the coconut milk, the water and the Thai curry paste in a bowl.
2. Put the pork meat and Thai curry sauce into the instant pot.
3. Secure the lid and select the 'manual' function. Set to high pressure and cook for 35 minutes.
4. 'Natural release' the steam for 10 minutes, then remove the lid.
5. Serve immediately.

Nutrition Values (Per Serving)

- Calories: 309
- Carbohydrate: 4.8g
- Protein: 25.4g
- Fat: 21.3g
- Sugar: 2.5g
- Sodium: 407mg

Jamaican Pork Roast

(**Serves**: 6 / **Prep Time:** 10 minutes / **Cooking Time**: 55 minutes)

- Ingredients
- 2 lbs pork shoulder
- ¾ tablespoon olive oil
- ¼ cup Jamaican jerk spice blend
- ¼ cup beef broth

How to

1. Use Jamaican jerk spice with olive oil to marinate the pork for 10 minutes.
2. Select the 'sauté' function on the instant pot and place the marinated pork inside.
3. Sear each side for 4 minutes, then add the broth.
4. Secure the lid and cook for 45 minutes at high pressure on the 'manual' setting.
5. 'Natural release' the steam for 10 minutes, then remove the lid.
6. Serve hot.

Nutrition Values (Per Serving)

- Calories: 226
- Carbohydrate: 0g (Zero gram)
- Protein: 35.4g
- Fat: 111.7g
- Sugar: 0g
- Sodium: 135mg

Smokey BBQ Pork Ribs

(**Serves**: 4 / **Prep Time:** 10 minutes / **Cooking Time**: 1 hour 35 minutes)

Ingredients

- 2 lbs baby back pork ribs
- 2 tablespoons apple cider vinegar
- 2 cups apple juice
- 1 tablespoon liquid smoke
- ½ teaspoon ground cumin
- ½ teaspoon brown sugar
- ½ teaspoon garlic powder
- ½ teaspoon black pepper
- 1 teaspoon salt
- ¼ cup BBQ sauce
- ¼ cup tomato ketchup
- 1 tablespoon Worcestershire sauce

How to

1. Combine the salt, pepper, brown sugar, cumin and garlic powder in a bowl to prepare the seasoning.
2. Add the pork to the mixture and mix well.
3. Now put the seasoned pork, apple cider vinegar, liquid smoke and apple juice into the instant pot.
4. Cook for 20 minutes at high pressure using the 'meat stew' function.
5. 'Natural release' the steam for 15 minutes, then remove the lid.
6. Stir in the Worcestershire sauce, the BBQ sauce and the tomato ketchup.
7. Let it sit for 15 minutes, then serve hot.

Nutrition Values (Per Serving)

- Calories: 746
- Carbohydrate: 25.2g
- Protein: 36.6g
- Fat: 54.5g
- Sugar: 20.7g
- Sodium: 1141mg

Cauliflower Tourtiere

(**Serves**: 10 / **Prep Time:** 5 minutes / **Cooking Time**: 55 minutes)

Ingredients

- 2 (9 inch) pie crust, frozen, ready-to-bake
- 2 lbs pork meat
- 1 cup water
- ½ teaspoon black pepper
- 2 teaspoons salt
- ½ teaspoon ground nutmeg
- 1 tablespoon ground sage
- 4 tablespoons butter
- 2 small onions, sliced
- 2 cups cooked cauliflower

How to

1. Put the meat, the onions, salt and water into the instant pot.
2. Secure the lid and cook for 20 minutes at high pressure using the 'meat stew' option.
3. 'Natural release' the steam for 5 minutes, then remove the lid.
4. In a blender, blend the cooked cauliflower and add this mixture to the pot.
5. Stir in the butter and all the spices.
6. Mix well and pour the mixture over the pie crust.
7. Bake the pie for 30 minutes at 350º F in an oven.
8. Serve warm.

Nutrition Values (Per Serving)

- Calories: 425
- Carbohydrate: 33.8g
- Protein: 20.3g
- Fat: 23g
- Sugar: 19.4g
- Sodium: 846mg

All Spice Pork Ribs

(**Serves**: 3 / **Prep Time:** 10 minutes / **Cooking Time**: 1 hour 45 minutes)

Ingredients

- 2 lbs pork ribs
- ¾ teaspoon erythritol
- ½ teaspoon garlic powder
- ½ teaspoon all spice
- ½ teaspoon salt
- ¼ teaspoon black pepper
- ½ teaspoon onion powder
- ¼ teaspoon coriander powder
- ¼ cup tomato ketchup
- ¾ tablespoon red wine vinegar
- ½ teaspoon ground mustard
- ¼ teaspoon liquid smoke

How to

1. Add all the dry spices to the pork and marinate for 1 hour.
2. In a separate bowl, combine the vinegar, mustard, ketchup and liquid smoke to prepare a sauce.
3. Place the marinated ribs in the instant pot and pour the sauce over it.
4. Secure the lid and select the 'manual' function. Cook for 35 minutes at high pressure.
5. 'Natural release' the steam for 5 minutes, then remove the lid.
6. Transfer the ribs to a platter.
7. Cook the remaining sauce in the pot on the 'sauté' setting for 5 minutes.
8. To serve, drizzle the sauce over the ribs.

Nutrition Values (Per Serving)

- Calories: 852
- Carbohydrate: 7.3g
- Protein: 80.7g
- Fat: 53.8g
- Sugar: 6.1g
- Sodium: 834mg

Delicious Pork Bo Kho

(**Serves**: 3 / **Prep Time:** 15 minutes / **Cooking Time**: 1 hour 35 minutes)

Ingredients

- 1¼ lbs pork briskets
- 1 tablespoon ghee
- ½ small onion, diced
- 1 tablespoon fresh ginger, grated
- 1 tablespoon red boat fish sauce
- ½ large stalk lemongrass, cut into 3-inch lengths
- ½ bay leaf
- ½ cup diced tomatoes
- ½ lb carrots, peeled and chopped
- 1 teaspoon Madras curry powder
- 1 tablespoon apple sauce
- 1 whole star anise
- ½ cup bone broth
- ½ teaspoon salt

How to

1. Select 'sauté' function on the instant pot and add the ghee to it.
2. Stir-fry the briskets in the pot in batches.
3. Transfer the briskets to a plate and put the onions into the pot.
4. Sauté the onions for 3 minutes then add the ginger, carrots, diced tomatoes, curry powder, red boat fish sauce, and the seared pork.
5. Stir in the lemongrass, bay leaf, broth, apple sauce and star anise.
6. Cook on "the 'manual' function for 35 minutes at high pressure.
7. Release the pressure naturally for 30 minutes then remove the lid.
8. Serve immediately.

Nutrition Values (Per Serving)

- Calories: 304
- Carbohydrate: 17.1g
- Protein: 46.9g
- Fat: 7.1g
- Sugar: 7.3g
- Sodium: 1691mg

Cheese Pork Schnitzel

(**Serves**: 6 / **Prep Time:** 10 minutes / **Cooking Time**: 30 minutes)

Ingredients

- 2 lbs boneless pork chops, thinly sliced
- 2 teaspoons water
- 2 eggs
- 4 tablespoons oil
- ¼ cup parmesan cheese, grated
- ½ teaspoon garlic powder
- 1 teaspoon salt
- 1 teaspoon black pepper
- ½ cup coconut flour
- 1 cup breadcrumbs

How to

1. Crack the eggs into a bowl and whisk them together with the water.
2. Stir in the coconut flour, salt, pepper and garlic powder.
3. Heat the oil using the 'sauté' function on the instant pot.
4. Take the pork chops, dip them into the egg mix, then dredge them through the breadcrumbs.
5. Place the chops in the pot and secure the lid.
6. Cook for 10 minutes on 'manual' setting at high pressure.
7. Release the steam, open the lid and flip the pork chops over. Secure the lid again.
8. Cook for another 10 minutes at the same settings
9. Release the pressure, remove the lid and serve.

Nutrition Values (Per Serving)

- Calories: 445
- Carbohydrate: 20.3g
- Protein: 46.7g
- Fat: 18.8
- Sugar: 1.3g
- Sodium: 670mg

Saucy Pork Brisket

(**Serves**: 8 / **Prep Time:** 10 minutes / **Cooking Time**: 1 hour)

Ingredients

- 4 lbs pork brisket, flat cut
- ½ teaspoon celery salt
- ½ teaspoon garlic salt
- ½ teaspoon Lowry's seasoned salt
- 2 tablespoons Worcestershire sauce
- 2 cups barbecue sauce
- 4 tablespoons liquid smoke
- 1 cup water

How to

1. Season the pork brisket with salt, garlic salt, celery salt, liquid smoker and Worcestershire sauce.
2. Marinate the seasoned pork overnight.
3. Put the barbecue sauce, water and marinated pork into the instant pot.
4. Select 'manual' and cook for 60 minutes at high pressure.
5. After the beep, 'natural release' the steam for 15 minutes.
6. Remove the lid and serve hot.

Nutrition Values (Per Serving)

- Calories: 321
- Carbohydrate: 27.6g
- Protein: 48.6g
- Fat: 3.2g
- Sugar: 19.1g
- Sodium: 1613mg

Pork Sausages with Mushrooms

(**Serves**: 2 / **Prep Time:** 10 minutes / **Cooking Time**: 45 minutes)

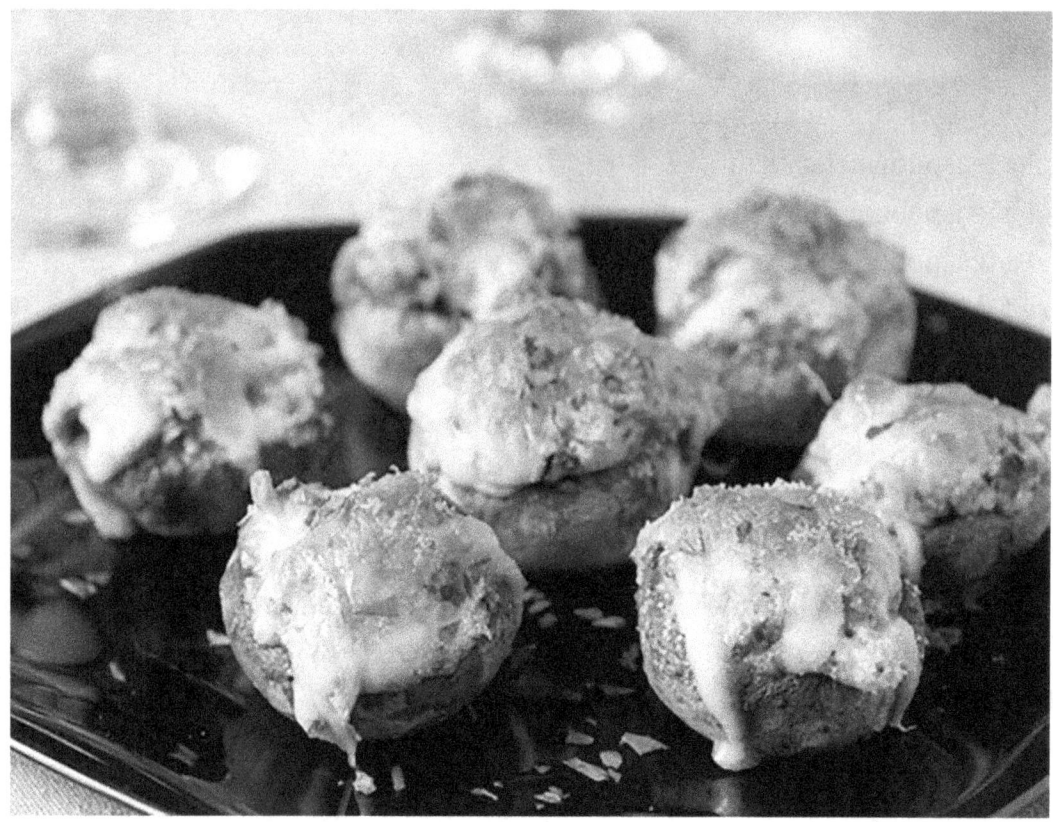

Ingredients

- 2 large Portobello mushrooms
- 6 oz. pork sausages
- ½ cup marinara sauce
- ½ cup whole milk ricotta cheese
- ½ cup whole milk mozzarella cheese, shredded
- ¼ cup parsley, chopped

How to

1. Stuff each mushroom with pork sausage.
2. Place the ricotta cheese over the sausages and carve a dent in the center.
3. Drizzle the marinara sauce over the ricotta cheese.
4. Cover with mozzarella cheese on top, and place the mushrooms in the instant pot.
5. Secure the lid, select the 'manual' function and cook for 35 minutes at high pressure.
6. 'Natural release' the steam, then remove the lid.
7. Serve immediately.

Nutrition Values (Per Serving)

- Calories: 624
- Carbohydrate: 27.2g
- Protein: 34.9g
- Fat: 41.7g
- Sugar: 7.8g
- Sodium: 1954mg

Peppercorns Beef

(**Serves**: 2 / **Prep Time:** 15 minutes / **Cooking Time**: 1 hour 45 minutes)

Ingredients

- 2 lbs corned beef, flat cut
- 4 whole peppercorns
- ½ small onion, quartered
- ½ cup water
- 2 large bay leaves
- 1 teaspoon dried thyme
- 1 cup low-sodium chicken broth

How to

1. Put the pork in the instant pot.
2. Add all the remaining ingredients and secure the lid.
3. Cook for 90 minutes at high pressure on 'manual' function.
4. 'Natural release' the steam and remove the lid.
5. Serve hot.

Nutrition Values (Per Serving)

- Calories: 797
- Carbohydrate: 4.9g
- Protein: 62g
- Fat: 56.8g
- Sugar: 0.8g
- Sodium: 4047mg

Pork Taco bowl

(**Serves**: 8 / **Prep Time:** 5 minutes / **Cooking Time**: 1 hour 5 minutes)

Ingredients

- 2 lbs pork sirloin roast, thickly sliced
- 2 teaspoons garlic powder
- 2 tablespoons olive oil
- 2 teaspoons cumin powder
- 2 teaspoons salt
- 2 teaspoons black pepper
- 20 oz green chili tomatillo salsa, without added sugar

How to

1. Put the garlic powder, salt, pepper and ground cumin in a bowl and mix together.
2. Put the pork in the bowl and dredge it in the spice mixture.
3. Pour the oil into the instant pot and select the 'sauté' function.
4. Place the pork in the oil then add the tomatillo salsa.
5. Secure the lid and cook for 45 minutes at high pressure using the 'manual' function.
6. Release the steam naturally for 15 minutes, then remove the lid.
7. Serve warm.

Nutrition Values (Per Serving)

- Calories: 295
- Carbohydrate: 6.1g
- Protein: 32.6g
- Fat: 14.3g
- Sugar: 2.7g
- Sodium: 872mg

Pork Roast Tacos

(**Serves**: 6 / **Prep Time:** 10 minutes / **Cooking Time**: 1 hour 5 minutes)

Ingredients

- 2 lbs pork sirloin tip roast
- 8 low-carb whole wheat tortillas
- 6 tablespoons olive oil
- 4 tablespoons lemon juice
- 1 cup chicken stock
- 1 cup Greek salsa
- 2 tablespoons Greek seasoning
- 1 teaspoon Greek oregano

How to

1. Pour the oil into the instant pot and select the 'sauté' function.
2. Add the pork roast to the heated oil and cook until it turns brown on both sides.
3. Add all the remaining ingredients, except the tortillas, and secure the lid.
4. Cook for 50 minutes at high pressure on the 'manual' setting.
5. 'Natural release' the steam for 15 minutes, then remove the lid.
6. Stuff the tortillas with cooked pork and serve.

Nutrition Values (Per Serving)

- Calories: 432
- Carbohydrate: 22g
- Protein: 37.9g
- Fat: 21g
- Sugar: 3g
- Sodium: 1094mg

POULTRY AND CHICKEN

Green Chilli Adobo Chicken

(**Serves**: 6 / **Prep time:** 6 minutes / **Cooking time**: 25 minutes)

Ingredients

- 6 boneless, skinless chicken breasts
- ½ cup water
- 1 tablespoon turmeric
- 1 tablespoon GOYA Adobo all-purpose seasoning with pepper
- two cups diced tomatoes
- 1 cup diced green chillies

How to

1. Place the chicken breasts in the inner pot.
2. Add Adobo seasoning pepper to the chicken. Sprinkle on both sides.
3. Add the sliced tomatoes to the chicken.
4. Pour half-cup of water over the chicken.
5. Cover and lock the lid. Use manual settings and set the time to 25 minutes.
6. When cooking is complete at the beep, use 'natural release' to vent the steam for 15 minutes.
7. Use quick the release option to vent all remaining steam.
8. Remove the pot and shred the chicken inside using two forks.
9. Serve with rice, or fill the tacos with the shredded chicken.

Nutrition Values (Per Serving)

- Calories: 204
- Carbohydrate: 7.6g
- Protein: 32.9g
- Fat: 4.2g
- Sugar: 2.2g
- Sodium: 735mg

Curry Chicken with Honey

(**Serves**: 4 / **Prep time:** 6 minutes / **Cooking time**: 25 minutes)

Ingredients

- ¼ cup yellow mustard
- ¼ cup unsalted butter, melted
- ¼ teaspoon cayenne pepper
- 1½ lbs boneless, skinless chicken thighs or breasts
- 1½ teaspoons hot curry powder
- 1 teaspoon salt
- ½ cup honey

How to

1. Put the mustard, curry powder, honey, cayenne pepper, salt, and melted butter into the inner pot.
2. Mix all the ingredients well. Place the pot in the cooker with the trivet.
3. Place the chicken pieces on the trivet.
4. Use 'manual' settings to set the cooker to high pressure for 18 minutes.
5. After cooking is complete, use the 'natural release' for 10 minutes to vent the steam.
6. Remove the chicken and trivet. Shred the pieces and put them to one side.
7. Leave the remaining ingredients in the pot and set the sauté option for 5 minutes.
8. Boil the sauce until it thickens.
9. Pour the sauce over the shredded chicken and stir well.
10. Serve with boiled rice.

Nutrition Values (Per Serving)

- Calories: 1895
- Carbohydrate: 41.3g
- Protein: 132.8g
- Fat: 133.6g
- Sugar: 34.9g
- Sodium: 894mg

Orange Spice Chicken

(**Serves**: 6 / **Prep time:** 15 minutes / **Cooking time**: 15 minutes)

Ingredients

- 2 lb chicken breast cut into two-inch pieces
- 2 tablespoons vegetable oil
- Two garlic heads, minced
- 1 cup tomato sauce
- 1 cup orange juice
- 4 tablespoons corn starch
- ¼ cup granulated sugar
- ¼ cup brown sugar
- ¼ cup soy sauce
- Salt and pepper to taste
- 4 green onions and orange zest

How to

1. Dry the chicken pieces with a paper towel.
2. Add oil and chicken to the pot of the cooker.
3. Press the 'sauté' key, and cook the chicken on a medium-high heat for 2-3 minutes, stirring constantly.
4. When the chicken turns golden brown, add the rest of the ingredients to the pot.
5. Mix all the ingredients well. Cover and lock the cooker lid.
6. Select the 'poultry' option and set the timer for 7 minutes.
7. After the completion beep, use 'natural release' to vent the steam for 10 minutes. Then open the lid.
8. Mix the corn-starch with the orange juice in a separate bowl and add it to the pot.
9. Select the 'sauté' function and cook the chicken in the sauce for 5 minutes. Stir constantly until it thickens.
10. Garnish with chopped green onions and orange zest on top.

Nutrition Values (Per Serving)

- Calories: 818
- Carbohydrate: 23.7g
- Protein: 128.2g
- Fat: 19.6g
- Sugar: 19.6g
- Sodium: 1120g

Chicken Bowl with Smoked Paprika

(**Serves**: 6 / **Prep Time:** 10 minutes / **Cooking Time**: 10 minutes)

Ingredients

- 1 teaspoon olive oil
- 3 strips bacon, chopped
- 1 small onion, chopped
- 2 garlic cloves, minced.
- 1 small red bell pepper, chopped
- 2 teaspoons smoked paprika
- 1 teaspoon salt
- 1 (12 oz.) can of beer.
- 1½ lb chicken breasts cut into small pieces
- 1 cup white rice
- 2 strips bacon, cooked (topping)

How to

1. Put the oil and bacon in the pot. Sauté it, without covering the lid, for 3 minutes.
2. Add the bell pepper to the oil and bacon and sauté for 3 more minutes.
3. Add the chopped onion and sauté for 2 minutes.
4. Add garlic and cook for 1 minute.
5. Add all the seasoning to the pot and turn off the 'sauté' function.
6. Add the beer to the mixture. Mix all the ingredients well.
7. Add the chicken and rice to the pot and select 'manual settings'.
8. Set to high pressure for 10 minutes and leave it to cook.
9. Use 'quick release' to vent all the steam, then remove the lid.
10. Serve the dish with the bacon strips on top.

Nutrition Values (Per Serving)

- Calories: 524
- Carbohydrate: 29.3g
- Protein: 68.5g
- Fat: 10.3g
- Sugar: 1.2g
- Sodium: 310mg

Instant Dumplings

(**Serves**: 4 / **Prep Time:** 10 minutes / **Cooking Time**: 10 minutes)

Ingredients

- 1 cup water
- 2 cups chicken broth
- 1½ lbs chicken breast, cubed
- 1 cup chopped carrots
- 1 teaspoon olive oil
- 1 cup frozen peas
- 2 teaspoons oregano
- 1 teaspoon onion powder
- 1 tube (16 oz.) refrigerated biscuits
- 1 teaspoon basil
- ½ teaspoon salt
- 2 cloves minced garlic
- ½ teaspoon pepper

How to

1. Press the biscuits to flatten them, then cut them into 2-inch strips with a sharp knife.
2. Put the olive oil, onion powder, oregano, chicken, garlic, salt, pepper and basil into the pot and mix them well.
3. Select the 'sauté' function on your pressure cooker and allow it to cook until the chicken turns brown.
4. Cancel the 'sauté' function when the cooking is finished.
5. Add the water, peas, carrots and chicken broth to the pot. Add the biscuits then stir well.
6. Cover with the lid and lock it.
7. Select the 'manual' function, and set the timer for 5 minutes.
8. After the beep, use the 'natural release' for 10 minutes to vent all steam.
9. Press 'cancel' to turn the cooker off, then remove the lid.
10. Serve the cooked chicken in a bowl.

Nutrition Values (Per Serving)

- Calories: 610
- Carbohydrate: 13.6g
- Protein: 100.5g
- Fat: 12.1g
- Sugar: 4.4g
- Sodium: 777mg

Sesame Chicken Teriyaki

(**Serves**: 4 / **Prep Time:** 10 minutes / **Cooking Time**: 10 minutes)

Ingredients

- 1 lb boneless, skinless chicken breasts.
- ½ cup soy sauce
- 1/3 cup honey
- 2 tablespoons apple cider vinegar.
- 1 teaspoon sesame oil
- 2 garlic cloves, minced
- 2 teaspoons minced ginger
- 2 tablespoons corn starch
- 3 tablespoons water
- Garnish: sliced green onions, sesame seeds

How to

1. Place the chicken in the pressure cooker pot.
2. In a separate small bowl, mix the soy sauce, sesame oil, ginger, garlic, vinegar and honey. Mix the ingredients well.
3. Pour the prepared mixture over the chicken in the pot.
4. Close the cooker lid and lock it.
5. Select the 'manual' function and set on high pressure for 5 minutes. Let it cook.
6. When the completion beep sounds, use the 'natural release' to vent all the pressure. This should take around 15 minutes.
7. Remove the chicken from the pot and shred it using two forks. Put it to one side.
8. Select the 'sauté function and add corn-starch and water to the remaining mixture.
9. Cook the sauce while stirring until it thickens.
10. Now add the chicken to the sauce and mix well.
11. Serve it with sprinkled sesame seeds and green onions on top.

Nutrition Values (Per Serving)

- Calories: 645
- Carbohydrate: 30.9g
- Protein: 97.2g
- Fat: 12.4g
- Sugar: 23.8g
- Sodium: 2027mg

Chicken with Lettuce Wrap

(**Serves**: 4 / **Prep Time:** 10 minutes / **Cooking Time**: 15 minutes)

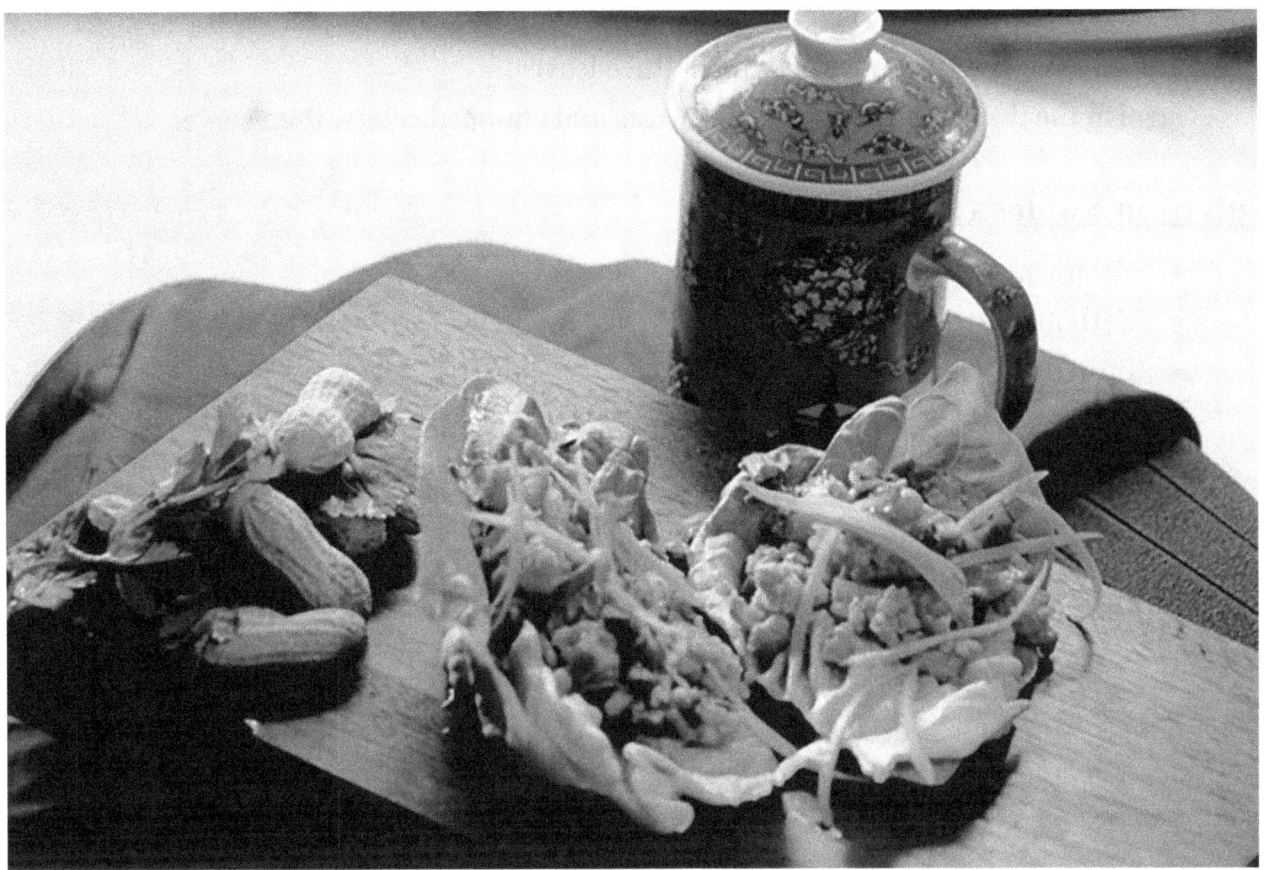

Ingredients

- 1 celery stalk
- 1 clove garlic
- 1 medium onion, chopped.
- 2 cups chicken broth
- large lettuce leaves
- ½ cup buffalo wing sauce
- 1 large boneless, skinless chicken breast
- ½ cup shredded carrots

How to

1. Put the chopped onions, minced garlic, chicken broth, buffalo wing sauce and chicken into the inner pot of the pressure cooker.
2. Cover with the cooker lid and lock it.
3. Select the 'poultry' function. Do not change the pressure and time settings.

4. Wait for the completion beep. Then use the 'natural release' method to vent the steam.

5. Then use the 'quick release' function to release the remaining pressure.

6. Shred the chicken while still in the pot using two forks.

7. Mix the chicken well with all the other ingredients.

8. Pour the chicken and sauce over the lettuce leaves.

9. Garnish the dish with the shredded carrots and chopped celery, then serve.

Nutrition Values (Per Serving)

- Calories: 564
- Carbohydrate: 6.2g
- Protein: 99.2g
- Fat: 11.9g
- Sugar: 4.3g
- Sodium: 883mg

Chicken with Black Beans

(**Serves**: 6 / **Prep Time:** 10 minutes / **Cooking Time**: 6 minutes)

Ingredients

- 1 small onion chopped
- 4 cups diced tomatoes with juice
- 1 lb boneless, skinless chicken breasts
- 1 tablespoon chipotle peppers
- ½ cup water
- 1 cup jasmine rice (uncooked)
- ½ lime, juiced
- 2 teaspoons sea salt.
- ½ teaspoon ground black pepper
- 2 tablespoons butter.
- 1 can organic black beans drained and rinsed

How to

1. Put the chicken, tomatoes, peppers, water, rice, salt, lemon juice, butter and onion in your electric cooker pot.
2. Use 'manual' settings and adjust pressure to high for 6 minutes.
3. Let it cook until the cooker beeps.
4. Use the 'quick pressure release' to vent the steam.
5. Add black beans to the chicken then stir well.
6. Add salt and pepper to taste.
7. Serve with shredded cheese and sour cream on top.

Nutrition Values (Per Serving)

- Calories: 447
- Carbohydrate: 15.2g
- Protein: 66.2g
- Fat: 11.7g
- Sugar: 3.9g
- Sodium: 188mg

Steamed Garlic Chicken Breasts

(**Serves**: 3 / **Prep Time:** 5 minutes / **Cook Time**: 9 minutes)

Ingredients

- ¼ teaspoon garlic powder
- 3 boneless chicken breasts
- 1 teaspoon black pepper
- ⅛ teaspoon dried oregano
- ⅛ teaspoon dried basil
- 1 tablespoon olive oil
- 1 cup water
- Salt to taste

How to

1. Add the oil to the pot and select the 'sauté function. Let it up heat without the lid on.
2. Sprinkle seasonings on both sides of the chicken.
3. Put the seasoned chicken into the pot with the oil, and cook each side for 3-4 minutes until they turn golden brown.
4. Add the water to the pot then set the trivet in the pot.
5. Place the chicken pieces on the trivet.
6. Select 'manual' settings, high pressure, and 5 minutes on the timer. Let it cook.
7. Use the 'natural release', after the beep, to release the steam. Use 'quick release' afterwards to make sure all the steam has been vented.
8. Remove the lid. Transfer the chicken to a platter.
9. Wait 5 minutes and serve with lime wedges, sprinkled oregano, and basil on top.

Nutrition Values (Per Serving)

- Calories: 155
- Carbohydrate: 0.3g
- Protein: 21.3g
- Fat: 7.2g
- Sugar: 4.3g
- Sodium: 51mg

Scrumptious Spicy Chicken

(**Serves**: 4 / **Prep Time:** 10 minutes / **Cooking Time**: 8 minutes)

Ingredients

- 3 large boneless, skinless chicken breasts
- ½ an onion, chopped.
- 1 can full-fat coconut milk
- 2 teaspoons smoked paprika
- 1½ teaspoons ground cumin
- 3 cloves garlic, minced
- 1½ teaspoons black pepper
- 1 teaspoon turmeric
- ½ cup of water
- 1 tablespoon olive oil
- Sea salt to taste

How to

1. Place the chicken and water in the instant pot. Cover with the lid and lock.
2. Use manual settings for high pressure and set timer to 15minutes.
3. When the timer beeps, use 'natural pressure' to release the steam.
4. Remove the chicken from the pot and shred it using two forks.
5. Add the oil, the onion and garlic to the instant pot, keeping the 'sauté' mode on.
6. Let the ingredients cook for 3 minutes, stirring constantly.
7. Turn the 'sauté' function off then add the shredded chicken, cumin, turmeric, coconut milk, smoked paprika, black pepper, and salt to the pot.
8. Mix all the ingredients well with the chicken.
9. Serve with steaming boiled rice.

Nutrition Values (Per Serving)

- Calories: 270
- Carbohydrate: 6.6g
- Protein: 17.9g
- Fat: 20.1g
- Sugar: 2.8g
- Sodium: 50mg

Chicken with Cashew Butter

(**Serves**: 6 / **Prep Time:** 5 minutes / **Cooking Time**: 8 minutes)

Ingredients

- 2 lbs chicken breasts
- ¼ cup rice vinegar
- ½ cup smooth cashew butter
- ¼ cup Soy Sauce
- 1 tablespoon chilli sauce
- ½ cup chicken broth
- ¼ cup honey
- 3 cloves garlic minced
- 3 tablespoons cilantro (chopped)
- 3 tablespoons cashews (chopped)

How to

1. Cut the chicken breasts into small, 2-inch chunks. Put the pieces in the cooker pot.
2. Put the cashew butter, honey, rice, soy sauce, chilli sauce, vinegar, chicken broth and garlic in a separate bowl and mix all the ingredients well.
3. Pour the butter mixture over the chicken pieces. Then cover with the lid.
4. After securing the lid select 'manual' function, set high pressure and 7 minutes on the timer.
5. Let it cook till it beeps. Then use the 'quick release' method to vent the steam.
6. Serve the chicken on a platter with the chopped cashews on top.

Nutrition Values (Per Serving)

- Calories: 640
- Carbohydrate: 26.3g
- Protein: 69.9g
- Fat: 27.6g
- Sugar: 13.7g
- Sodium: 854mg

Lime Chicken with chillies

(**Serves**: 6 / **Prep Time:** 5 minutes / **Cooking Time**: 10 minutes)

Ingredients

- 2 lb chicken breasts
- 1 teaspoon sea salt
- 1 onion, diced
- 1 tablespoon olive oil.
- 5 garlic cloves, minced
- ½ cup organic chicken broth
- 1 teaspoon dried parsley
- ¼ teaspoon paprika
- ¼ cup white wine.
- 1 large lemon juiced.
- 4 teaspoons arrowroot flour

How to

1. Put the cooking oil and chopped onion in the instant pot. Select the 'sauté' function to cook the onion for 5-10 minutes, until it turns light brown.
2. Add all the remaining ingredients to the pot and select the 'poultry' function without changing the settings.
3. Allow it cook. Release the steam after the beep.
4. Remove the lid. Check the sauce is thick enough.
5. If not, add dissolved arrowroot flour into the sauce to increase thickness.
6. Transfer the cooked chicken onto a platter and serve immediately.

Nutrition Values (Per Serving)

- Calories: 697
- Carbohydrate: 2.9g
- Protein: 127.3g
- Fat: 15.1g
- Sugar: 0.7
- Sodium: 401mg

Instant Tso's Chicken

(**Serves**: 6 / **Prep Time:** 5 minutes / **Cooking Time**: 8 minutes)

Ingredients

- 1/3 cup white wine vinegar
- 2 tablespoons tomato paste
- 3 tablespoons arrowroot powder
- 1½ lb chicken breast (cut into 2-inch pieces)
- 1 tablespoon honey
- ½ cup soy sauce
- 2 tablespoons olive oil
- 1 tablespoon almond butter
- ¼ cup coconut sugar
- 2 cloves garlic crushed
- 2 tablespoons minced ginger
- 3 tablespoons red hot chilli pepper
- ½ cup water
- 2 tablespoons sesame seeds
- ¼ cup chopped green onion

How to

1. Roll the chicken pieces in the arrowroot powder until each one is covered with a uniform layer.
2. Select the 'sauté' option on your instant cooker. Add the oil, garlic and chicken to the pot.
3. Let it cook, stirring occasionally, until the chicken turns golden brown. Don't forget to cancel the sauté function.
4. Mix all the remaining ingredients together in a separate bowl and whisk them to make a smooth paste.
5. Add this mixture to the pot then secure the cooker lid.
6. Use 'manual' settings, with high pressure and 8 minutes cooking time.
7. After the beep, carefully release the steam and open the lid.
8. Sprinkle sesame seeds and green onion over the dish, then serve.

Nutrition Values (Per Serving)

- Calories: 617
- Carbohydrate: 15g
- Protein: 96.6g
- Fat: 16.1g
- Sugar: 9.4g
- Sodium: 1432g

Mustard Chicken with Lime Juice

(**Serves**: 6 / **Prep Time:** 20 minutes / **Cooking Time**: 15 minutes)

Ingredients

- 2 tablespoons olive oil
- ¼ cup lemon juice
- ¾ cup chicken broth
- 2 lb chicken thighs, boneless.
- 2 tablespoons Italian seasoning
- 3 lb red potatoes, quartered
- 3 tablespoons Dijon mustard
- Salt and pepper

How to

1. Place the oil and the chicken in the instant pot. Sprinkle salt and pepper to taste.
2. In a separate bowl, combine the lemon juice, the chicken broth and the Dijon mustard, and mix them well.
3. Now add the potatoes, cut into 4 pieces, along with the remaining seasoning.
4. Secure the lid and select the 'manual' option - 15 minutes at high pressure.
5. Let it cook until the beep. Release the steam over 15 minutes using the 'natural release' method.
6. Serve.

Nutrition Values (Per Serving)

- Calories: 748
- Carbohydrate: 4.3g
- Protein: 127.5g
- Fat: 19.9g
- Sugar: 4.4g
- Sodium: 656mg

Chicken with Grape Tomatoes

(**Serves**: 2 / **Prep Time:** 20 minutes / **Cooking Time**: 15 minutes)

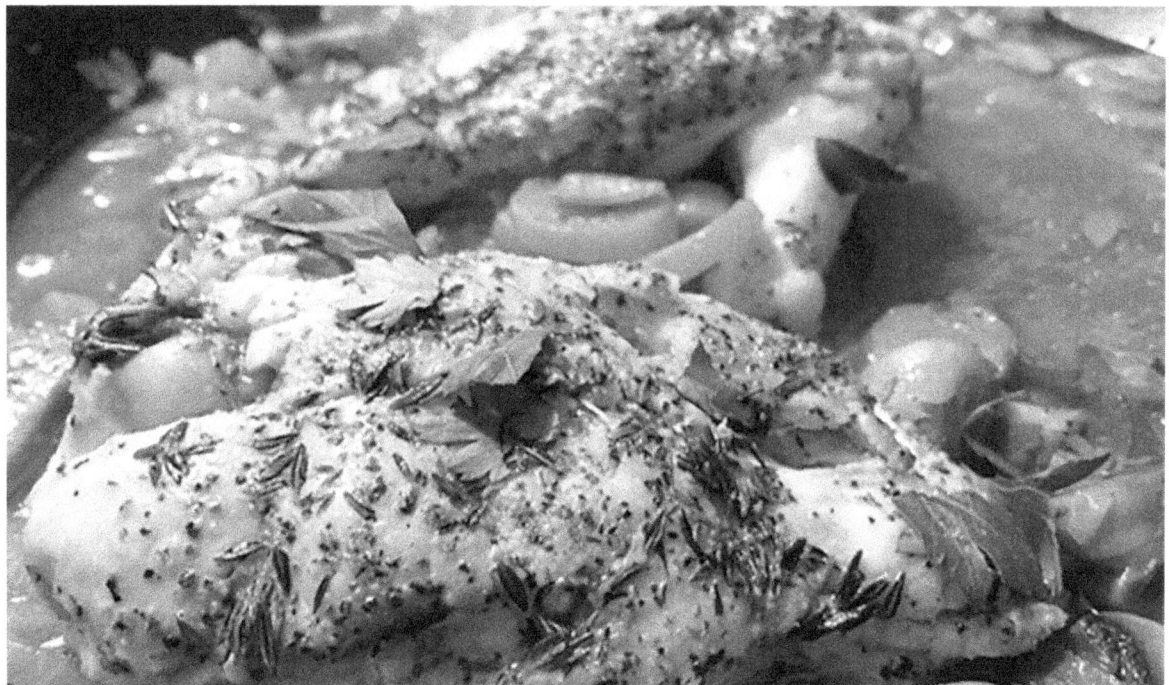

Ingredients

- 3 cups of cold water
- ½ tsp salt
- 2/3 lb boneless, skinless chicken breast
- 1 tablespoon Dijon mustard
- 1 tablespoon honey
- 1 tablespoon balsamic vinegar
- 3 cloves garlic, finely minced
- 3 tablespoons olive oil
- Field greens.
- Grape tomatoes, cut in half

How to

1. Take a large bowl and put two cups of water and the chicken pieces into it. Let it refrigerate for 45 minutes.
2. Pour 1 cup of water into the instant pot and place a trivet over it.
3. Place the chicken pieces on the trivet and select 'manual' function to set high pressure for 5 minutes.

4. After the completion beep, release the steam naturally, then let the chicken stay for 5 minutes.
5. Meanwhile, put the Dijon mustard, olive oil, garlic, balsamic vinegar and honey into a bowl and mix them all together.
6. Slice the chicken and add the field greens and tomatoes.
7. Pour the honey mixture over the chicken and serve.

Nutrition Values (Per Serving)

- Calories: 407
- Carbohydrate: 11g
- Protein: 32g
- Fat: 25g
- Sugar: 9g
- Sodium: 262mg

Turkey with Gravy

(**Serves**: 2 / **Prep Time:** 5 minutes / **Cooking Time**: 1 hr 5 Min)

Ingredients

- 1¼ cup chicken broth
- 1 lb turkey breast (boneless)
- 4 tablespoons butter, melted
- 2 tablespoons turkey herb rub
- 1 large onion, quartered
- 4 stalks celery, cut into large pieces
- 5 cloves garlic, crushed
- A few sprigs of fresh herbs - rosemary, sage and thyme
- 2 (0.87 oz.) packets turkey gravy mix

How to

1. Pour the chicken broth into the instant pot. Set the trivet in the pot.
2. Put the turkey roast on the trivet and pour melted butter over it.
3. Sprinkle all the herbs and seasoning over the top of the turkey.
4. Add the garlic, onion and celery to the pot and cover with the lid.
5. Set 'manual' function to high pressure for 55 minutes.
6. After the program has terminated, use the 'natural release' function to release the steam.
7. Open the cooker and remove the turkey roast. Slice it and set it aside.
8. Add the gravy packets to the instant pot and select the 'sauté' option. Boil the ingredients for 5 minutes until the mixture thickens.
9. Pour the gravy over the sliced turkey and serve.

Nutrition Values (Per Serving)

- Calories: 220
- Carbohydrate: 12.9g
- Protein: 12.3g
- Fat: 13.4g
- Sugar: 6.1g
- Sodium: 1104mg

Turkey Breasts

(**Serves**: 8/ **Prep Time:** 10 minutes / **Cooking Time**: 40minutes)

Ingredients

- 6½ lb bone-in, skin-on turkey breast
- Spices: Salt, pepper, garlic powder, onion powder, and paprika
- 1 (14 oz.) can turkey or chicken broth
- 1 large onion, quartered
- 1 stock of celery, cut into large pieces
- 1 sprig of thyme
- 3 cloves of garlic
- 3 tablespoons corn-starch
- 3 tablespoons cold water

How to

1. Add all the spices to the turkey breast and cover with a thin layer of seasoning.
2. Stuff garlic, thyme celery and onion inside the turkey breast.
3. Put the butter in the instant pot and select 'sauté' function. Add the turkey breast to the pot.
4. Let it cook until the turkey is golden brown on both sides. Turn off the 'sauté' function.
5. Leave the turkey breast with its side up and add the chicken broth to it.
6. Cover and lock the lid. Select 'manual' settings at high pressure for 30 minutes and leave to cook.
7. After the beep, switch the cooker off. Use 'natural release' for 10 minutes to release the steam, and then 'quick release'.
8. Remove the lid and add the corn-starch (dissolved in water) to the pot.
9. Let it cook on 'sauté' function until broth thickens.
10. Add pepper and salt to taste. Slice the turkey breast and serve with the steaming broth.

Nutrition Values (Per Serving)

- Calories: 360
- Carbohydrate: 3g
- Protein: 49g
- Fat: 16g
- Sugar: 0.9g
- Sodium: 869mg

Maple Mustard Turkey Thighs

(**Serves**: 4 / **Prep Time:** 20 minutes / **Cooking Time**: 40 minutes)

Ingredients

- ½ cup butter, unsalted
- 1 teaspoon fresh rosemary, chopped
- 1 teaspoon fresh thyme, chopped
- 1 tablespoon smoked paprika
- 2 tablespoons Dijon mustard
- ½ cup maple syrup
- 2 (3 lb) turkey thighs bone-in skin-on, washed and dried (3 lb)
- 1 teaspoon salt
- ½ teaspoon pepper
- 1 cup water
- 1 large onion, chopped
- 5 stalks celery, chopped
- 5 carrots, chopped
- 4 sprigs rosemary
- 2 sprigs thyme

How to

1. Add the melted butter, thyme, rosemary, maple syrup, smoked paprika and Dijon mustard to the instant pot.
2. Boil the mixture on 'sauté' function, stirring occasionally.
3. Add the salt, pepper, and half the maple syrup mixture to the turkey thighs. Toss it well.
4. Add the water, celery, onion, rosemary, thyme, and carrots to the instant pot.
5. Place the trivet in the pot then place turkey thighs over the trivet.
6. Pour the remaining maple syrup mixture over the thighs.
7. Select 'manual' and set to high pressure for 30 minutes and let it cook.
8. After the beep, vent the steam, using 'natural release' for 10 minutes, then use 'quick release'.
9. Remove the lid and take out the turkey thighs. Leave for 10 minutes then cut them into slices.
10. Pour the maple mustard mixture over the sliced thighs and serve.

Nutrition Values (Per Serving)

- Calories: 633
- Carbohydrate: 41g
- Protein: 44g
- Fat: 34g
- Sugar: 30g
- Sodium: 1810mg

Turkey with Cranberry Sauce

(**Serves**: 6 / **Prep Time:** 10 minutes / **Cooking Time**: 40 minutes)

Ingredients

- 3 cups cranberries, fresh or frozen
- 1 cup orange juice
- 1 cup apple jelly
- ½ teaspoon five-spice
- 3 tablespoons corn-starch
- 4 lb turkey breast with skin
- 1 tablespoon fresh rosemary, chopped
- ½ teaspoon dried thyme
- ½ cup chicken broth
- Salt and pepper to taste
- 4 tablespoons unsalted butter
- 2 medium onions, chopped

How to

1. Put the 2 cups of cranberries, apple jelly, Five Spice, orange juice and corn-starch into a blender. Blend well to form a smooth paste.
2. Add the melted butter and the prepared mixture to the instant pot. Select the 'sauté' function to boil, then keep it aside.
3. Sprinkle salt, pepper, thyme and rosemary generously over the turkey breasts.
4. Add butter to the instant pot. Select 'sauté' function, then add the turkey to the pot.
5. Let it cook until it turns brown on both sides. Then keep it aside.
6. Add butter, onion, salt and pepper to the pot and 'sauté' for 5 minutes.
7. Add the cranberry mixture to the pot and bring it to the boil while stirring constantly.
8. Add the remaining cup of cranberries to the sauce and mix well.
9. Add the chicken broth and place the turkey breasts in the pot. Secure the cooker lid.
10. Select 'manual' function to high pressure for 25 minutes.
11. After the beep, release the steam completely, then remove the lid.
12. Serve the steaming hot turkey breasts with cranberry sauce.

Nutrition Values (Per Serving)

- Calories: 600
- Carbohydrate: 51.8g
- Protein:70.8g
- Fat: 9.6g
- Sugar: 32.2g
- Sodium: 195mg

Turkey Breasts with Tomato and Basil Sauce

(**Serves**: 4 / **Prep Time:** 10 minutes / **Cooking Time**: 25 Min)

Ingredients

- 3 tablespoons olive oil
- 1 lb turkey breast cut into long strips
- Salt and pepper to taste
- 5 cloves garlic, minced
- 8 leaves basil, chopped
- 15 oz. fire roasted tomatoes
- ½ cup heavy cream, 125 mL

How to

1. Put the roasted tomatoes in a blender and blend to form a smooth puree. Put it to one side.
2. Sprinkle salt and pepper over the chicken breasts for seasoning.
3. Add olive oil to the instant pot and select the 'sauté' function. Add the turkey breasts to the pot and cook until golden brown.
4. Now remove the turkey breasts and put them aside.
5. Add the oil, garlic and basil to the pot and 'sauté' for 1 minute.
6. Pour the tomato paste and heavy cream into the pot and let it cook for 2-3 minutes.
7. Now put the turkey breasts into the sauce and secure the lid.
8. Select 'manual' function to high pressure for 15 minutes.
9. After the beep, release the steam and remove the lid.
10. Garnish with basil leaves.

Nutrition Values (Per Serving)

- Calories: 355
- Carbohydrate: 11.5g
- Protein: 36.5g
- Fat: 18.3g
- Sugar: 5.6g
- Sodium: 624mg

Turkey Lettuce Stacks

(**Serves**: 4 / **Prep Time:** 15 minutes / **Cooking Time**: 20 minutes)

Ingredients

- 1 lb ground turkey
- Salt and pepper to taste
- ¼ teaspoon cayenne pepper
- 1 teaspoon Herbs de Provence
- 1 tablespoon olive oil
- 4 slices Swiss cheese
- 4 eggs
- 1 tomato cut into 4 slices
- 4 slices turkey bacon
- 4 lettuce leaves

How to

1. Put the ground turkey, cayenne pepper, salt, herbs de Provence and pepper into a bowl and mix all the ingredients well.
2. Make 4 burger patties using this mixture.
3. Add olive oil to the instant pot and select the 'sauté' function. Carefully place the turkey patties in the pot.
4. Cook them from both sides until they turn golden brown.
5. Remove the patties from the pot and put them aside.
6. Add 1 cup of water to the pot and place the trivet in it.
7. Place the fried patties on the trivet and cover each one with a cheese slice. Place the turkey bacon strips on the trivet too.
8. Secure the lid and select 'manual' function, setting at high pressure for 5 minutes.
9. After the beep, release the steam completely and remove the lid.
10. To serve, take the lettuce leaves and stack them up with a tomato slice, a turkey patty, bacon and fried egg on top.

Nutrition Values (Per Serving)

- Calories: 720
- Carbohydrate: 1.7g
- Protein: 122.3g
- Fat: 18.9g
- Sugar: 0.7g
- Sodium: 534mg

Turkey with Garlic Herb Sauce

(**Serves**: 4 / **Prep Time:** 5 minutes / **Cooking Time**: 20 minutes)

Ingredients

- 4 turkey thighs with skin and bones
- Salt and pepper to taste
- 2 tablespoons olive oil
- 8 cloves garlic, minced
- 2 teaspoons fresh thyme, chopped
- 2 teaspoons fresh oregano, chopped
- ½ cup sherry, or dry red wine
- ½ cup chicken broth

How to

1. Add salt and pepper seasoning to the turkey thighs.
2. Select the 'sauté' function on the instant pot, and add the olive oil to it.
3. Place the turkey thighs in the pot and let them cook for 5 minutes on both sides.
4. Remove the turkey thighs when they turn golden brown.
5. Now, put the oil, garlic, thyme and oregano into the pot and 'sauté' for 2 minutes.
6. Add the sherry (or wine), the chicken broth and fried turkey thighs to the pot.
7. Secure the lid and select the 'manual' function, high pressure for 20minutes.
8. After the beep, use the 'natural release' to vent the steam.
9. Serve with fresh herbs sprinkled on top.

Nutrition Values (Per Serving)

- Calories: 545g
- Carbohydrate: 3.2g
- Protein: 66.7g
- Fat: 24.1g
- Sugar: 0.7g
- Sodium: 229mg

Stuffed Pepper with Turkey

(**Serves**: 4 / **Prep Time:** 5 minutes / **Cooking Time**: 20 minutes)

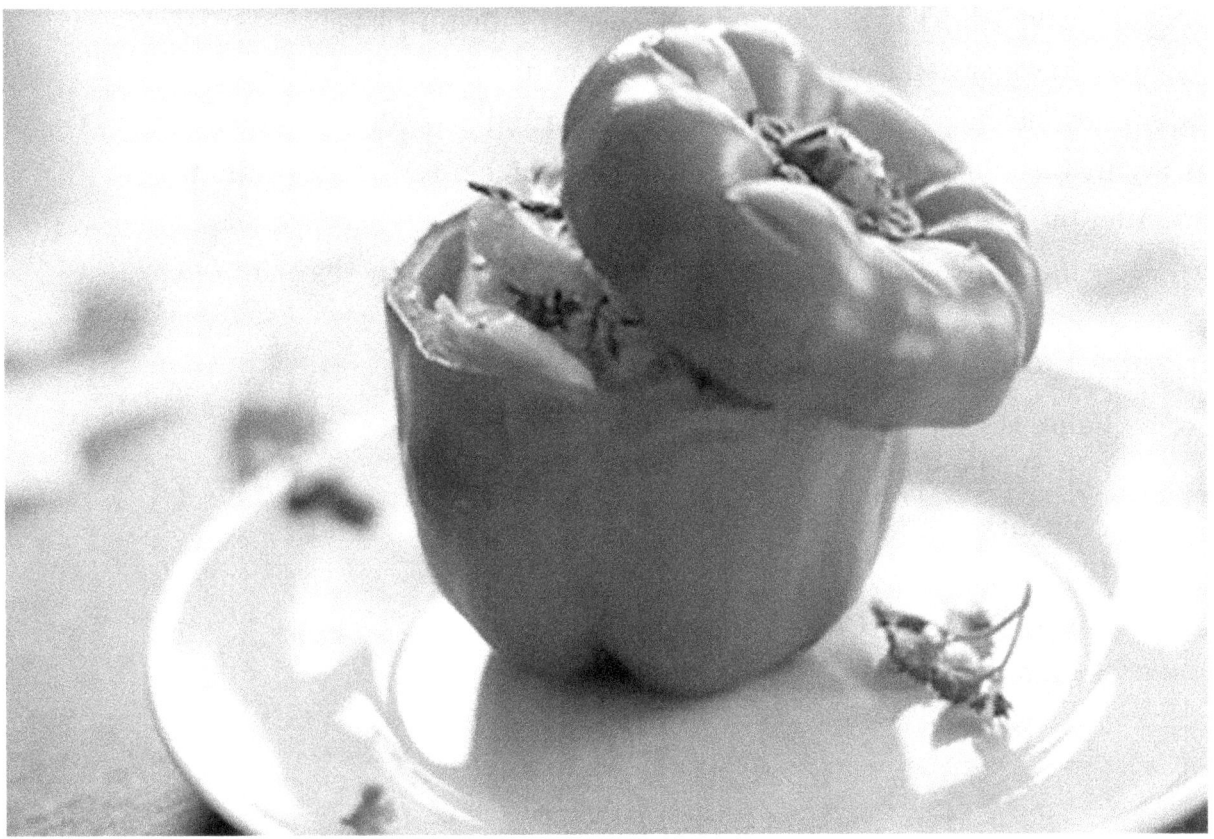

Ingredients

- 4 red bell peppers
- 1 tablespoon olive oil
- 1 medium onion, chopped
- 5 cloves garlic, minced
- ½ cup boiled rice
- 1 lb. ground turkey
- Salt and pepper to taste
- 1 tablespoon dry basil
- ½ cup cheddar cheese, shredded
- ½ cup water

How to

1. Slice all the bell peppers from the top and clean them from inside.
2. Chop down the top portion and put to one side.
3. Pour the oil into the instant pot and select the 'sauté' function.

4. Add the garlic, onion, dry basil, pepper, chopped bell pepper, and ground turkey to the pot.
5. Stir and cook all the ingredients well for 10 minutes.
6. Add the boiled rice to the pot and stir. Keep this mixture aside.
7. Now add water to the pot and place a trivet in it.
8. Stuff the bell pepper cups with turkey stuffing and place them on the trivet.
9. Secure the lid and set the 'manual' function at high pressure for 5 minutes.
10. After the beep, release the steam and remove the lid.
11. Serve the stuffed bell peppers with sprinkled cheese and herbs on top.

Nutrition Values (Per Serving)

- Calories: 825
- Carbohydrate: 15.5g
- Protein: 93.7g
- Fat: 43.9g
- Sugar: 5.4g
- Sodium: 931mg

Turkey Meatballs with Marinara Sauce

(**Serves**: 6 / **Prep Time:** 5 minutes / **Cooking Time**: 20 minutes)

Ingredients

- 1.3 lb. ground turkey breast
- ¼ Panko breadcrumbs
- ¼ cup grated Parmigiano-Reggiano cheese
- ¼ cup parsley, chopped
- 1 large clove garlic, crushed
- 1 onion, chopped
- Salt and pepper (seasoning)
- 2½ cups marinara sauce

How to

1. Put all the ingredients, except the marinara sauce, into a large bowl.
2. Mix the ingredients well with the ground turkey.
3. Use this mixture to make 30 turkey meatballs about 2 inches in diameter.
4. Add the marinara sauce to the instant pot and select the 'sauté' function.
5. Bring it to the boil then add the turkey meatballs.
6. Cover with the lid and lock.
7. Select 'manual' settings to high pressure and 20 minutes on the timer.
8. After the completion beep, use the 'natural release' to vent the steam.
9. Remove the lid and serve with fresh herbs sprinkled on top.

Nutrition Values (Per Serving)

- Calories: 545
- Carbohydrate: 3.2g
- Protein: 66.7g
- Fat: 24.1g
- Sugar: 0.7g
- Sodium: 229mg

Kung Pao Turkey

(**Serves**: 4 / **Prep Time:** 5 minutes / **Cooking Time**: 20 minutes)

Ingredients

Turkey marinade:
- 2 tablespoons soy sauce
- 2 tablespoons cornstarch
- 2 tablespoons red wine vinegar
- 3 cloves garlic minced
- 1 tablespoon sesame oil
- Salt and pepper to taste

Main ingredients:
- 1 large yellow bell pepper, chopped
- 1½ lb. turkey breast cut into cubes
- 1 cucumber, chopped
- ½ cup pistachios
- 5 green onions, chopped
- 3 tablespoons olive oil
- 5 cloves of garlic, minced
- Salt and pepper to taste

Sauce:
- 4 tablespoons soy sauce
- 2 tablespoons red wine vinegar
- 1 tablespoon chili garlic sauce
- 1 tablespoon brown sugar
- 2 tablespoons hot and spicy ketchup
- ½ cup water
- 2 tablespoons cornstarch

How to

1. Put all the ingredients for the marinade into a large bowl and mix.
2. Add the turkey pieces to the marinade. Let them soak for 20 minutes.
3. Pour the olive oil into the instant pot and select the 'sauté' function.
4. Add the minced garlic and let it cook for 30 seconds.
5. Now add the marinated turkey and let it cook for 10 minutes.
6. Add all the vegetables, except green onions, to the pot.

7. Allow the dish to cook for 3 minutes then add all the ingredients for the sauce.
8. Keep cooking until the sauce thickens.
9. Stir the pistachios and green onions into the turkey sauce.
10. Switch off the instant pot and serve.

Nutrition Values (Per Serving)

- Calories: 1245
- Carbohydrate: 23.2g
- Protein: 96.7g
- Fat: 24.1g
- Sugar: 0.7g
- Sodium: 956mg
-

Turkey Stuffed Tacos

(**Serves**: 6 / **Prep Time:** 5 minutes / **Cooking Time**: 20 minutes)

Ingredients

- 2 tablespoons olive oil
- 1 medium onion
- 3 cloves garlic
- 3/4 lb. chopped white turkey meat
- 1 jalapeno pepper, diced
- 1 teaspoon cumin
- Salt and pepper to taste
- ½ bottle of any dark beer
- 4 diced tomatoes
- 8 taco shells

Toppings:

- Tomatoes
- Lettuce
- Cheddar cheese
- Salsa

How to

1. Put the olive oil, chopped onion and garlic into the instant pot.
2. Select the 'sauté' function and let it cook for 5 minutes.
3. Add the jalapeno pepper and chopped turkey to the pot.
4. Let it cook for 5 minutes.
5. Now add the salt, pepper, cumin and diced tomatoes.
6. After 5 minutes more cooking, pour in the beer.
7. Now cover the lid and lock it properly. Select the 'manual' function - 5 minutes at high pressure.
8. After the beep, use the 'natural release' to release all the steam.
9. Remove the cooker lid but leave the prepared filling to one side.
10. To serve, stuff the filling in a taco wrap, and add cheese on top.

Nutrition Values (Per Serving)

- Calories: 675
- Carbohydrate: 8.2g
- Protein: 78.7g
- Fat: 19.1g
- Sugar: 3.7g
- Sodium:8945mg

Greek Style Turkey Breast

(**Serves**: 3 / **Prep Time:** 10 minutes / **Cooking Time**: 1 Hr)

Ingredients

- 1 cup water
- 1 turkey breast, sliced
- 2 tablespoons olive oil
- 3 cloves garlic, minced
- ½ Poblano pepper, minced
- ½ teaspoons chili flakes
- 3 tablespoons sliced olives
- ½ cup canned, diced tomatoes
- ½ cup crumbled feta cheese
- 2 tablespoons lemon juice
- Salt and pepper to taste
- Rosemary
- Basil
- Chopped parsley

How to

1. Take a large bowl and put the olive oil, Poblano pepper, garlic, lemon juice, salt, chilli flakes, rosemary, basil and pepper in it.
2. Mix all the ingredients well, then immerse the turkey in the mixture to marinate. Let it simmer in the marinade.
3. Cover the bowl with a plastic wrap and put it in a refrigerator for 3 hours.
4. Add water to the instant pot and place a trivet in it.
5. Now place the turkey pieces on the trivet. Pour the marinade generously over the turkey.
6. Secure the cooker lid. Select the 'manual' function and set high pressure for 50 minutes.
7. Release all the steam after the beep and remove the lid.
8. Top each piece with a tomato slice, sliced olives and cheese, then grill them for 10 minutes in an oven.
9. Garnish with fresh parsley and serve.

Nutrition Values (Per Serving)

- Calories: 932
- Carbohydrate: 15.7g
- Protein: 84.7g
- Fat: 32.2g
- Sugar: 2.3g
- Sodium: 678mg

Turkey Noodle Soup

(**Serves**: 8 / **Prep Time:** 10 minutes / **Cooking Time**: 20 minutes)

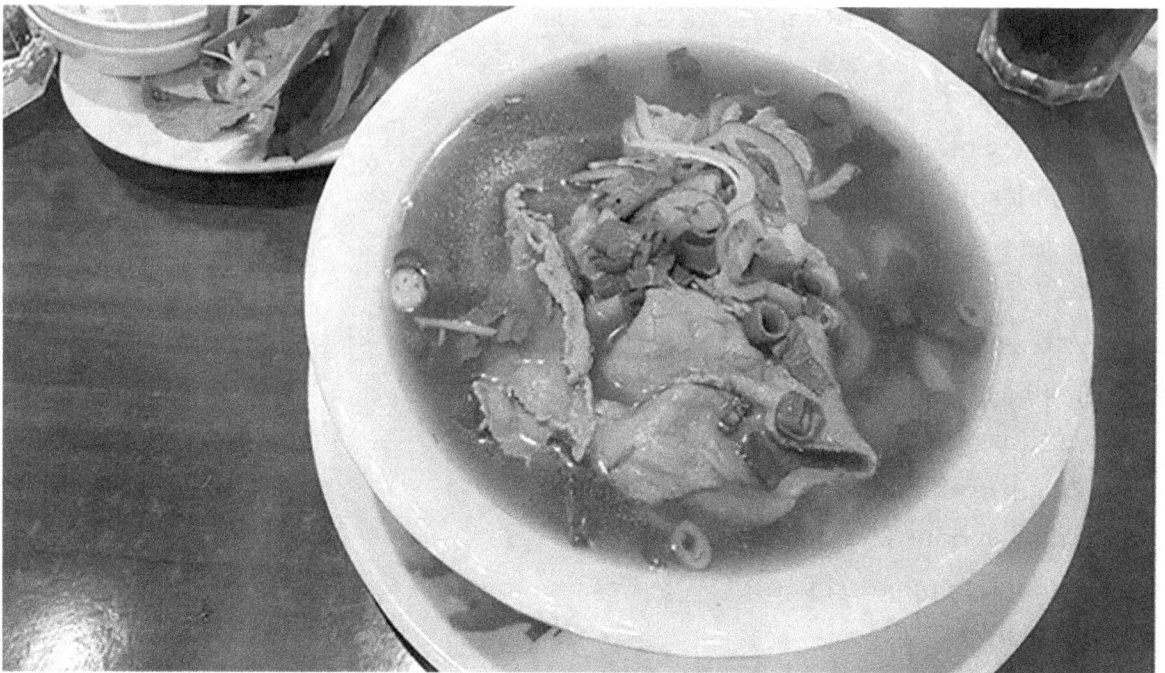

Ingredients

Broth:
- 1 turkey carcass left over from a carved turkey
- 1 cup shredded turkey
- 14 cups water
- 1 large onion, peeled
- 3 carrots, peeled and cleaned
- 2 stalks celery, washed
- Salt and pepper to taste

Soup:
- 3 cups turkey meat, chopped, white or dark
- 8 oz. egg noodles (cooked)
- Salt and pepper to taste
- Scallions, chopped

How to

1. Put the, water, onion, celery sticks, carrots, salt, pepper and turkey pieces into the instant pot. Secure the lid and select the 'soup' function.
2. Let the mixture cook until the cooker beeps. Release the steam using 'natural release'.
3. Strain the turkey broth to separate the liquid from the solid.
4. Pour the broth back into the pot.
5. Add the shredded turkey, the carrots and the celery. Select the 'sauté' function. Allow the soup to boil.
6. Add the precooked noodles.
7. Cook for 1 more minute then serve with scallions garnishing.

Nutrition Values (Per Serving)

- Calories: 458
- Carbohydrate: 9.4g
- Protein: 76.7g
- Fat: 11.6g
- Sugar: 2.7g
- Sodium: 671mg

Turkey with Smoked Paprika

(**Serves**: 6 / **Prep Time:** 10 minutes / **Cooking Time**: 50 minutes)

Ingredients

- 1 lb turkey thighs.
- ½ cup olive oil
- 8 cloves garlic minced
- 2 tablespoons smoked paprika
- ½ teaspoon red pepper flakes
- ¼ cup parsley fresh, chopped
- 2 tablespoons oregano fresh, chopped
- ½ teaspoon salt.
- ½ teaspoon black pepper.
- ½ cup water

How to

1. Pour the oil into the instant pot. Select the 'sauté' function.
2. Add the garlic, smoked paprika, herbs, and red pepper flakes. Cook for 1 minute.
3. Add salt and pepper to taste.
4. Pour this mixture over the turkey thighs, generously coating them.
5. Add the water to the pot. Place a trivet inside.
6. Put the coated turkey thighs on the trivet.
7. Secure the lid. Set the 'manual' function to high pressure for 50 minutes.
8. After the beep, release the steam naturally, then remove the lid.
9. Take out the turkey thighs and slice them.
10. Sprinkle fresh parsley and oregano to serve.

Nutrition Values (Per Serving)

- Calories: 903
- Carbohydrate: 5.4g
- Protein: 96.4g
- Fat: 13.2g
- Sugar: 0.4g
- Sodium: 498mg

Turkey Cheese Gnocchi

(**Serves**: 6 / **Prep Time:** 10 minutes / **Cooking Time**: 20 minutes)

Ingredients

- 2 tablespoons olive oil
- 1 lb turkey boneless pieces.
- ½ teaspoon salt
- ½ teaspoon black pepper
- ¼ cup shallots chopped
- 2 cloves garlic minced
- ¼ cup sun-dried tomatoes.
- 1 cup cream
- 2 cups chicken broth
- 2 lbs gnocchi
- 2 cups fresh spinach chopped
- 2 cups mozzarella cheese shredded
- ½ cup parmesan cheese shredded

How to

1. Select the 'sauté' option on your instant pot. Pour in the oil and heat.
2. Add the turkey, with salt and pepper. Let it cook for 3 minutes on each side.
3. Now add the garlic, the tomatoes and the shallots to the pot. Cook for 2 minutes while stirring.
4. Add the cream and chicken broth to the pot. Secure the cooker lid.
5. Select 'manual' settings at high pressure for 10 minutes.
6. After the beep, release the steam naturally, then remove the lid.
7. Add the gnocchi to the mixture.
8. Select the sauté' function and let it all cook for 5 minutes until gnocchi is tender.
9. Switch off the appliance then add the cheese to the pot.
10. Serve immediately.

Nutrition Values (Per Serving)

- Calories: 1033
- Carbohydrate: 32.6g
- Protein: 99.2g
- Fat: 19.9g
- Sugar: 2.3g
- Sodium: 890mg

Chicken Bourbon with Honey

(**Serves**: 4 / **Prep Time:** 10 minutes / **Cooking Time**: 20 minutes)

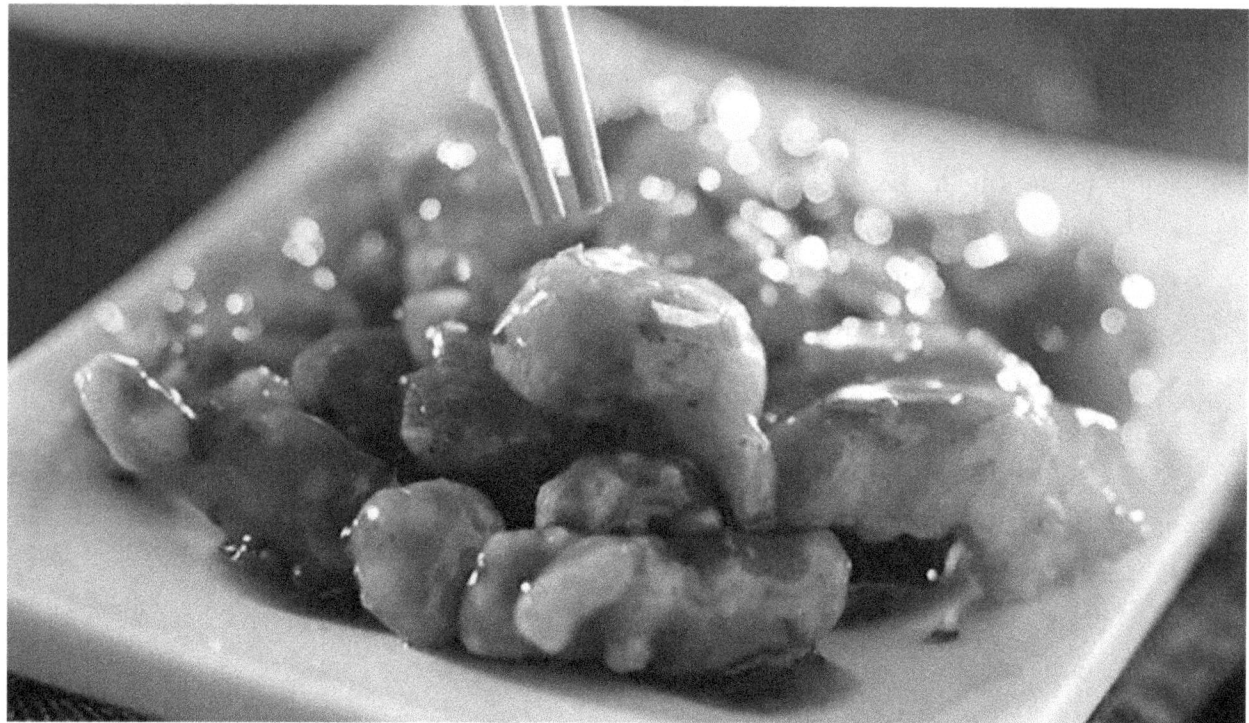

Ingredients

- 2 tablespoons vegetable oil
- ½ lb chicken thighs, boneless/skinless
- ⅛ teaspoon black pepper
- ½ cups diced onion
- ½ cups soy sauce
- ¼ cups ketchup
- 2 teaspoons minced garlic cloves
- ¼ tablespoon red pepper flakes
- ⅛ teaspoon salt
- 1 cup honey
- Parsley (Garnish)

How to

1. Put all the ingredients, except the corn-starch and water, into the instant pot.
2. Cover with the cooker lid and secure it.
3. Select the 'poultry' function and set the timer for 15 minutes.

4. Let it cook till you hear the beep. Now run 'natural release' for 5 minutes to vent the steam.
5. Use 'quick release' to vent any remaining pressure.
6. Remove the chicken from the sauce and dice it.
7. Select the 'sauté' function.
8. Mix the corn starch and water in a bowl. Add this mixture to the pot while stirring.
9. Put the chicken back into the pot and cook for 3 minutes.
10. Garnish with parsley and serve.

Nutrition Values (Per Serving)

- Calories: 961
- Carbohydrate: 22.3g
- Protein: 65.7g
- Fat: 11.1g
- Sugar: 5.4g
- Sodium: 1121mg

Chicken Thighs with Potatoes

(**Serves**: 6 / **Prep Time:** 10 minutes / **Cooking Time**: 20 minutes)

Ingredients

Spice Mixture:
- ¼ teaspoon Onion Powder
- ¼ teaspoon Black Pepper
- ¼ teaspoon Poultry Seasoning
- ½ teaspoon Garlic Powder
- ½ teaspoon Paprika
- ½ teaspoon Kosher Salt

Chicken Thighs and Potatoes:
- 2 tablespoons olive oil
- 6 chicken thighs (I use skin on, bone in)
- 1½ cups chicken broth low sodium
- 3 large red potatoes cut into quarters
- 1 tablespoon butter
- 1 small sprig rosemary
- ½ lemon

How to

1. In a medium-sized bowl, add all the spices to the chicken thighs and mix well.
2. Select the 'sauté' function on the cooker. Put the olive oil and the seasoned chicken into the pot.
3. Let it cook for 4 minutes on each side until the chicken turns golden brown.
4. Remove the chicken from the pot and add the broth to it.
5. Add the potatoes, the rosemary and the butter.
6. Place a trivet in the pot and put the chicken thighs on it.
7. Pour lime juice over the chicken thighs, then secure the lid.
8. Switch the 'sauté' function to 'poultry', and set the timer to 13 minutes.
9. After the completion beep, use 'natural release' for 10 minutes, and then quickly release any remaining steam.
10. Remove the chicken, the trivet and the potatoes from the pot.
11. Select the 'sauté' function and cook the remaining gravy in the pot, adding corn starch (mixed in water) to it.
12. Keep stirring until it thickens.
13. Pour the gravy over the cooked potatoes and chicken thighs. Serve.

Nutrition Values (Per Serving)

- Calories: 1231
- Carbohydrate: 36.15g
- Protein: 26.7g
- Fat: 15.8g
- Sugar: 3.7g
- Sodium: 938mg

Chicken Marsala

(**Serves**: 4 / **Prep Time:** 10 minutes / **Cooking Time**: 20 minutes)

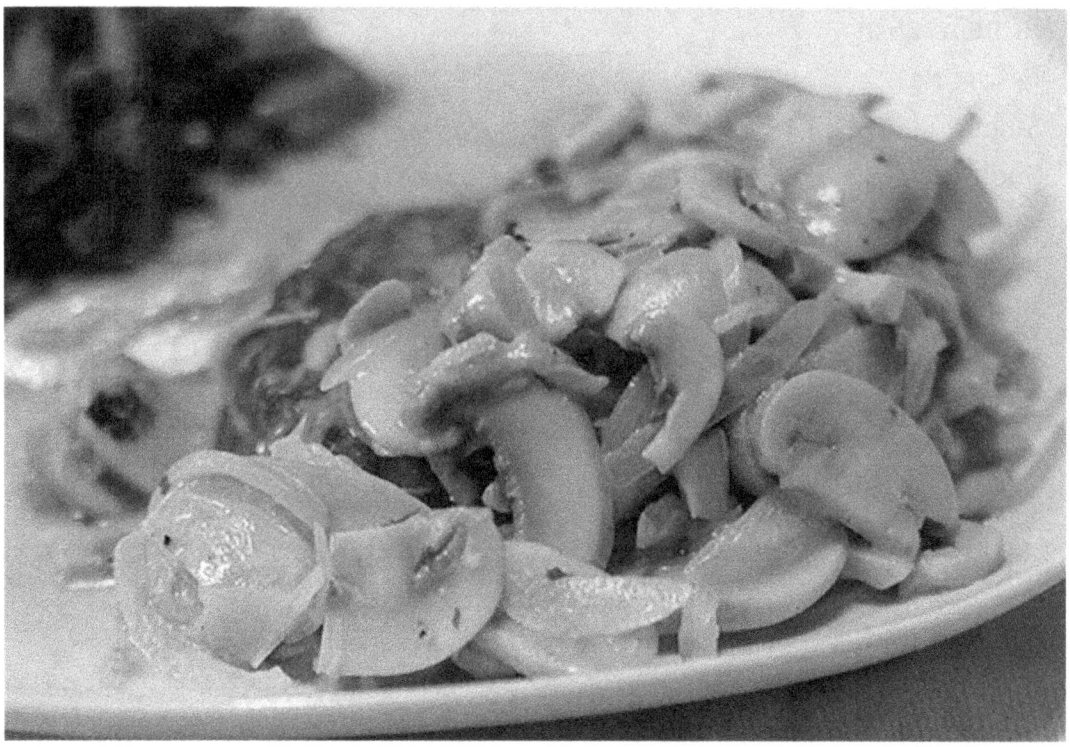

Ingredients

- 3 tablespoons olive oil
- ½ cup potato starch
- ½ teaspoon black pepper
- 2 boneless/skinless chicken breasts, cut in half
- ½ cup chicken broth
- 3 oz. Prosciutto, diced
- 2 tablespoons butter
- 3 cloves fresh garlic, minced
- 1 lb Cremini mushrooms, sliced
- 1 cup dry Marsala wine
- 1/2 teaspoon Herbs de Provence
- 2 large shallots
- 3 sprigs fresh thyme
- 1 tablespoon kosher salt
- Parsley for garnish

How to

1. In a shallow bowl, mix the potato starch, pepper and salt. Add the chicken slices to the mix.
2. Coat the chicken evenly with the starch mix.
3. Select the 'sauté' function on your instant pot. Add the oil and chicken to the pot.
4. Cook the chicken cutlets on each side until they turn golden brown.
5. Remove the chicken from the pot. Add the Prosciutto, ¼ cup of marsala wine, the mushrooms and the shallots to the pot.
6. Sauté the ingredients for 3 minutes. Then add the garlic.
7. Stir in remaining the Marsala wine to and cook until it bubbles.
8. Add the chicken stock, the thyme and the Herb de Provence, then secure the lid.
9. Cook at high pressure for 2 minutes using the 'manual' function.
10. Switch off the cooker and release the steam naturally.
11. Garnish the chicken with parsley and serve.

Nutrition Values (Per Serving)

- Calories: 1315
- Carbohydrate: 30.9g
- Protein: 78.6g
- Fat: 0.8g
- Sugar: 2.7g
- Sodium: 873mg

Chicken Salsa

(**Serves**: 2 / **Prep Time:** 5 minutes / **Cooking Time**: 15 minutes)

Ingredients

- 1 lb frozen, skinless, boneless chicken breast halves
- 1(1 oz.) packet taco seasoning mix
- ½ cup salsa
- ½ cup chicken broth.

How to

1. Place the chicken breasts in the instant pot.
2. Sprinkle taco seasoning uniformly over both sides of the chicken breasts.
3. Add the salsa and chicken broth to the pot.
4. Secure the lid.
5. Set the 'poultry' function on your pressure cooker to cook for 15 minutes.
6. After the beep, release the steam naturally for 20 minutes. Use 'quick release' to vent any remaining steam.
7. Remove the chicken and shred it.
8. Serve the shredded chicken with the steaming hot sauce.

Nutrition Values (Per Serving)

- Calories: 387
- Carbohydrate: 4.5g
- Protein: 21.7g
- Fat: 3.4g
- Sugar: 1.4g
- Sodium: 568mg

Crack Chicken

(**Serves**: 6 / **Prep Time:** 10 minutes / **Cooking Time**: 20 minutes)

Ingredients

- 1 cup mayonnaise
- 4 chicken breasts
- ½ cup chicken broth
- 1 packet ranch dressing mix
- 1 lb. bacon, diced, raw
- 8 oz. cream cheese
- 2 cups shredded cheddar cheese
- ¼ cup chopped green onions

How to

1. Select the 'sauté' function on your instant pot. Put the chopped bacon into the pot and cook for 5 minutes.
2. Clean the pot then add the chicken breasts and cream cheese.
3. Add the chicken broth to the pot.
4. Secure the lid. Select 'manual' function and set to high pressure with 15 minutes on the timer.
5. After the beep, release the steam over 5 minutes using 'natural release'.
6. Use the 'quick release' to discharge any remaining steam.
7. Remove the lid and take the chicken out of the pot.
8. Shred the chicken and put it aside.
9. Use the 'sauté' function to cook the remaining cream cheese. Keep stirring until it thickens.
10. Stir in the mayonnaise, the shredded chicken, cheese, green onions and bacon.
11. Serve and enjoy.

Nutrition Values (Per Serving)

- Calories: 910
- Carbohydrate: 19.4g
- Protein: 86.7g
- Fat: 14.8g
- Sugar: 1.7g
- Sodium: 792mg

Chicken Garlic Delight

(**Serves**: 6 / **Prep Time:** 10 minutes / **Cooking Time**: 15 minutes)

Ingredients

- 1 tablespoon olive oil
- 1 tablespoon butter
- 6 bone-in chicken thighs
- 1½ teaspoons kosher salt
- ½ teaspoon ground black pepper
- 40 peeled garlic cloves
- 2 thyme sprigs
- ¼ cup dry white wine
- ¼ cup chicken broth
- Chopped parsley leaves (garnish)

How to

1. Select the 'sauté' function on your instant pot. After 5 minutes, pour in the oil.
2. Season the chicken thighs with salt and pepper, then put them into the oil.
3. Let the chicken cook on each side for 3 minutes until it turns golden brown.
4. Remove the chicken from the pot, then add garlic and thyme to it.
5. Let it cook for one minute with occasional stirring. Then add the broth and the wine to the pot.
6. Put the chicken back in the pot and secure the lid.
7. Use 'manual' settings at high pressure and 15 minutes cooking time.
8. When it's done, let it stay for 5 minutes, then use the 'natural release' to vent the steam.
9. Serve it with parsley sprinkled on top.

Nutrition Values (Per Serving)

- Calories: 925
- Carbohydrate: 16.2g
- Protein: 53.7g
- Fat: 9.1g
- Sugar: 0.9g
- Sodium: 772mg

Juicy Mojo Chicken Tacos

(**Serves**: 12 / **Prep Time:** 5 minutes / **Cooking Time**: 30 minutes)

Ingredients

- 4 skinless, boneless chicken breasts

Mojo:
- ¼ cup olive oil
- 2/3 cup fresh lime juice
- 8 garlic cloves, minced
- 1 tablespoon dried oregano
- 2/3 cup orange juice
- 2 teaspoons ground cumin
- 1 tablespoon grated orange peel
- ¼ teaspoon ground black pepper
- 2 teaspoons kosher salt
- ½ cup chopped fresh cilantro

Serve:
- 12 organic corn tortillas
- ½ cup red onion, finely diced
- 1 avocado, sliced
- Chopped cilantro.

How to

1. Put all the ingredients of mojo into a small bowl and mix together.
2. Put the chicken in the pot and pour the mojo mix over it.
3. Cover with the cooker lid and select the 'poultry' function with 20 minutes on the timer.
4. After the beep, use 'natural release' for 10 minutes, then 'quick release' to remove all the steam.
5. Remove the lid carefully. Shred the chicken inside the pot using two forks.
6. To make the chicken crispier, broil it in an oven for 8 minutes.
7. Serve it with tacos, onion, avocado and fresh cilantro on top.

Nutrition Values (Per Serving)

- Calories: 110
- Carbohydrate: 13.3g
- Protein: 10.8g
- Fat: 1.7g
- Sugar: 0.7g
- Sodium: 421mg

Tasty Taco Bowls

(**Serves**: 6 / **Prep Time:** 10 minutes / **Cooking Time**: 15 minutes)

Ingredients

- 5 chicken breasts (boneless, skinless)
- 2 tablespoons taco seasoning
- 1 (12 oz.) bag frozen corn
- ½ cup shredded cheddar cheese
- 1 (15.5 oz.) jar salsa
- 3 cups uncooked jasmine rice, rinsed
- 3 cups chicken broth
- 1 (15 oz.) can black beans
- cilantro
- sour cream

How to

1. Pour one cup of chicken broth into the instant pot.
2. Add the chicken, the rice, taco seasoning, salsa, corns, and beans to the pot.
3. Select the 'manual' function on your cooker, setting it to high pressure and 12 minutes cooking time.
4. Let it cook until it beeps.
5. Use 'quick release' to vent the steam.
6. Remove the lid when pressure is completely released.
7. Shred the chicken in the pot.
8. Serve it with cheddar cheese, sour cream, and cilantro on top.

Nutrition Values (Per Serving)

- Calories: 957
- Carbohydrate: 44.2 g
- Protein: 140.g
- Fat: 19.8g
- Sugar: 1.5g
- Sodium: 993mg

Instant BBQ Chicken Wings

(**Serves**: 6 / **Prep Time:** 10 minutes / **Cooking Time**: 15 minutes)

Ingredients

- 2 lbs. chicken wings
- ¾ cup favourite barbecue sauce
- 2 tablespoons seasoned salt
- ¾ cup cold water
- ¼ cup hot sauce

How to

1. Place chicken wings in a medium-sized bowl and add seasoned salt to it.
2. Toss the wings in the bowl to add more flavour.
3. Put the seasoned chicken wings in an instant pot and add the barbecue sauce to it.
4. Add 1 cup of water to the pot then secure the lid.
5. Select the 'manual' function on the pressure cooker and set to high pressure with 10 minutes cooking time.
6. After the completion beep, release the steam carefully with 'quick release'.
7. Remove the lid and let the wings stay for 2 minutes.
8. Now stir the sauce in with the chicken wings to enrich their flavour.
9. Serve the dish with red pepper slices and celery sticks.

Nutrition Values (Per Serving)

- Calories: 206
- Carbohydrate: 16.7 g
- Protein: 9.7g
- Fat: 10.8g
- Sugar: 8.1g
- Sodium: 550mg

Potatoes with BBQ Chicken

(**Serves**: 6 / **Prep Time:** 10 minutes / **Cooking Time**: 15 minutes)

Ingredients

- 2 lb chicken breasts
- 1 large, red onion, sliced
- 1 cup BBQ sauce
- ½ cup water
- 1 tablespoon minced garlic
- 1 tablespoon Italian seasoning
- 2-3 large potatoes, chopped

How to

1. Place all the ingredients in the instant pot.
2. Cover with the cooker lid and lock.
3. Select the 'poultry' function on the cooker, and set it for 15 minutes cooking time.
4. After it's done, use the 'natural release' for 10 minutes to discharge the steam.
5. Remove the lid and shred the chicken with two forks.
6. Stir the sauce well to 'simmer' the shredded chicken into it.
7. Serve immediately.

Nutrition Values (Per Serving)

- Calories: 878
- Carbohydrate: 45.6g
- Protein: 129.9g
- Fat: 15.3g
- Sugar: 13.6g
- Sodium: 854mg

Chicken Cacciatore

(**Serves**: 4 / **Prep Time:** 10 minutes / **Cooking Time**: 30 minutes)

Ingredients

- 2 tablespoons olive oil.
- 4 chicken thighs, with the bone, skinless
- ½ can crushed tomatoes.
- ¼ cup diced red bell pepper
- ½ teaspoon dried oregano
- ½ cup diced onion
- ½ cup diced green bell pepper
- 1 bay leaf
- kosher salt and fresh pepper to taste
- 2 tablespoons parsley (garnish)

How to

1. Add salt and pepper to the chicken. Sprinkle it on both sides.
2. Select the 'sauté' function on the instant pot.
3. Spray the base of the pot with a light layer of oil. Allow it heat, then add the chicken.
4. Cook the chicken until it turns golden brown.
5. Add more oil along with peppers and onions. Let it cook for 5 minutes.
6. Now add the tomatoes, bay leaf, pepper, oregano and salt.
7. Secure the lid and select the 'manual' function for 25 minutes of cooking at high pressure.
8. When its finished, use the 'natural release' method to vent the steam.
9. Garnish with parsley and serve over pasta.

Nutrition Values (Per Serving)

- Calories: 249
- Carbohydrate: 6.6g
- Protein: 20.1g
- Fat: 17.2g
- Sugar: 3g
- Sodium: 86mg

Chicken Noodle Pho

(**Serves**: 4 / **Prep Time:** 10 minutes / **Cooking Time**: 15 minutes)

Ingredients

Broth:
- 2 lb chicken pieces, bones-in
- 3 whole cloves
- 1 large yellow onion, sliced
- 4 cups just-boiled water
- 1 small Fuji apple, sliced
- ¾ cup chopped cilantro sprigs
- 2¼ teaspoons sea salt
- 2-inch ginger, sliced
- 1 tablespoon coriander seeds
- 1½ tablespoons fish sauce
- 2 teaspoons maple syrup

Bowls:
- 10 oz. flat rice noodles, boiled
- ½ small yellow onions, thinly sliced
- 2 thinly sliced green onions, green parts
- Freshly ground black pepper.
- ¼ cup chopped fresh cilantro, leafy tops only

How to

1. Select the 'sauté' function on your instant pot, and add the coriander seeds and the cloves.
2. Let them roast for 60 seconds, then add 4 cups of water, the chicken, salt, apple, cilantro, and salt.
3. Secure the lid and set the cooker on 'manual' to cook for 15 minutes at high pressure.
4. After the beep, use 'natural release' for 20 minutes to vent all the steam.
5. Remove the chicken from the broth. Pull the meat from the bones and put it aside as thin slices.
6. Strain the remaining chicken broth and discard all the solids.
7. Place all the vegetables, the boiled noodles and chicken slices in a serving bowl.
8. Pour the hot broth into the bowl, sprinkle black pepper, and serve immediately.

Nutrition Values (Per Serving)

- Calories: 546
- Carbohydrate: 8g
- Protein: 95.6g
- Fat: 11.5g
- Sugar: 4.9g
- Sodium: 752mg

Instant Thai Chicken

(**Serves**: 8 / **Prep Time:** 10 minutes / **Cooking Time**: 17 minutes)

Ingredients

- 3 lb boneless chicken breasts
- 1 can full-fat coconut milk
- 1 medium yellow onion, thinly sliced
- 1/3 cup tomato paste
- 2 tablespoons coconut aminos*
- 2 teaspoons fresh lime juice
- 2 cloves garlic, minced
- 3/4 teaspoon ground ginger
- ½ cup Thai red curry paste
- 2 tablespoons fish sauce
- 4 cups mixed vegetables
- 2 teaspoons sea salt
- fresh cilantro, garnish

How to

1. Place the chicken, along with all the other ingredients, into the instant pot.
2. Whisk all the ingredients well to coat the chicken evenly.
3. Cover with the cooker lid and lock.
4. Select the 'poultry' function on the pressure cooker, and set 15 minutes on the timer.
5. Let it cook until it beeps. Release the pressure with 'quick release'.
6. Remove the lid and take the chicken out of the pot.
7. Dice the chicken and replace it in the pot.
8. Now add the vegetables and secure the lid again.
9. Use 'manual' settings to cook at high pressure for 2 minutes.
10. After the beep, release the steam completely, then remove the lid.
11. Stir the sauce well. Garnish with cilantro sprinkled on top.

Nutrition Values (Per Serving)

- Calories: 871
- Carbohydrate: 5.9g
- Protein: 143.9g
- Fat: 6.9g
- Sugar: 2.6g
- Sodium: 968mg

(**Note:** Coconut Aminos* - Coconut-based sauce satisfies, awesome tasting and healthy coconut sugar mixed with mineral-rich sea Salt-Aged to perfection)

Traditional Country Chicken

(**Serves**: 6 / **Prep Time:** 20 minutes / **Cooking Time**: 15 minutes)

Ingredients

- 2 tablespoons olive oil
- 3 lbs. chicken pieces (with bones and skin)
- ½ teaspoon black pepper
- 1 cup chicken stock
- 1 celery stalk, cut into quarters
- 1 cup carrots, chopped.
- ½ teaspoon gravy seasoning.
- 4 sprigs fresh, flat-leaf parsley
- 2 sprigs rosemary
- ½ cup onion, sliced.
- 1½ cups frozen green peas, thawed
- 3 tablespoons melted butter
- 5 baby red potatoes, cut in half
- 2 sprigs thyme
- 5 tablespoons all-purpose flour
- 1 teaspoon salt

How to

1. Season the chicken pieces with the salt, pepper and oil. Put them to one side.
2. Put the chicken stock and gravy mix into the instant pot.
3. Put the steam rack over the pot then place the chicken, potatoes, celery, carrots, onions, and tied up herbs, over the rack.
4. Secure the lid and cook on high pressure for 12 minutes using the 'manual' function on your pressure cooker.
5. After the beep, use the 'quick release' to relieve the pressure.
6. Remove the chicken and vegetables. Discard all the herbs.
7. Add the peas to the hot chicken broth in the pot. Select the 'sauté' function for cooking.
8. In a separate bowl, whisk melted butter with flour, then add the mix to the instant pot.
9. Let it cook for 3 minutes, stirring constantly.
10. Pour over the chicken and vegetables and serve.

Nutrition Values (Per Serving)

- Calories: 1845
- Carbohydrate: 37.4g
- Protein: 292.2g
- Fat: 49.8g
- Sugar: 6.9g
- Sodium: 1021mg

Instant Scampi Chicken

(**Serves**: 6 / **Prep Time:** 10 minutes / **Cooking Time**: 10 minutes)

Ingredients

- 3 chicken breasts, cut into strips
- 1/2 red onion sliced
- 1 red bell pepper sliced
- 3 cloves of garlic minced
- 1 cup white wine
- ½ cup parmesan cheese
- ½ teaspoon pepper
- ½ teaspoon Italian seasoning
- 1 yellow bell pepper sliced
- ½ cup chicken broth
- ½ teaspoon garlic powder
- 1/2 cup flour
- 1 teaspoon salt
- 2 tablespoons olive oil

How to

1. Select the 'sauté' function on your instant pot pressure cooker. Allow it to preheat for 5 minutes.
2. Meanwhile put the flour, salt and pepper into a shallow container. Add the chicken strips to the dry mix and dredge it through to get an even coating.
3. Now put the oil into the preheated cooker, and place chicken in it.
4. Let it cook for 3 minutes, from each side, until it turns golden brown.
5. Add the peppers, garlic cloves, onions, chicken broth and wine.
6. Cover with the cooker lid. Using the 'manual' function, set the timer for 5 minutes and cook at high pressure.
7. After the beep, do a 'quick release', then open the lid.
8. Add parmesan cheese to the pot immediately. Stir it well in.
9. Serve over pasta.

Nutrition Values (Per Serving)

- Calories: 480
- Carbohydrate: 12.5g
- Protein: 68g
- Fat: 14.3g
- Sugar: 1.9g
- Sodium: 332mg

FISH AND SEAFOOD

Delicious Seafood Jambalaya

(**Serves**: 3 / **Prep time:** 20 minutes / **Cooking time**: 4 hrs. 45 min)

Ingredients

- 4 oz. catfish (cut into 1-inch cubes)
- 4 oz. shrimp (peeled and deveined)
- 1 tablespoon olive oil
- 2 bacon slices, chopped
- 1 1/5 cups vegetable broth
- ¾ cup sliced celery stalk
- ¼ teaspoon minced garlic
- ½ cup chopped onion
- 1 cup canned diced tomatoes
- 1 cup uncooked long-grain white rice
- ½ tablespoon Cajun seasoning
- ¼ teaspoon dried thyme
- ¼ teaspoon cayenne pepper
- ½ teaspoon dried oregano
- Salt and freshly ground black pepper, to taste

How to

1. Select the "Sauté" function on your Instant Pot and add the oil into it.
2. Put the onion, garlic, celery, and bacon to the pot and cook for 10 minutes.
3. Add all the remaining ingredients to the pot except seafood.
4. Stir well, then secure the cooker lid.
5. Select the "Slow Cook" function on a medium mode.
6. Keep the pressure release handle on "venting" position. Cook for 4 hours.
7. After it is done, remove the lid and add seafood to the gravy.
8. Secure the lid again, keep the pressure handle in the venting position.
9. Cook for another 45 minutes then serve.

Nutrition Values (Per Serving)

- Calories: 505
- Carbohydrate: 58.6g
- Protein: 27.4g
- Fat: 16.8g
- Sugar: 3.1g
- Sodium: 848mg

Luscious Shrimp Creole

(**Serves**: 4 / **Prep time:** 20 minutes / **Cooking time**: 7 hrs. 10 min)

Ingredients

- 1 lb. shrimp (peeled and deveined)
- 1 tablespoon olive oil
- 1 (28 oz.) can crush whole tomatoes
- 1 cup celery stalk (sliced)
- ¾ cup chopped white onion
- ½ cup green bell pepper (chopped)
- 1 (8 oz.) can tomato sauce
- ½ teaspoon minced garlic
- ¼ teaspoon ground black pepper
- 1 tablespoon Worcestershire sauce
- 4 drops hot pepper sauce
- Salt, to taste

How to

1. Put the oil to the Instant Pot along with all the ingredients except shrimp.
2. Secure the cooker lid and keep the pressure handle valve turned to the venting position.
3. Select the "Slow Cook" function on your cooker and set it on medium heat.
4. Let the mixture cook for 6 hours.
5. Remove the lid afterwards and add shrimp to the pot.
6. Stir and let the shrimp cook for another 1 hour on "Slow Cook" function.
7. Keep the lid covered with pressure release handle in the venting position.
8. To serve, pour the juicy shrimp creole over steaming white rice.

Nutrition Values (Per Serving)

- Calories: 146
- Carbohydrate: 13.5g
- Protein: 19.5g
- Fat: 1.7g
- Sugar: 0.9g
- Sodium: 894mg

Mouth-Watering Casserole

(**Serves**: 4 / **Prep time:** 20 minutes / **Cooking time**: 4 hrs.)

Ingredients

- ½ cup milk
- 2 teaspoons olive oil
- 12 oz. water-packed tuna
- 15 oz. cream of mushroom soup
- 8 oz. egg noodles (cooked and drained)
- 8 oz. thawed frozen mixed vegetables
- 2 tablespoons dried parsley
- Salt and ground black pepper, to taste
- ¼ cup toasted almonds (sliced)

How to

1. Add the tuna, mushroom soup, salt, pepper, parsley, milk, and vegetables in a medium-sized bowl and whisk it well.
2. Add the oil to the Instant Pot and grease its base properly.
3. Add the tuna mixture to the pot and sprinkle sliced almonds on top.
4. Secure the lid and keep its steam release handle to the venting position.
5. Select the "Slow Cook" function on your cooker and set its heat to "High."
6. Cook the mixture for 4 hours.
7. Remove the lid and serve hot.

Nutrition Values (Per Serving)

- Calories: 236
- Carbohydrate: 24.6g
- Protein: 25.5g
- Fat: 7.1g
- Sugar: 19.6g
- Sodium: 1120mg

Scrumptious Salmon Casserole

(**Serves**: 4 / **Prep Time:** 20 minutes / **Cooking Time**:8 hrs.)

Ingredients

- ½ tablespoon olive oil
- 8 oz. cream of mushroom soup
- ¼ cup water
- 3 medium potatoes (peeled and sliced)
- 3 tablespoons flour
- 1 (16 oz.) can salmon (drained and flaked)
- ½ cup chopped scallion
- ¼ teaspoon ground nutmeg
- Salt and freshly ground black pepper, to taste

How to

1. Pour mushroom soup and water in a separate bowl and mix it well.
2. Add the olive oil to the Instant Pot and grease it lightly.
3. Place half of the potatoes in the pot and sprinkle salt, pepper, and half of the flour over it.
4. Now add a layer of half of the salmon over potatoes, then a layer of half of the scallions.
5. Repeat these layers and pour mushroom soup mix on top.
6. Top it with nutmeg evenly.
7. Secure the lid and set its pressure release handle to the venting position.
8. Select the "Slow Cook" function with "Medium" heat on your Instant Pot.
9. Let it cook for 8 hours then serve.

Nutrition Values (Per Serving)

- Calories: 235
- Carbohydrate: 27.5g
- Protein: 18g
- Fat: 6.3g
- Sugar: 1.2g
- Sodium: 310mg

Flavorsome Tuna Chowder

(**Serves**: 3 / **Prep Time:** 20 minutes / **Cooking Time**: 7hrs)

Ingredients

- 6 oz. water-packed tuna (drained chunks)
- 1 (8 oz.) can diced tomatoes with juice
- ½ teaspoon crushed dried thyme
- ½ cup chopped celery
- ½ cup chopped onion
- ½ cup peeled and roughly shredded carrot
- 7 oz. chicken broth
- ½ teaspoon. cayenne pepper
- ½ teaspoon. freshly ground black pepper
- Salt to taste
- 1 chopped medium red potato

How to

1. Add all the ingredients except tuna to the Instant Pot and mix them well.
2. Secure the lid with its pressure release handle on the venting position.
3. Select the "Slow Cook" function with "Medium" heat for 7 hours.
4. Remove the lid after 7 hours and add tuna chunks to the pot.
5. Cover the lid immediately and let tuna stay in the steaming hot gravy for 5 minutes.
6. Serve sizzling hot chowder immediately.

Nutrition Values (Per Serving)

- Calories: 158
- Carbohydrate: 18.7g
- Protein: 18.3g
- Fat: 1.2g
- Sugar: 4.4g
- Sodium: 777mg

Nutritious Salmon Soup

(**Serves**: 4 / **Prep Time:** 20 minutes / **Cooking Time**: 17 minutes)

Ingredients

- 1 lb. salmon fillets
- 1 tablespoon coconut oil
- 1 cup carrots, peeled and chopped
- ½ cup celery stalk, chopped
- ½ cup yellow onion, chopped
- 1 cup cauliflower, chopped
- 2 cups homemade chicken broth
- 1 ½ cups half-and-half cream
- Salt and freshly ground black pepper, to taste
- 2 tablespoons fresh parsley, chopped

How to

1. Add 1 cup of water to the Instant Pot, then place the trivet in it.
2. Arrange a single layer of salmon fillets over the trivet.
3. Secure the lid and turn the pressure release handle to the "Sealed" position.
4. Select the "Manual" function on your cooker with high pressure and 9 minutes cooking time
5. After the beep, release the steam with a Quick release.
6. Remove salmon, trivet, and water from the pot.
7. Dice down salmon into edible chunks
8. Now add the coconut oil to the Instant Pot and select the "Sauté" function for cooking.
9. Add the celery, carrots, and onions to the pot and cook for 5 minutes with occasional stirring.
10. Add chicken broth and cauliflower to the pot then secure the lid.
11. Select the "Manual" settings with high pressure for 8 minutes.
12. After the completion beep, do a Natural release.
13. Remove the lid and add salmon chunks along with salt and pepper to the soup.
14. Serve with parsley sprinkled on top.

Nutrition Values (Per Serving)

- Calories: 284
- Carbohydrate: 41.3g
- Protein: 132.8g
- Fat: 16.4g
- Sugar: 23.8g
- Sodium: 508mg

Nourishing Salmon Curry

(**Serves**: 8 / **Prep Time:** 10 minutes / **Cooking Time**: 12 minutes)

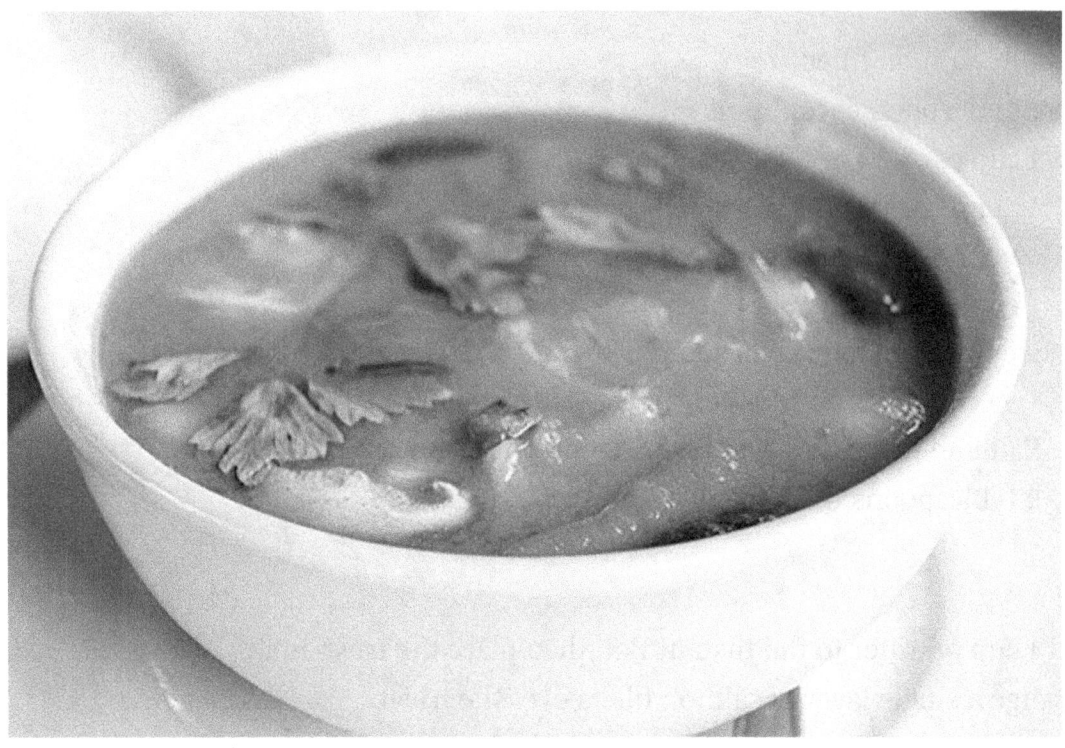

Ingredients

- 3 lbs. salmon fillets (cut into pieces)
- 2 tablespoons olive oil
- 2 Serrano peppers, chopped
- 1 teaspoon ground turmeric
- 4 tablespoons curry powder
- 4 teaspoons ground cumin
- 4 curry leaves
- 4 teaspoons ground coriander
- 2 small yellow onions, chopped
- 2 teaspoons red chili powder
- 4 garlic cloves, minced
- 4 cups unsweetened coconut milk
- 2 ½ cups tomatoes, chopped
- 2 tablespoons fresh lemon juice
- Fresh cilantro leaves (Garnish)

How to

1. Put the oil and curry leaves to the insert of the Instant Pot. Select the "Sauté" function to cook for 30 secs.
2. Add the garlic and onions to the pot, cook for 5 minutes.
3. Stir in all the spices and cook for another 1 minute.
4. Put the fish, Serrano pepper, coconut milk, and tomatoes while cooking.
5. Cover and lock the lid. Seal the pressure release valve.
6. Select the "Manual" function at low pressure for 5 minutes.
7. After the beep, do a "Natural" release to release all the steam.
8. Remove the lid and squeeze in lemon juice.
9. Garnish with fresh cilantro leaves and serve.

Nutrition Values (Per Serving)

- Calories: 559
- Carbohydrate: 12.2g
- Protein: 36.9g
- Fat: 43.2g
- Sugar: 6.5g
- Sodium: 106mg

Super-Easy Salmon Fillets

(**Serves**: 3 / **Prep Time:** 10 minutes / **Cooking Time**: 03 minutes)

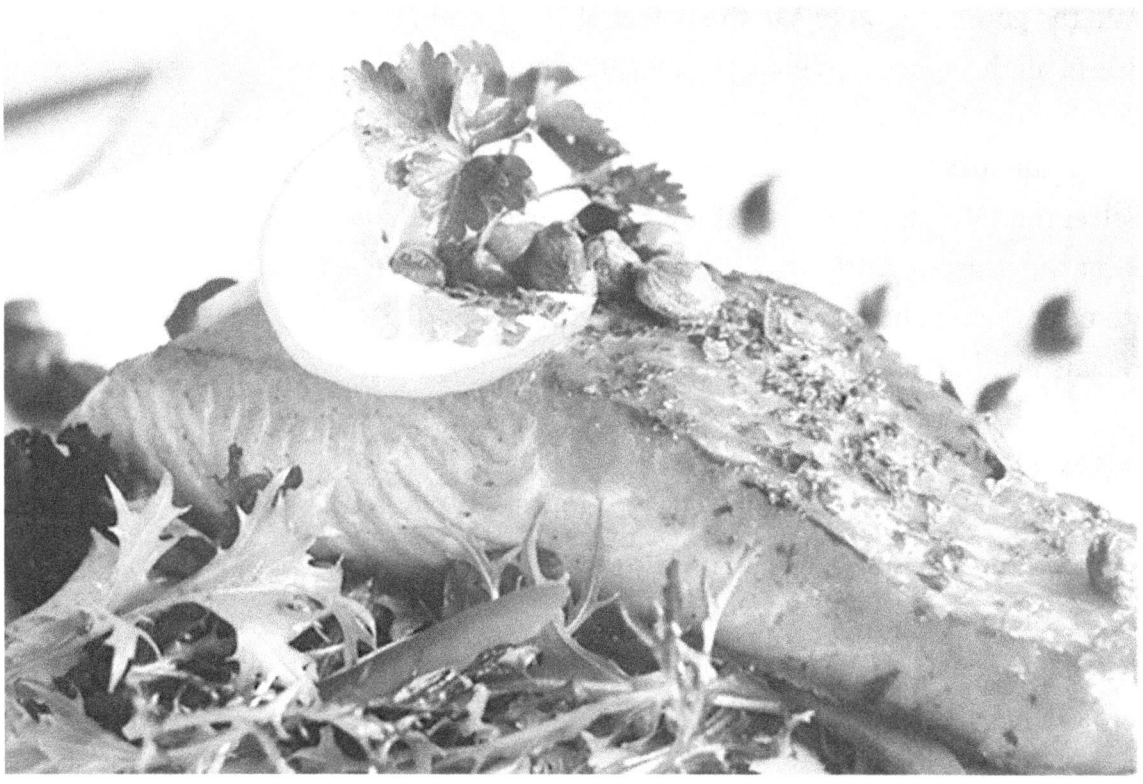

Ingredients

- 1 cup water
- 3 lemon slices
- 1 (5-oz.) salmon fillet
- 1 teaspoon fresh lemon juice
- Salt and ground black pepper, to taste
- Fresh cilantro (Garnish)

How to

1. Add the water to the Instant pot and place a trivet inside.
2. In a shallow bowl, place the salmon fillet. Sprinkle salt and pepper over it.
3. Squeeze some lemon juice on top then place a lemon slice over the salmon fillet.
4. Cover the lid and lock it. Set its pressure release handle to "Sealing" position.
5. Use "Steam" function on your cooker for 3 minutes to cook.
6. After the beep, do a Quick release and release the steam.
7. Remove the lid, then serve with the lemon slice and fresh cilantro on top.

Nutrition Values (Per Serving)

- Calories: 63
- Carbohydrate: 0.2g
- Protein: 9.2g
- Fat: 2.9g
- Sugar: 0.1g
- Sodium: 48mg

Lime-filled Salmon Fillet

(**Serves**: 2 / **Prep Time:** 20 minutes / **Cooking Time**: 5 minutes)

Ingredients

- 2 (4 oz.) salmon fillets
- ½ tablespoon olive oil
- ½ teaspoon garlic, minced
- ½ cup homemade chicken broth
- ½ teaspoon lemon zest (freshly grated)
- 1 tablespoon fresh lemon juice
- Salt and black pepper, to taste

How to

1. Put all the ingredients to the Instant pot and mix them well.
2. Secure the lid and turn its pressure release handle to "Sealing" position.
3. Select the "Manual" function at high pressure for 5 minutes.
4. After the beep, release the steam naturally for 10 minutes.
5. Remove the lid and dish out the salmon fillets along with their sauce.
6. Serve.

Nutrition Values (Per Serving)

- Calories: 192
- Carbohydrate: 0.7g
- Protein: 23.3g
- Fat: 10.9g
- Sugar: 0.4g
- Sodium: 281mg

Spicy Salmon Meal

(**Serves**: 8 / **Prep Time:** 10 minutes / **Cooking Time**: 02 minutes)

Ingredients

- 2 cups water
- 2 garlic cloves, minced
- 2 teaspoons powdered stevia
- 2 tablespoons red chili powder
- 2 teaspoons ground cumin
- Salt and freshly grated black pepper, to taste
- 2 lbs. salmon fillet, cut into 8 pieces

How to

1. Pour two cups of water in the insert of the Instant Pot. Set the trivet in it.
2. In a separate bowl, add all the ingredients and mix well.
3. Pour this mixture over the salmon fillets and rub it all over it.
4. Place the salmon slices over the trivet in a single layer.
5. Top each fillet with a lemon slice.
6. Secure the lid and select "Steam" function for 2 minutes.
7. After the beep, do a Quick release and then remove the lid.
8. Serve immediately.

Nutrition Values (Per Serving)

- Calories: 159
- Carbohydrate: 1.5g
- Protein: 22.4g
- Fat: 7.4g
- Sugar: 0.2g
- Sodium: 109mg

Rich Cheese Salmon

(**Serves**: 6 / **Prep Time:** 05 minutes / **Cooking Time**: 03 minutes)

Ingredients

- 1 ½ lbs. salmon fillets
- 1 ½ cup water
- ¼ cup olive oil
- 1 ½ garlic clove, minced
- 1 ½ tablespoon feta cheese, crumbled
- ½ teaspoon dried oregano
- 3 tablespoons fresh lemon juice
- Salt and freshly ground black pepper, to taste
- 3 fresh rosemary sprigs
- 3 lemon slices

How to

1. Take a large bowl and add garlic, feta cheese, salt, pepper, lemon juice, and oregano. Whisk all the ingredients well.
2. Add water to the Instant pot then place steamer trivet in it.
3. Arrange the salmon fillets over the trivet in a single layer.
4. Pour the cheese mix over these fillets.
5. Place a lemon slice and a rosemary sprig over each fillet.
6. Secure the lid.
7. Select the "Steam" function on your cooker and set 3 minutes cooking time.
8. After it is done, do a Quick release carefully. Remove the lid.
9. Serve hot.

Nutrition Values (Per Serving)

- Calories: 270
- Carbohydrate: 1.1g
- Protein: 22.5g
- Fat: 20.3g
- Sugar: 0.3g
- Sodium: 117mg

Tangy Mahi-Mahi

(**Serves**: 4 / **Prep Time**: 15 minutes / **Cooking Time**: 7 minutes)

Ingredients

- 1 ½ cup water
- 4 (4-oz.) mahi-mahi* fillets
- Salt and freshly ground black pepper, to taste
- 4 garlic cloves, minced
- 4 tablespoons fresh lime juice
- 4 tablespoons erythritol*
- 2 teaspoons red pepper flakes, crushed

How to

1. Sprinkle salt and pepper over Mahi-Mahi fillets for seasoning.
2. In a separate bowl add all the remaining ingredients and mix well.
3. Add the water to the Instant pot and place the trivet in it.
4. Arrange the seasoned fillets over the trivet in a single layer.
5. Pour the prepared sauce on top of each fillet.
6. Cover and secure the lid.
7. Set the "Steam" function on your cooker for 5 minutes.
8. After the completion beep, do a quick release then remove the lid.
9. Serve the steaming hot Mahi-Mahi and enjoy.

Nutrition Values (Per Serving)

- Calories: 108
- Carbohydrate: 18.6g
- Protein: 21.4g
- Fat: 1.2g
- Sugar: 15.1g
- Sodium: 189mg

(**Note: Mahi-Mahi*** -Mahi-mahi is the Hawaiian name for the species Coryphaena hippurus, also known in Spanish as the Dorado or the dolphin fish in English. Now don't worry. We are not talking about Flipper, the bottlenose dolphin, an air-breathing mammal.)

(**Erythritol*** - Erythritol is a sugar alcohol that has been approved for use as a food additive in the United States and throughout much of the world. It was discovered in 1848 by Scottish chemist John Stenhouse.)

Mahi-Mahi with Tomatoes

(**Serves**: 3 / **Prep Time:** 05 minutes / **Cooking Time**: 14 minutes)

Ingredients

- 3 (4 oz.) mahi-mahi fillets
- 1 ½ tablespoons butter
- ½ yellow onion, sliced
- ½ teaspoon dried oregano
- 1 tablespoon fresh lemon juice
- Salt and freshly ground black pepper, to taste
- 1 (14 oz.) can sugar-free diced tomatoes

How to

1. Put the butter to the Instant Pot. Select the "Sauté" function on it.
2. Add all the ingredient to the pot except the fillets. Cook them for 10 minutes.
3. Press the "Cancel" key, then add mahi-mahi fillets to the sauce.
4. Cover the fillets with sauce by using a spoon.
5. Secure the lid and set the "Manual" function at high pressure for 4 minutes.
6. After the beep, do a Quick release then remove the lid.
7. Serve the fillets with their sauce, poured on top.

Nutrition Values (Per Serving)

- Calories: 184
- Carbohydrate: 8.2g
- Protein: 22.6g
- Fat: 7.1g
- Sugar: 4.4g
- Sodium:187mg

Delicious Cod Wrap

(**Serves**: 6 / **Prep Time:** 15 minutes / **Cooking Time**: 05 minutes)

Ingredients

- 2 (4 oz.) cod fillets
- ½ teaspoon garlic powder
- Salt and black pepper, to taste
- 2 fresh dill sprigs
- 4 lemon slices
- 1 ½ tablespoons butter

How to

1. Place two large squares of parchment paper over a plain surface.
2. Arrange a layer of cod fillets at the center of each parchment piece.
3. Sprinkle salt, pepper, and garlic powder over the fillets.
4. Now place 1 dill sprig and 2 lemon slices over each fillet. Top these with a tablespoon of butter.
5. Wrap around the parchment paper to seal the cod with its filling.
6. Now add a cup of water to the instant pot. Place the trivet in it.
7. Arrange the wrapped cod parcel over the trivet in a layer. Then secure the lid.
8. Select the "Manual" function with high pressure for 5 minutes.
9. After the beep, do a Quick release then remove the lid.
10. Remove the parchment paper from each fish parcel then serve.

Nutrition Values (Per Serving)

- Calories: 196
- Carbohydrate: 0.8g
- Protein: 20.5g
- Fat: 12.6g
- Sugar: 0.3g
- Sodium: 230mg

Inviting Cod Platter

(**Serves**: 6 / **Prep Time:** 20 minutes / **Cooking Time**: 05 minutes)

Ingredients

- 1 ½ lbs. cherry tomatoes, halved
- 2 ½ tablespoons fresh rosemary, chopped
- 6 (4-oz.) cod fillets
- 3 garlic cloves, minced
- 2 tablespoons olive oil
- Salt and freshly ground black pepper, to taste

How to

1. Add the olive oil, half of the tomatoes and rosemary to the insert of the Instant Pot.
2. Place cod fillets over these tomatoes. Then add more tomatoes to the pot.
3. Add the garlic to the pot. Then secure the lid.
4. Select the "Manual" function with high pressure for 5 minutes.
5. After the beep, use the quick release to discharge all the steam.
6. Serve cod fillets with tomatoes and sprinkle a pinch of salt and pepper on top.

Nutrition Values (Per Serving)

- Calories: 149
- Carbohydrate: 6g
- Protein: 21.4g
- Fat: 5g
- Sugar: 3g
- Sodium: 116mg

Ready-to-Eat Dinner Mussels

(**Serves**: 8 / **Prep Time:** 10 minutes / **Cooking Time**: 07 minutes)

Ingredients

- 2 tablespoons olive oil
- 2 medium yellow onions, chopped
- 1 teaspoon dried rosemary, crushed
- 2 garlic cloves, minced
- 2 cups chicken broth
- 4 lbs. mussels, cleaned and debearded
- ¼ cup fresh lemon juice
- Salt and ground black pepper, to taste

How to

1. Put the oil to the Instant Pot and select the "Sauté" function for cooking.
2. Add the onions and cook for 5 minutes with occasional stirring.
3. Add the rosemary and garlic to the pot. Stir and cook for 1 minute.
4. Pour chicken broth and lemon juice into the cooker, sprinkle some salt and black pepper over it.
5. Place the trivet inside the cooker insert and arrange mussels over it.
6. Select the "Manual" function at low pressure for 1 minute.
7. Secure the lid and let the mussels cook.
8. After the beep, do a Quick release then remove the lid.
9. Serve the mussels with its steaming hot soup in a bowl.

Nutrition Values (Per Serving)

- Calories: 249
- Carbohydrate: 11.7g
- Protein: 28.6g
- Fat: 9g
- Sugar: 1.5g
- Sodium: 881mg

Butter-Dipped Lobsters

(**Serves**: 4 / **Prep Time:** 20 minutes / **Cooking Time**: 03 Min)

Ingredients

- 1 cup water.
- 4 lbs. lobster tails, cut in half
- 4 tablespoons unsalted butter, melted
- Salt to taste
- Black pepper to taste

How to

1. Pour 1 cup of water into the insert of Instant pot and place trivet inside it.
2. Place all the lobster tails over the trivet with their shell side down.
3. Cover the lid and lock it. Select the "Manual" function at low pressure for 3 minutes.
4. After the beep, press cancel and do a Quick release.
5. Remove the lid and the trivet from the pot.
6. Transfer the lobster to a serving plate.
7. Pour the melted butter over lobster tails to add more flavor.
8. Sprinkle some salt and pepper on top, then serve.

Nutrition Values (Per Serving)

- Calories: 507
- Carbohydrate: 0g (Zero gram)
- Protein: 86.3g
- Fat: 15.3g
- Sugar: 0g
- Sodium: 2000mg

Nourishing Creamy Lobster

(**Serves**: 4 / **Prep Time:** 20 minutes / **Cooking Time**: 03 minutes)

Ingredients

- 1½ cups water
- 4 lbs. fresh lobster tails
- 2 teaspoons old bay seasoning
- 1 cup mayonnaise
- 2 scallions, chopped
- ¼ cup unsalted butter, melted
- 4 tablespoons fresh lemon juice

How to

1. Put the water and Old Bay seasoning to the instant pot. Place the steamer trivet inside.
2. Arrange the lobster tails over the trivet with their meat side up.
3. Pour lemon juice over lobster tails.
4. Set the "Manual" settings at high pressure for 3 minutes.
5. Secure the lid and let it cook.
6. After the beep, do a Quick release.
7. Remove the lobster tails and add them to an ice bath. Let them sit for 1 minute.
8. Use a pair of sharp scissors to cut the underside of the tail down to its center.
9. Pull out the meat and dice it into small chunks.
10. In a serving bowl, add lobster meat, mayonnaise, scallions, butter, lemon juice and seasoning. Mix them well.
11. Refrigerate for 15 minutes, then serve.

Nutrition Values (Per Serving)

- Calories: 740
- Carbohydrate: 14.4g
- Protein: 87g
- Fat: 35g
- Sugar: 4.1g
- Sodium: 3,000mg

Special Crab Legs Delight

(**Serves**: 6 / **Prep Time:** 20 minutes / **Cooking Time**: 04 Min)

Ingredients

- 3 lbs. frozen crab legs
- 4 tablespoons butter, melted
- 2 teaspoons salt.
- 1 cup water

How to

1. Put the water to the Instant pot with a teaspoon of salt.
2. Set the trivet in the pot. Place crab legs over it.
3. Sprinkle some salt over, then secure the lid.
4. Select the "Manual" function at high pressure for 4 minutes.
5. After the beep, cancel the program then do a Quick release.
6. Transfer the crab legs to a platter.
7. Pour the melted butter on top and serve.

Nutrition Values (Per Serving)

- Calories: 313
- Carbohydrate: 20.5 g
- Protein: 23.6g
- Fat: 15.2g
- Sugar: 0g
- Sodium: 1128mg

Citrus Enriched Salmon

(**Serves**: 6 / **Prep Time:** 10 minutes / **Cooking Time**: 07 Min)

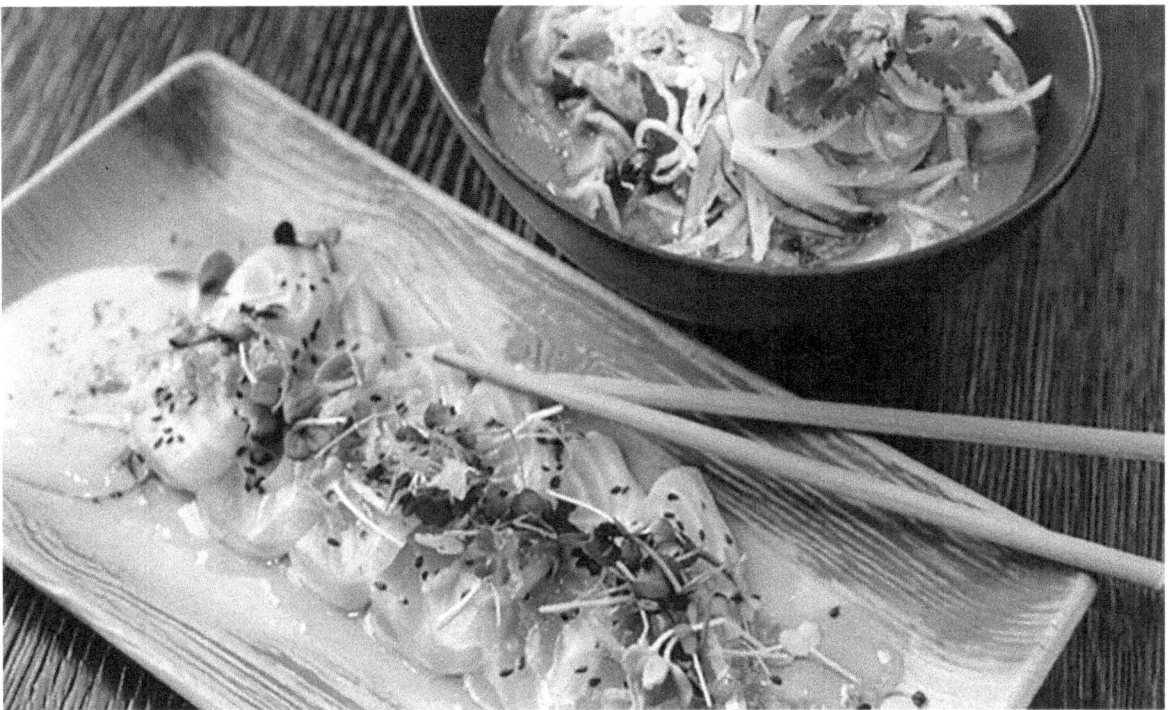

Ingredients

- 6 (4-oz.) salmon fillets
- 1 ½ teaspoon fresh ginger, minced
- 1 ½ tablespoon olive oil
- 1 ½ cup white wine
- 4 tablespoons fresh orange juice
- 2 ½ teaspoons fresh orange zest, grated finely
- Freshly ground black pepper, to taste
- Fresh herbs (garnish)

How to

1. Add all the ingredients to the insert of the Instant Pot. Mix them well.
2. Cover and secure the cooker lid.
3. Select the "Manual" function at high pressure for 7 minutes.
4. After the beep, do a "Natural" release to remove all the steam.
5. Remove the lid and transfer the Salmon fillets to the serving platter.
6. Pour the remaining sauce over them and garnish with fresh herbs.
7. Serve.

Nutrition Values (Per Serving)

- Calories: 236
- Carbohydrate: 3.2g
- Protein: 22.2g
- Fat: 10.6g
- Sugar: 1.4g
- Sodium: 53mg

Wine-Sauce Glazed Cod

(**Serves**: 2 / **Prep Time:** 05 minutes / **Cooking Time**: 02 Min)

Ingredients

- 7 (4 oz.) cod fillets
- 1 tablespoon fresh parsley
- 1 garlic clove, chopped
- ¼ teaspoon paprika
- ½ cup white wine
- 1 cup water

How to

1. Put the water to the Instant Pot and set the steamer trivet in it.
2. Place the cod fillets over the trivet in a single layer.
3. Cover and secure the lid. Select the "Manual" function with high pressure for 2 minutes.
4. After the beep, hit "Cancel" then do a Quick release. Remove the lid afterwards.
5. Meanwhile, add the remaining ingredients to a blender and blend well to form a smooth mixture.
6. Pour this mixture into a bowl, then add cooked cod.
7. Stir, then serve.

Nutrition Values (Per Serving)

- Calories: 368
- Carbohydrate: 2.4g
- Protein: 70.2g
- Fat: 3.6g
- Sugar: 0.5g
- Sodium: 253mg

Fish Curry Delight

(**Serves**: 8 / **Prep Time:** 05 minutes / **Cooking Time**: 12 Min)

Ingredients

- 3 lbs. cod fillets, cut into bite-sized pieces
- 2 tablespoons olive oil
- 4 curry leaves
- 4 medium onions, chopped
- 2 tablespoons fresh ginger, grated finely
- 4 garlic cloves, minced
- 4 tablespoons curry powder
- 4 teaspoons ground cumin
- 4 teaspoons ground coriander
- 2 teaspoons red chili powder
- 1 teaspoon ground turmeric
- 4 cups unsweetened coconut milk
- 2 ½ cups tomatoes, chopped
- 2 Serrano peppers, seeded and chopped
- 2 tablespoons fresh lemon juice

How to

1. Put the oil to the Instant Pot and select "Sauté" function for cooking.
2. Add curry leaves and cook for 30 seconds. Stir onion, garlic, and ginger into the pot and cook 5 minutes.
3. Add all the spices to the mixture and cook for another 1 ½ minutes.
4. Hit "Cancel" then add coconut milk, Serrano pepper, tomatoes, and fish to the pot.
5. Secure the lid and select the "Manual" settings with low pressure and 5 minutes cooking time.
6. After the beep, do a Quick release and remove the lid.
7. Drizzle lemon juice over the curry then stir.
8. Serve immediately.

Nutrition Values (Per Serving)

- Calories: 758
- Carbohydrate: 47.3g
- Protein: 29.8g
- Fat: 54.1g
- Sugar: 8.2g
- Sodium: 940mg

Shrimp and Beans Mix

(**Serves**: 4 / **Prep Time:** 10 minutes / **Cooking Time**: 25 Min)

Ingredients

- 1 ½ tablespoons olive oil
- 1 medium onion, chopped
- ½ small green bell pepper, seeded and chopped
- ½ celery stalk, chopped
- 1 garlic clove, minced
- 1 tablespoon fresh parsley, chopped
- ½ teaspoon red pepper flakes, crushed
- ½ teaspoon cayenne pepper
- ½ lb. great northern beans, rinsed, soaked, and drained
- 1 cup chicken broth
- Water, as required
- 1 bay leaf
- ½ lb. medium shrimp, peeled and deveined

How to

1. Select the "Sauté" function on your Instant pot, then add the oil, onion, celery, bell pepper and cook for 5 minutes.
2. Now add the parsley, garlic, spices, and bay leaf to the pot and cook for another 2 minutes.
3. Pour in the chicken broth then add beans to it. Secure the cooker lid.
4. Select the "Manual" function for 15 minutes with medium pressure.
5. After the beep, do a Natural release in 10 minutes and remove the lid.
6. Add shrimp to the beans and cook them together on the "Manual" function for 2 minutes at high pressure.
7. Do a Quick release, keep it aside for 10 minutes, then remove the lid.
8. Serve hot.

Nutrition Values (Per Serving)

- Calories: 320
- Carbohydrate: 39.9g
- Protein: 26.3g
- Fat: 7g
- Sugar: 3.4g
- Sodium: 331mg

Delectable Shrimp Curry

(**Serves**: 8 / **Prep Time:** 05 minutes / **Cooking Time**: 09 Min)

Ingredients

- 2 tablespoons olive oil
- 1 ½ medium onion, chopped
- 1 ½ teaspoons ground cumin
- 2 teaspoons red chili powder
- 2 teaspoons ground turmeric
- 3 medium white rose potatoes, diced
- 6 medium tomatoes, chopped
- 1/2 cup water
- 2 lbs. medium shrimp, peeled and deveined
- 1 ½ tablespoons fresh lemon juice
- Salt to taste
- ½ cup fresh cilantro, chopped

How to

1. Select the "Sauté" function on your Instant Pot. Add the oil and onions then cook for 2 minutes.
2. Add the tomatoes, potatoes, cilantro, and all the spices into the pot and secure the lid.
3. Select the "Manual" function at medium pressure for 5 minutes.
4. Do a natural release then remove the lid. Stir shrimp into the pot.
5. Secure the lid again then set the "Manual" function with high pressure for 2 minutes.
6. After the beep, use "Natural" release and let it stand for 10 minutes.
7. Remove the lid and serve hot.

Nutrition Values (Per Serving)

- Calories: 227
- Carbohydrate: 19.2g
- Protein: 27.1g
- Fat: 5.4g
- Sugar: 4.4g
- Sodium: 298mg

Rice-Mixed Shrimp

(**Serves**: 2 / **Prep Time:** 05 minutes / **Cooking Time**: 12 Min)

Ingredients

- ½ tablespoon olive oil
- 1 lb. shrimp, peeled and deveined
- 1/8 teaspoon red pepper flakes, crushed
- Freshly ground black pepper, to taste
- ½ small onion, chopped
- ½ large red bell pepper, chopped
- 1 celery stalk, chopped
- 1 garlic clove, minced
- ½ jalapeño pepper, seeded and chopped
- 1 cup tomatoes, chopped very finely
- ½ cup long grain white rice
- ½ cup chicken broth
- Salt, to taste
- 1/8 cup scallion (green part), chopped

How to

1. Select the "Sauté" settings on your Instant pot then add oil, shrimp, salt, half of the red pepper and black pepper. Let it cook for 3 minutes then transfer mixture to a bowl.
2. Put the garlic, jalapeno, remaining black pepper and red pepper to the pot, then cook for 1 minute.
3. Stir in chicken broth, rice, and tomatoes then secure the lid.
4. Select the "Manual" settings with high pressure and 8 minutes cooking time.
5. After the beep, do a Quick release then remove the lid.
6. Immediately add shrimp to the pot, stir then cover the lid and let it stay for 5 minutes.
7. Serve hot.

Nutrition Values (Per Serving)

- Calories: 259
- Carbohydrate: 24.8g
- Protein: 28.6g
- Fat: 4.2g
- Sugar: 2.6g
- Sodium: 419mg

Irresistible Seafood Gumbo

(**Serves**: 4 / **Prep Time:** 10 minutes / **Cooking Time**: 22Min)

Ingredients

- 4 tablespoons olive oil, divided
- 1 red bell pepper, seeded and chopped
- ½ onion, chopped
- 1 ½ celery stalks, chopped
- 2 garlic cloves, minced
- 1 smoked sausage, chopped
- 1 tablespoon dried thyme, crushed
- Freshly ground black pepper, to taste
- 3 ½ cups low-sodium chicken broth, divided
- 1/4 cup all-purpose flour
- ½ lb. crabmeat
- ½ lb. large shrimp, peeled and deveined
- ½ lb. scallops

How to

1. Select the "Sauté" function on your Instant Pot, then add the oil, onion, celery, bell pepper, garlic and cook for 5 minutes.
2. Hit "cancel" then stir in 3 cups chicken broth, black pepper, sausage, and thyme.
3. Secure the cooker lid then select the "Manual" function with medium pressure for 10 minutes.
4. After the beep, do a Quick release then remove the lid.
5. Meanwhile, add the oil to a skillet and set it on a medium-low heat. Add flour to the oil then cook for 5 minutes while stirring constantly.
6. Turn off the heat, then stir in remaining chicken broth to the flour. Mix well to avoid lumps.
7. Now add this flour mixture and seafood to the Instant Pot and secure the lid.
8. Cook on the "Manual" function at medium pressure for 2 minutes.
9. After the beep, do a Quick release then remove the lid.
10. Serve immediately.

Nutrition Values (Per Serving)

- Calories: 429
- Carbohydrate: 25.4g
- Protein: 35g
- Fat: 20.3g
- Sugar: 5.8g
- Sodium:9685mg

Omega Rich Seafood Soup

(**Serves**: 4 / **Prep Time:** 10 minutes / **Cooking Time**: 1 hrs. 45 Min)

Ingredients

- 1 ½ tablespoons olive oil
- 1 lb. sea scallops
- ½ medium onion, chopped
- 1 lb. mussels, cleaned and debearded
- ¼ cup carrot, peeled and chopped
- ¼ cup celery stalk, chopped
- 3 cups fresh spinach, chopped
- 8 cups chicken broth
- 1 garlic clove, minced
- ½ cup fresh parsley, chopped
- ½ lb. large shrimp, peeled and deveined
- ½ cup fresh tomatoes, chopped finely
- 1 ½ tablespoons fresh lime juice
- Sea salt and ground black pepper, to taste

How to

1. Select the "sauté" function on your Instant pot and add oil with all the vegetables except parsley.
2. Sauté for 1 minute then add parsley. Then secure the lid.
3. Select the "Slow Cook" for 1 hour. Keep the pressure release handle to the "Venting" position.
4. Place shrimp, mussels, and scallops over vegetables and cover the lid.
5. Secure the lid and "Slow Cook" for another 45 minutes.
6. Serve hot.

Nutrition Values (Per Serving)

- Calories: 391
- Carbohydrate: 15.7g
- Protein: 54.3g
- Fat: 11.6g
- Sugar: 3.4g
- Sodium: 2138mg

Salmon Zucchini Stew

(**Serves**: 2 / **Prep Time:** 10 minutes / **Cooking Time**: 6 hrs.)

Ingredients

- ½ lb. salmon fillet, cubed
- ½ tablespoon coconut oil
- ½ medium onion, chopped
- ½ garlic clove, minced
- ½ zucchini, sliced
- ½ green bell pepper, seeded and cubed
- ¼ cup tomatoes, chopped
- ½ cup fish broth
- 1/8 teaspoon dried oregano, crushed
- 1/8 teaspoon dried basil, crushed
- Salt and ground black pepper, to taste

How to

1. Add all the ingredients to the Instant pot and mix well.
2. Secure the lid and select "Slow Cook" for 6 hrs.
3. Keep the pressure release handle to the "venting" position.
4. After complete cooking, stir the stew well.
5. Serve immediately.

Nutrition Values (Per Serving)

- Calories: 223
- Carbohydrate: 7.9g
- Protein: 24.7g
- Fat: 11g
- Sugar: 4.3g
- Sodium: 249mg

Sardines Curry

(**Serves**: 4 / **Prep Time:** 10 minutes / **Cooking Time**: 8 hrs. 5 Min)

Ingredients

- 1 tablespoon olive oil
- 1 lb. fresh sardines, cubed
- 2 plum tomatoes, chopped finely
- ½ large onion, sliced
- 1 garlic clove, minced
- ½ cup tomato puree
- Salt and ground black pepper, to taste

How to

1. Select the "Sauté" function on your Instant pot then add oil and sardines to it.
2. Let it sauté for 2 minutes then add all the remaining ingredients.
3. Cover the lid and select "Slow cook" function for 8 hours.
4. Remove the lid and stir the cooked curry.
5. Serve warm.

Nutrition Values (Per Serving)

- Calories: 296
- Carbohydrate: 6.6g
- Protein: 29.2g
- Fat: 16.6g
- Sugar: 4.3g
- Sodium: 587mg

Filling Salmon Teriyaki

(Serves: 4 / **Prep Time:** 10 minutes / **Cooking Time**: 08 Min)

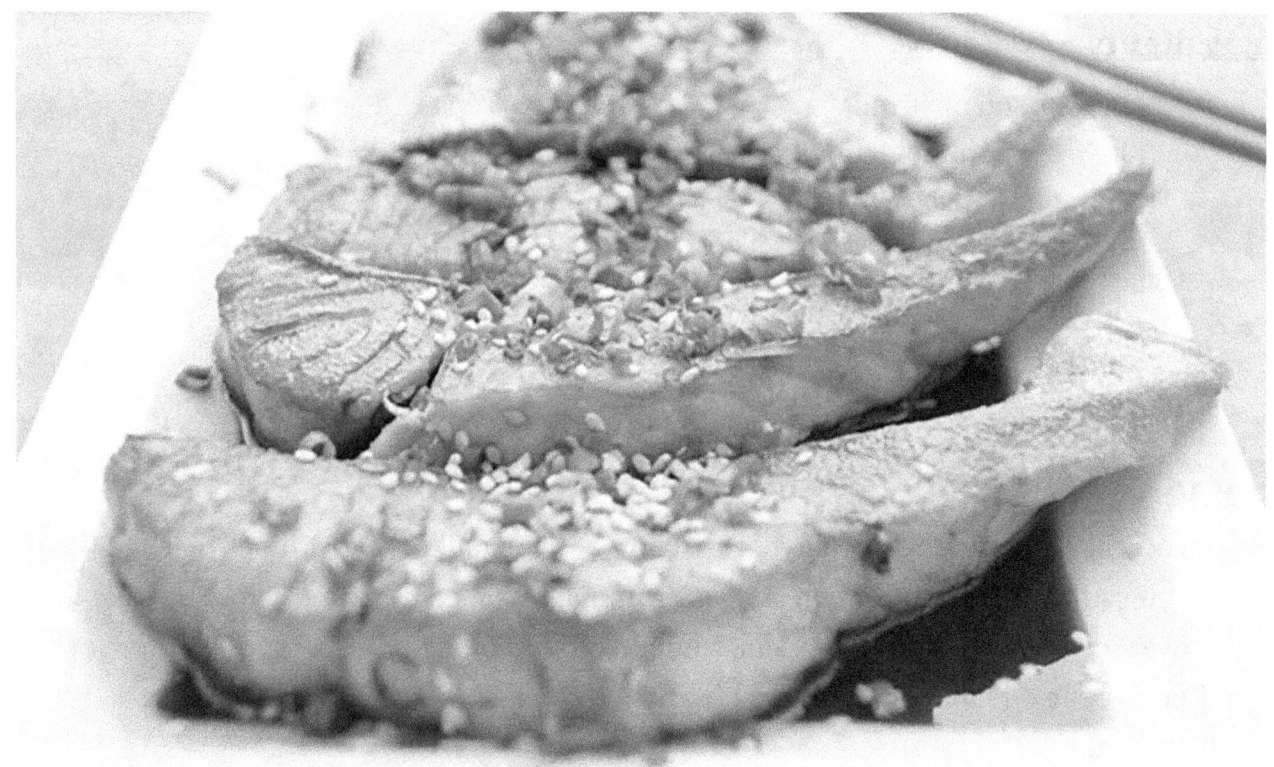

Ingredients

- 4 (8 oz.) thick salmon fillets.
- 1 cup soy sauce
- ½ cup water
- ½ cup mirin
- 2 tablespoons sesame oil
- 4 teaspoons sesame seeds
- 2 cloves garlic, minced
- 2 tablespoons freshly grated ginger
- 4 tablespoons brown sugar
- 1 tablespoon corn starch
- 4 green onions, minced

How to

1. Put the soy sauce, sesame oil, sesame seeds, mirin, ginger, water, garlic, green onions, and brown sugar to a small bowl. Mix them well.
2. In a shallow dish place the salmon fillets and pour half of the prepared mixture over the fillets. Let it marinate for 30 minutes in a refrigerator.
3. Pour 1 cup of water into the insert of your Instant pot and place trivet inside it.
4. Arrange the marinated salmon fillets over the trivet and secure the lid.
5. Select the "Manual" settings with high pressure and 8 minutes cooking time.
6. Meanwhile, take a skillet and add the remaining marinade mixture in it.
7. Let it cook for 2 minutes, then add corn starch mixed with water. Stir well and cook for 1 minute.
8. Check the pressure cooker, do a Quick release if it is done.
9. Transfer the fillets to a serving platter and pour the sesame mixture over it.
10. Garnish with chopped green chilies then serve hot.

Nutrition Values (Per Serving)

- Calories: 491
- Carbohydrate: 33.7g
- Protein: 46.2g
- Fat: 20.5g
- Sugar: 18.3g
- Sodium: 3955mg

Creamy Shrimp Grits

(**Serves**: 8 / **Prep Time:** 05 minutes / **Cooking Time**: 15 Min)

Ingredients

- 1 tablespoon oil
- 2 cups Quick Grits
- 12 oz. parmesan shredded cheese
- 1 stick butter
- 2 cups heavy cream
- 24 oz. tail-on Shrimp
- 2 tablespoons Old Bay seasoning
- Pinch of ground black pepper
- 4 cups water

How to

1. Add a tablespoon of oil to the Instant Pot. Select "Sauté" function for cooking.
2. Add the shrimp to the oil and drizzle old bay seasoning over it.
3. Cook the shrimp for 3-4 minutes while stirring then set them aside.
4. Now add water, cream, and quick grits to the pot. Select the "Manual" function for 3 minutes at high pressure.
5. After the beep, do a Quick release then remove the lid.
6. Add the shredded cheese and butter to the grits then stir well.
7. Take a serving bowl, first pour in the creamy grits mixture then top it with shrimp.
8. Sprinkle black pepper on top then serve hot.

Nutrition Values (Per Serving)

- Calories: 637
- Carbohydrate: 34.6g
- Protein: 39.2g
- Fat: 37.8g
- Sugar: 0g
- Sodium: 1505mg

Alfredo Tuscan Shrimp

(**Serves**: 4 / **Prep Time:** 05 minutes / **Cooking Time**: 15 Min)

Ingredients

- 1 lbs. of shrimp
- 1 jar of alfredo sauce
- 1 ½ cups of fresh spinach
- 1 cup of sun-dried tomatoes
- 1 box of penne pasta
- 1 ½ teaspoon Tuscan seasoning
- 3 cups water

How to

1. Add water and pasta to a pot over a medium heat, boil until it cooks completely. Then strain the pasta and keep it aside.
2. Select the "Sauté" function on the Instant Pot and add tomatoes, shrimp, Tuscan seasoning, and alfredo sauce into it.
3. Stir and cook until shrimp turn pink in color.
4. Now add spinach leaves to the pot and cook for 5 minutes.
5. Add pasta to the pot and stir well.
6. Serve hot.

Nutrition Values (Per Serving)

- Calories: 593
- Carbohydrate: 75.9g
- Protein: 42.8g
- Fat: 11.7g
- Sugar: 7.1g
- Sodium: 1132mg

Butter Shrimp Risotto

(**Serves**: 3 / **Prep Time:** 05 minutes / **Cooking Time:** 10 Min)

Ingredients

- ½ cup jasmine rice
- ½ cup water
- 1 tablespoon melted butter
- ½ tablespoon lemon juice
- ¼ cup frozen vegetables
- ½ lb. frozen raw shrimp
- ¼ cup shredded Parmesan cheese
- Salt, to taste
- Pepper, to taste

How to

1. Add butter, salt, pepper, lemon juice, water, and rice to the insert of the Instant Pot.
2. Place frozen vegetables and frozen shrimp in the pot. Secure the cooker lid.
3. Only use "frozen" shrimp and vegetables to match the cooking time for rice.
4. Now select the "Manual" function for 5 minutes at high pressure.
5. After the beep, do a Quick release then remove the lid.
6. Stir in Parmesan cheese then serve.

Nutrition Values (Per Serving)

- Calories: 240
- Carbohydrate: 26.8g
- Protein: 19g
- Fat: 5.7g
- Sugar: 0.5g
- Sodium: 221mg

Appetizing Shrimp Corn Chowder

(**Serves**: 8 / **Prep Time:** 15 minutes / **Cooking Time**: 7 Min)

Ingredients

- 2 lbs. Shrimp
- 4 tablespoons melted butter
- 2 cups onions, chopped
- 6 cloves fresh garlic minced
- 3 cups corn kernels
- 4 cups carrots chopped
- 16 oz. cremini mushrooms cut in half
- 4 cups string beans cut in half
- 2 lbs. potatoes peeled and cubed
- 4 cups chicken broth
- ½ cup dry sherry wine
- 2 fresh lemons
- 1 cup heavy whipped cream
- ½ teaspoon ground black pepper
- 3 teaspoons sea salt
- ¼ teaspoon white pepper
- ¼ teaspoon crushed red pepper flakes

How to

1. Put the butter, onions, and garlic to the insert of the Instant Pot and "Sauté" for 3 minutes.
2. Add all the ingredients, except shrimp and cream, to the pot and secure the lid.
3. Select the "Manual" function with high pressure and 7 minutes cooking time.
4. After the beep, do a Natural release and remove the lid.
5. Stir in shrimp to the vegetable sauce. Cook on the "Sauté" function for 3 minutes.
6. Then add whipped cream into the cooking sauce.
7. Serve hot in a bowl.

Nutrition Values (Per Serving)

- Calories: 449
- Carbohydrate: 52.5g
- Protein: 36.4g
- Fat: 10.1g
- Sugar: 10g
- Sodium: 1471mg

Healthy Clam Meal

(**Serves**: 8 / **Prep Time:** 05 minutes / **Cooking Time**: 12 Min)

Ingredients

- 8 bacon slices., chopped
- 16 oz. clam juice
- 20 oz. Fancy Whole Baby Clam, drained
- 12 oz. minced clams
- 2 small chopped onion
- 2 celery sticks, chopped
- 4 garlic cloves, minced or pressed
- 3 cups chicken broth
- ½ teaspoon ground white pepper
- ½ teaspoon dried thyme
- 1 teaspoon kosher salt
- 2 cups heavy cream
- 16 oz. cream cheese

How to

1. Select the "Sauté" function on your Instant pot and add bacon to its insert.
2. Cook the bacon until it turns crispy. Remove the bacon and leave its fat in the pot.
3. Now add onion, celery, and garlic to the pot and cook for 5 minutes.
4. Stir in chicken broth, clam juice, clams, salt, thyme, cooked bacon, and white pepper.
5. Secure the lid and select the "Manual" function at high pressure for 5 minutes.
6. After the beep, do a Quick release then remove the lid.
7. Add cream cheese and heavy cream to the pot then stir well.
8. Serve and enjoy.

Nutrition Values (Per Serving)

- Calories: 991
- Carbohydrate: 75.5g
- Protein: 49.9g
- Fat: 54.9g
- Sugar: 19.2g
- Sodium: 4055mg

American Clam Chowder

(**Serves**: 2 / **Prep Time:** 5 minutes / **Cooking Time**: 07 Min)

Ingredients

- 2 pieces of bacon, chopped
- ½ onion, chopped
- ½ clove minced garlic
- ¼ cup green pepper, chopped
- 1 tablespoon flour
- 1 medium potatoes, peeled and diced
- ¼ cup chopped celery
- 1 teaspoon nutmeg
- 1 ½ tablespoons parsley
- 1 (8 oz.) can tomatoes, smashed
- 1 ½ cups clam juice
- 1 bay leaf
- ½ cup minced clam

How to

1. Add the bacon to the Instant Pot and cook on the "Sauté" settings until it gets crispy.
2. Now add onion, green pepper, and garlic to the pot. Cook for 3 minutes.
3. Add clam juice, tomatoes, potatoes, celery, parsley, bay leaf, salt, pepper, and nutmeg in the pot and stir well.
4. Secure the lid and select the "Manual" function for 5 minutes with high pressure.
5. After the beep, do a Quick release then remove the lid.
6. Remove the bay leaves from the mixture and add clams into it.
7. Let it stay for 5 minutes and then serve hot.

Nutrition Values (Per Serving)

- Calories: 381
- Carbohydrate: 54.7g
- Protein: 22.1g
- Fat: 9.2g
- Sugar: 12.2g
- Sodium: 1680mg

Coconut Cod curry

(Serves: 6 / Prep Time: 05 minutes / Cooking Time: 03 Min)

Ingredients

- 1 (28 oz.) can coconut milk
- Juice of 2 lemons
- 2 tablespoons red curry paste
- 2 teaspoons fish sauce
- 2 teaspoons honey
- 4 teaspoons Sriracha*
- 4 cloves garlic, minced
- 2 teaspoons ground turmeric
- 2 teaspoons ground ginger
- 1 teaspoon sea salt
- 1 teaspoon white pepper
- 2 lbs. codfish, cut into 1" cubes
- ½ cup chopped fresh cilantro (Garnish)
- 4 lime wedges (Garnish)

How to

1. Add all the ingredients, except cod cubes and garnish, to a large bowl and whisk them together.
2. Arrange the cod cube at the base of the Instant Pot and pour the coconut milk mixture over it.
3. Secure the lid and hit the "Manual" key, select high pressure with 3 minutes cooking time.
4. After the beep, do a Quick release then remove the lid.
5. Garnish with fresh cilantro and lemon wedges then serve.

Nutrition Values (Per Serving)

- Calories: 358
- Carbohydrate: 15.4 g
- Protein: 4.8g
- Fat: 33.3g
- Sugar: 6.6g
- Sodium: 783mg

(**Note: Sriracha*** - Sriracha is a type of hot sauce or chili sauce made from a paste of chili peppers, distilled vinegar, garlic, sugar, and salt)

Creamy Chipotle Soup

(**Serves**: 2 / **Prep Time:** 05 minutes / **Cooking Time**: 25 Min)

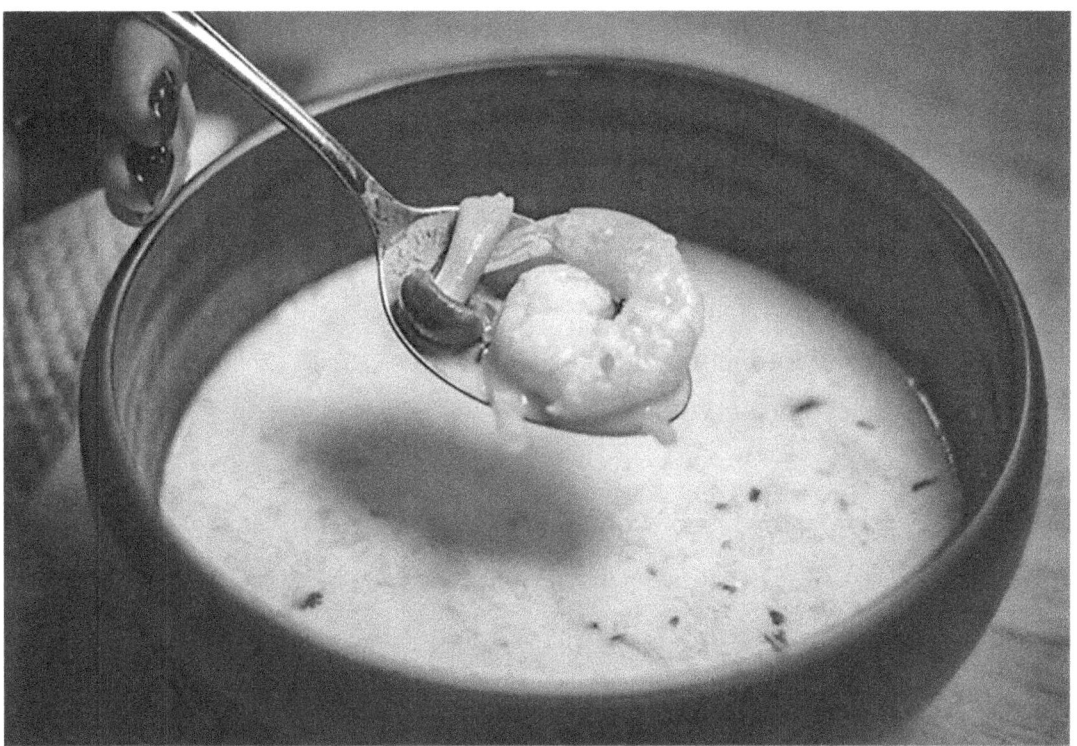

Ingredients

- 2 slices bacon, chopped
- ½ cup onion, diced
- ½ cup celery, chopped
- ½ teaspoon garlic
- ½ tablespoon flour
- ½ cup dry white wine
- 1 cup chicken broth
- ¼ cup whole milk
- 1 cup potatoes, cut into small (1/3-inch) cubes
- ½ cup frozen corn kernels
- 1 teaspoon diced Chipotle in Adobo Sauce
- ½ teaspoon salt (or to taste)
- ¼ teaspoon ground black pepper
- ¼ teaspoon dried thyme
- ¼ lb. shrimp, peeled and deveined
- 2 tablespoons heavy cream

How to

1. Select the "Sauté" function on your Instant pot then add bacon to its insert. Cook it for 3 minutes.
2. Add garlic, celery, and onions then cook again for 3 minutes,
3. Add flour to the vegetables and let it cook for 30 seconds.
4. Stir in chicken broth, corn, milk, potatoes, salt, thyme, black pepper, and Chipotle to the pot.
5. Secure the lid and cook on "Manual" with high pressure for 1 minute.
6. After the beep, do a Quick release then remove the lid.
7. Add shrimp followed by cream.
8. Mix well, close the lid and let it stand for 10 minutes.
9. Garnish with parsley and serve.

Nutrition Values (Per Serving)

- Calories: 424
- Carbohydrate: 30.6 g
- Protein: 27.3g
- Fat: 17.1g
- Sugar: 6.1g
- Sodium: 1750mg

Tuna with Noodles

(**Serves**: 2 / **Prep Time:** 05 minutes / **Cooking Time**: 04 Min)

Ingredients

- ½ can tuna drained
- 8 oz. egg noodles
- ½ cup frozen peas
- 14 oz. can cream mushroom soup
- 2 oz. shredded cheddar cheese
- 1 ½ cups water

How to

1. Add the water with egg noodles to the base of the Instant Pot.
2. Place tuna and peas over it. Then pour the mushroom soup on top.
3. Secure the lid and cook with the "Manual" function at high pressure for 4 minutes.
4. After the beep, do a Quick release then remove the lid.
5. Stir in shredded cheese to the tuna mix.
6. Serve warm.

Nutrition Values (Per Serving)

- Calories: 453
- Carbohydrate: 50.7g
- Protein: 27.2g
- Fat: 15.6g
- Sugar: 6.7g
- Sodium: 997mg

Mayo-Lobster Rolls

(**Serves**: 2 / **Prep Time:** 15 minutes / **Cooking Time**: 04 Min)

Ingredients

- ¼ teaspoons celery salt
- 4 tablespoons melted butter
- 2 teaspoons old bay seasoning
- 3 scallions, chopped
- ½ cup mayonnaise
- 1 lemon, cut in half
- 1 ½ cups chicken broth
- 2 lbs. Maine Lobster Tails
- 2 hot dog buns (sliced in half)

How to

1. Add chicken broth and a teaspoon of old bay seasoning to the insert of the Instant Pot. Set the steamer trivet inside it.
2. Place the lobster tails with their meat sides up, over the trivet.
3. Cook the lobster tails on the "Manual" function with high pressure for 4 minutes.
4. Meanwhile, prepare an ice bath for the tails. After the beep, do a quick release then remove the lid.
5. Transfer the lobster tails immediately to the ice bath and let them rest.
6. Use kitchen shears to cut the underbelly of each tail and remove the meat from it. Dice down the meat into edible chunks.
7. Add all the remaining ingredients, except the hot dog buns, into a bowl and whisk them together.
8. Add lobster to the mixture, mix then refrigerate it for 15 minutes.
9. Prepare the buns by heating them in a skillet greased with melted butter.
10. Use the refrigerated lobster mix to fill the buns. Serve.

Nutrition Values (Per Serving)

- Calories: 677
- Carbohydrate: 44.1g
- Protein: 8.1g
- Fat: 46.3g
- Sugar: 9.6g
- Sodium: 2519mg

Shrimps with Broccoli Florets

(**Serves**: 2 / **Prep Time:** 05 minutes / **Cooking Time**: 10 Min)

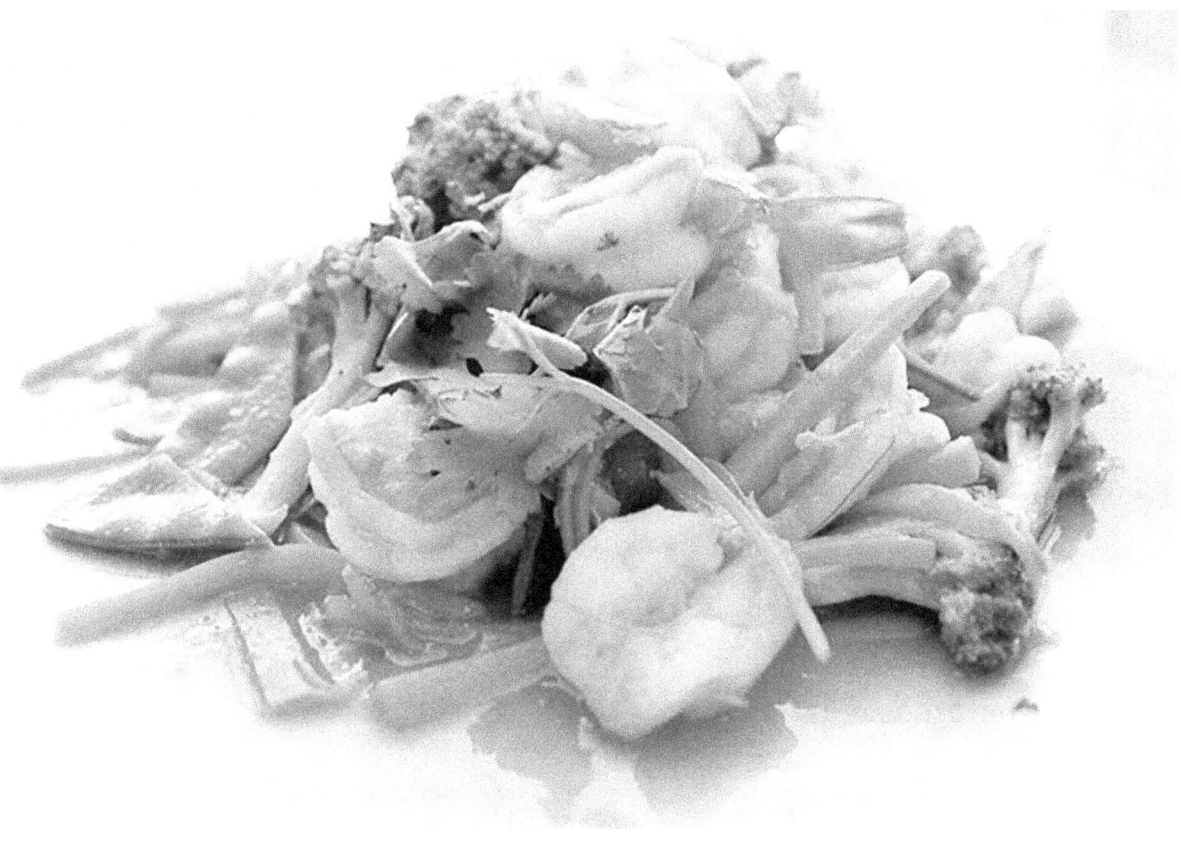

Ingredients

- 2 teaspoons vegetable oil
- 2 tablespoons corn starch
- 1 cup broccoli florets
- ¼ cup chicken broth
- 8 oz. large shrimp, peeled and deveined
- ¼ cup soy sauce
- ¼ cup water
- 2 tablespoons sugar
- ¼ cup sliced carrots
- 3 tablespoons rice vinegar
- 2 teaspoons sesame oil
- 1 tablespoon chili garlic sauce
- Coriander leaves for garnish

How to

1. Add 1 tablespoon of corn starch and shrimp to a bowl. Mix them well then set it aside.
2. In a small bowl, mix the remaining corn starch, chicken broth, carrots, chili garlic sauce, rice vinegar and soy sauce together. Keep the mixture aside.
3. Select the "Sauté" function on your Instant pot, add sesame oil and broccoli florets to the pot and sauté for 5 minutes.
4. Add water to the broccoli, cover the lid and cook for 5 minutes.
5. Stir in shrimp and vegetable oil to the broccoli, sauté it for 5 minutes.
6. Garnish with green onions on top.
7. Serve with rice or noodles.

Nutrition Values (Per Serving)

- Calories: 303
- Carbohydrate: 27.8g
- Protein: 25.4g
- Fat: 9.4g
- Sugar: 13.7g
- Sodium: 2100mg

Shrimp with Spaghetti Squash

(**Serves**: 4 / **Prep Time:** 05 minutes / **Cooking Time**: 25 Min)

Ingredients

- ½ cup dry white wine
- ¼ teaspoon crushed red pepper flakes
- 1 large shallot, finely chopped
- 1 lb. jumbo shrimp, peeled and deveined
- 1 (28 oz.) can crushed tomatoes
- 2 cloves of garlic, minced
- 2 ½ lbs. of spaghetti squash
- 1 teaspoon olive oil
- salt and pepper, to taste
- parsley leaves (garnish)

How to

1. At first, sprinkle some salt and pepper over the shrimp and keep them in a refrigerator until further use.
2. Hit the "Sauté" function on your Instant Pot, then add olive oil and red pepper into it. Sauté for 1 minute.
3. Add shallots and cook for 3 minutes. Then add garlic, cook for 1 minute.
4. Add dry wine, tomatoes, and whole spaghetti squash in the pot. Select "Manual" settings with medium pressure for 20 minutes.
5. After the beep, do a "Natural" release. Remove the lid and the spaghetti squash.
6. Cut squash in half, remove its seed and stab with a fork to form spaghetti strands out of it. Keep them aside.
7. Select the "Sauté" function on your cooker again, stir in shrimp.
8. Mix the shrimp with the sauce well.
9. To serve, top the spaghetti squash with shrimp and sauce. Garnish it with parsley.

Nutrition Values (Per Serving)

- Calories: 301
- Carbohydrate: 40.4g
- Protein: 27.5g
- Fat: 2.9g
- Sugar: 13.4g
- Sodium: 1751mg

Teriyaki Scallops

(**Serves**: 6 / **Prep Time:** 05 minutes / **Cooking Time:** 10 Min)

Ingredients

- 2 lbs. jumbo sea scallops
- 2 tablespoons olive oil
- 6 tablespoons 100% maple syrup
- 1 cup coconut aminos*
- 1 teaspoon ground ginger
- 1 teaspoon garlic powder
- 1 teaspoon sea salt

How to

1. Add olive oil to the Instant pot and heat it on "the Sauté" settings of your cooker.
2. Add the scallops to the pot and cook for a minute from each side.
3. Stir in all the remaining ingredients in the pot and mix them well.
4. Secure the lid and select the "Steam" function to cook for 2 minutes.
5. After the beep, do a Quick release then remove the lid.
6. Serve hot.

Nutrition Values (Per Serving)

- Calories: 258
- Carbohydrate: 48.9g
- Protein: 11.4g
- Fat: 2g
- Sugar: 34.5g
- Sodium: 618mg

(**Note: Coconut Aminos*** - Coconut aminos is a delicious sauce made from coconut sap. It is dark, rich, salty and slightly sweet in flavor. It resembles a light soy sauce or tamari (wheat free soy sauce), but it is soy free and gluten free)

Tomato Clam & Shrimps

(**Serves**: 2 / **Prep Time:** 05 minutes / **Cooking Time**: 15 Min)

Ingredients

- 4 cups Tomato Clam Cocktail
- 1 chopped onion
- 2 tablespoons butter
- 1 teaspoon dried oregano
- 1 tablespoon smoked paprika
- ½ teaspoon salt
- ½ cup grated Parmesan
- ½ teaspoon ground black pepper
- 1 ½ cup Arborio rice
- 1 cup shrimp, deveined

How to

1. Select the "Sauté" function on your Instant pot then add oil to its insert.
2. Add the onions to the heated oil, cook for 3 minutes then add all the seasoning.
3. Cook for another 2 minutes then add rice to the pot.
4. Pour in Tomato Clam Cocktail to the rice then cover the lid.
5. Secure the cooker lid and set it on the "Manual" settings at high pressure for 10 minutes.
6. After the beep, do a Quick release then remove the lid.
7. Stir in shrimp to the rice soup. Cover the lid and let it stay for 5 minutes.
8. Drizzled grated parmesan on top then serve.

Nutrition Values (Per Serving)

- Calories:490
- Carbohydrate: 60.4g
- Protein: 15.2g
- Fat: 20.8g
- Sugar: 22.4g
- Sodium: 1969mg

Seafood Platter

(**Serves**: 4 / **Prep Time:** 05 minutes / **Cooking Time**: 40 Min)

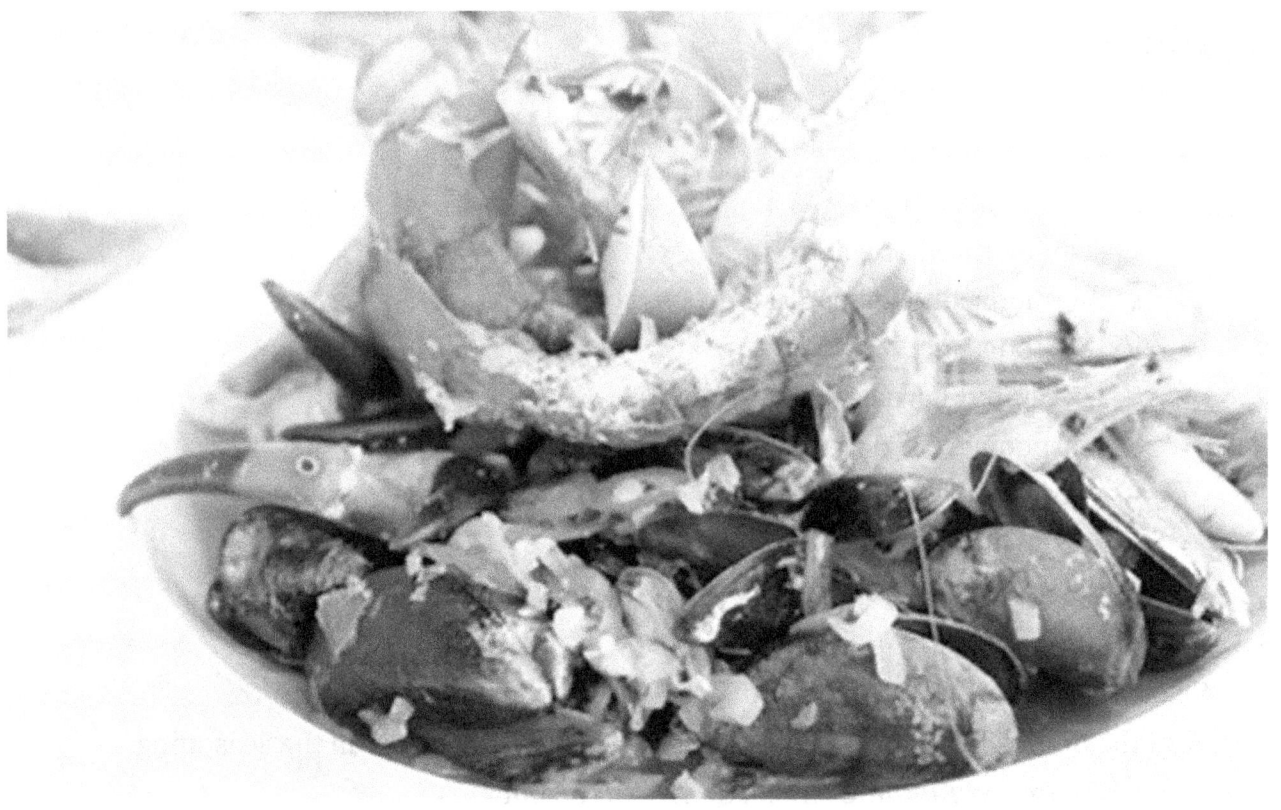

Ingredients

- ½ lb. medium sized red potatoes, halved
- 1 cup seafood stock
- 1 ½ tablespoons Cajun's shrimp boil
- ½ lb. clams, fresh frozen
- ½ lb. shell on shrimp, deveined
- ½ lb. mussels, fresh or frozen
- 1 lemon, quartered
- ½ lb. smoked Kielbasa, cut into 2-inch pieces
- 1 tablespoon chopped parsley
- Cilantro and lemon wedges (Garnish)

How to

1. Add the seafood stock, boiling spice, and potatoes to the Instant Pot.
2. Cover the lid and let it "Slow Cook" for 30 minutes till the potatoes get tender.
3. Remove the lid and add clams, shrimp, mussels, Kielbasa, and lemon to the pot.
4. Cook for 10 minutes if you are using frozen seafood, else cook for only 5 minutes.
5. Garnish with cilantro and lemon wedges on top.
6. Serve.

Nutrition Values (Per Serving)

- Calories: 432
- Carbohydrate: 30.7g
- Protein: 41.8g
- Fat: 15.9g
- Sugar: 3.9g
- Sodium: 1855mg

VEGETARIAN MAINS

Italian Vegetable Stew

(**Serves**: 4 / **Prep time:** 10 minutes / **Cooking time**: 18 minutes)

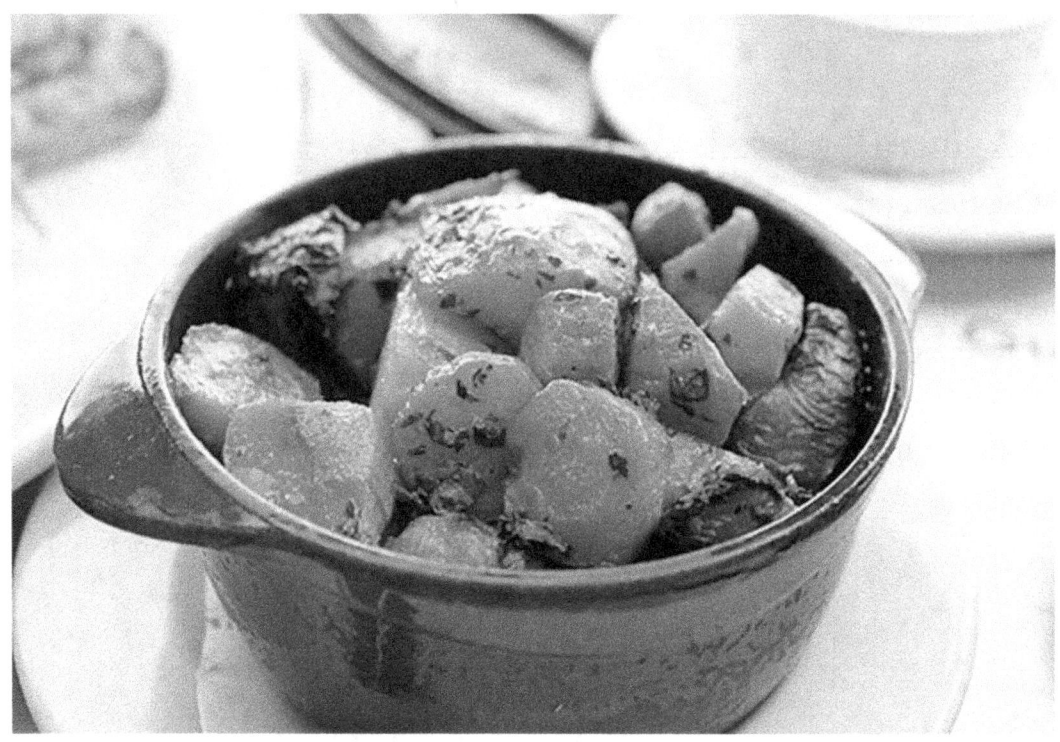

Ingredients

- ¾ large yellow or white onions, chopped
- 1½ medium carrots, diced
- 1½ ribs celery, chopped
- ¾ tablespoon garlic, chopped
- 1 tablespoon olive oil
- 2½ cups water
- 1 lb white potatoes, peeled and diced
- ¼ cup tomato paste
- ½ tablespoon Italian herbs
- ½ tablespoon paprika
- 1 teaspoon fresh rosemary
- ¾ cups peas
- ¼ cup fresh parsley, chopped

How to

1. Put the oil and all the vegetables into the instant pot and 'sauté' for 5 minutes.
2. Stir in the remaining ingredients and secure the lid.
3. Cook on 'manual' function for 13 minutes at high pressure.
4. After the beep, 'natural release' the steam and remove the lid.
5. Garnish with fresh parsley and serve hot.

Nutrition Values (Per Serving)

- Calories: 230
- Carbohydrate: 38.8g
- Protein: 6.9g
- Fat: 6.3g
- Sugar: 9.6g
- Sodium: 115mg

Brazilian Potato Curry

(**Serves**: 2 / **Prep Time:** 10 minutes / **Cooking Time**: 30 minutes)

Ingredients

- 1 large potato, peeled and diced
- 1 small onion, peeled and diced
- 8 oz fresh tomatoes
- 1 tablespoon olive oil
- 2 tablespoon garlic cloves grated
- ½ tablespoon rosemary
- ½ tablespoon cayenne pepper
- 1½ tablespoon thyme
- Salt and pepper to taste

How to

1. Pour a cup of water into the instant pot and place the steamer trivet inside.
2. Place the potatoes and half the garlic over the trivet and sprinkle some salt and pepper on top.
3. Secure the lid and cook on 'steam' function for 20 minutes.
4. After the beep 'natural release' the steam and remove the lid.
5. Put the potatoes to one side and empty the pot.
6. Add the remaining ingredients to the cooker and 'sauté' for 10 minutes.
7. Use an immerse blender to puree the cooked mixture.
8. Stir in the steamed potatoes and serve hot.

Nutrition Values (Per Serving)

- Calories: 176
- Carbohydrate: 26.4g
- Protein: 3.7g
- Fat: 7.9g
- Sugar: 5.2g
- Sodium: 181mg

Flavorsome Vegetable Chow Mein

(**Serves**: 2 / **Prep Time:** 10 minutes / **Cooking Time**: 21 minutes)

Ingredients

- ½ (1lb) pack noodles
- ½ large onion, chopped
- 2 large carrots, diced
- 2 celery sticks, chopped
- ½ small leek, chopped
- 1 tablespoon olive oil
- ½ tablespoon ginger paste
- ½ teaspoon garlic paste
- ½ tablespoon Worcester sauce
- 1½ tablespoon soy sauce
- 1 tablespoon Chinese five spice
- ½ tablespoon Oriental seasoning
- ½ teaspoon coriander
- ½ teaspoon parsley
- 2 cups water
- Salt and pepper to taste

How to

1. Put the oil, onion, ginger and garlic paste into the instant pot and 'sauté' for 5 minutes.
2. Stir in the remaining vegetables and stir-fry for 3 minutes.
3. Add the remaining ingredients and secure the lid.
4. Cook on 'manual' function for 13 minutes at high pressure.
5. After the beep, 'natural release' the steam and remove the lid.
6. Stir well and serve warm.

Nutrition Values (Per Serving)

- Calories: 392
- Carbohydrate: 65.1g
- Protein: 9.9g
- Fat: 10.8g
- Sugar: 7.4g
- Sodium: 780mg

Instant Ratatouille

(**Serves**: 4 / **Prep Time:** 10 minutes / **Cooking Time**: 6 minutes)

Ingredients

- 2 large zucchinis, sliced
- 2 medium eggplants, sliced
- 4 medium tomatoes, sliced
- 2 small red onions, sliced
- 4 cloves garlic, diced
- 2 tablespoons of thyme leaves
- 2 teaspoons sea salt
- 1 teaspoon black pepper
- 2 tablespoons balsamic vinegar
- 4 tablespoons olive oil
- 2 cups water

How to

1. Line a 6-inch springform pan with foil and place the chopped garlic in the bottom.
2. Now arrange the vegetable slices, alternately, in circles.
3. Sprinkle the thyme, pepper and salt over the vegetables. Top with oil and vinegar.
4. Pour a cup of water into the instant pot and place the trivet inside.
5. Secure the lid and cook on 'manual' function for 6 minutes at high pressure.
6. Release the pressure naturally and remove the lid.
7. Remove the vegetables along with the tin foil.
8. Serve on a platter and enjoy.

Nutrition Values (Per Serving)

- Calories: 250
- Carbohydrate: 29.2g
- Protein: 6g
- Fat: 15.1g
- Sugar: 14.5g
- Sodium: 970mg

Crowd-Pleasing Carrot Stew

(**Serves**: 4 / **Prep Time:** 10 minutes / **Cooking Time**: 15 minutes)

Ingredients

- 1½ tablespoons olive oil
- 1 cup homemade tomato sauce
- ½ teaspoon smoked paprika
- 1 cup vegetable broth
- 1 large onion, cut into bite-sized pieces
- ½ lb carrots, peeled and cut into bite-sized pieces
- ½ lb potatoes, peeled and cut into bite-sized pieces
- ½ garlic clove, minced
- ¼ cup fresh cilantro, chopped

How to

1. Put the oil and all the vegetables into the instant pot and 'sauté' for 5 minutes.
2. Stir in the paprika, the broth and tomato paste, then secure the lid.
3. Cook on 'manual' setting at high pressure for 10 minutes.
4. After the beep, 'natural release' the steam and remove the lid.
5. Stir well and serve with the fresh cilantro on top.

Nutrition Values (Per Serving)

- Calories: 169
- Carbohydrate: 21.5g
- Protein: 3.6g
- Fat: 8g
- Sugar: 7.3g
- Sodium: 410mg

Nutritious Vegetable Mix

(**Serves**: 3 / **Prep Time:** 10 minutes / **Cooking Time**: 28 minutes)

Ingredients

- 1 tablespoon olive oil
- ½ carrot, peeled and minced
- ½ celery stalk, minced
- ½ small onion, minced
- 1 garlic clove, minced
- ½ teaspoon dried sage, crushed
- ½ teaspoon dried rosemary, crushed
- 4 oz fresh Portabella mushrooms, sliced
- 4 oz fresh white mushrooms, sliced
- ¼ cup red wine
- 1 Yukon Gold potato, peeled and chopped
- ¾ cup fresh green beans, trimmed and chopped
- 1 cup tomatoes, chopped
- ½ cup tomato paste
- ½ tablespoon balsamic vinegar
- 1¼ cups water
- 1 tablespoon corn-starch
- ⅛ cup water
- Salt and freshly ground black pepper to taste
- 2 oz frozen peas

How to

1. Put the oil, onion, carrots and celery into the instant pot and 'sauté' for 5 minutes.
2. Stir in the herbs and garlic and cook for 1 minute.
3. Add the mushrooms and sauté for 5 minutes. Stir in the wine and cook for a further 2 minutes
4. Add the green beans, potatoes, carrots, tomato paste, water and vinegar.
5. Secure the lid and cook on 'manual' function for 15 minutes at high pressure.
6. After the beep, 'natural release' the steam and remove the lid.
7. Combine the corn-starch with water in a separate bowl and stir it into a slurry.
8. Add the corn-starch slurry, peas, onion, black pepper and salt to the pot.
9. 'Sauté' for 1 minute and serve hot.

Nutrition Values (Per Serving)

- Calories: 183
- Carbohydrate: 28.1g
- Protein: 6.7g
- Fat: 5.3g
- Sugar: 11g
- Sodium: 80mg

Barbeque Mushroom Tacos

(**Serves**: 3 / **Prep Time:** 10 minutes / **Cooking Time**: 13 minutes)

Ingredients

- 4 large guajillo chilies
- 2 teaspoons oil
- 2 bay leaves
- 2 large onions, sliced
- 2 garlic cloves
- 2 chipotle chillies in adobo sauce
- 2 teaspoons ground cumin
- 1 teaspoon dried oregano
- 1 teaspoon smoked hot paprika
- ½ teaspoon ground cinnamon,
- Salt to taste
- ¾ cup vegetable broth
- 1 teaspoon apple cider vinegar
- 3 teaspoons lime juice
- ¼ teaspoon sugar
- 8 oz mushrooms chopped
- Tacos to serve

How to

1. Put the oil, onion, garlic, salt and bay leaves into the instant pot and 'sauté' for 5 minutes.
2. Blend half of this mixture, in a blender, with all the spices and chillies.
3. Add the mushrooms to the remaining onions and 'sauté' for 3 minutes.
4. Pour the blended mixture into the pot and secure the lid.
5. Cook on 'manual' function for 5 minutes at high pressure.
6. 'Quick release' the steam and remove the lid.
7. Stir well and serve with tacos.

Nutrition Values (Per Serving)

- Calories: 160
- Carbohydrate: 22.9g
- Protein: 4.1g
- Fat: 6.7g
- Sugar: 8.2g
- Sodium: 519mg

Egg Plant Curry

(**Serves**: 4 / **Prep Time:** 10 minutes / **Cooking Time**: 22 minutes)

Ingredients

- ¾ cup lentils, soaked and rinsed
- 1 teaspoon olive oil
- ½ onion, chopped
- 4 garlic cloves, chopped
- 1 teaspoon ginger, chopped
- 1 hot green chile, chopped
- ¼ teaspoon turmeric
- ½ teaspoon ground cumin
- 2 tomatoes, chopped
- 1 cup eggplant, chopped
- 1 cup sweet potatoes, cubed
- ¾ teaspoon salt
- 2 cups water
- 1 cup baby spinach leaves
- Cayenne and lemon/lime to taste
- Pepper flakes (garnish)

How to

1. Put the oil, garlic, ginger, chili and salt into the instant pot and 'sauté' for 3 minutes.
2. Stir in the tomatoes and all the spices. Cook for 5 minutes.
3. Add all the remaining ingredients, except the spinach leaves.
4. Secure the lid and cook on 'manual' function for 12 minutes at high pressure.
5. After the beep, release the pressure naturally and remove the lid.
6. Stir in the spinach leaves and let the pot simmer for 2 minutes on 'sauté'.
7. Serve warm.

Nutrition Values (Per Serving)

- Calories: 212
- Carbohydrate: 38.7g
- Protein: 11.2g
- Fat: 1.9g
- Sugar: 3.8g
- Sodium: 458mg

Jack Fruit Stew

(**Serves**: 4 / **Prep Time:** 5 minutes / **Cooking Time**: 10 minutes)

Ingredients

- 2 teaspoons oil
- 1 teaspoon cumin seeds
- 1 teaspoon mustard seeds
- 1 teaspoon nigella seeds
- 2 bay leaves
- 4 dried red chillies
- 2 small onions, chopped
- 5 cloves of garlic, chopped
- 2-inch ginger, chopped
- 2 teaspoons coriander powder
- 2 teaspoons turmeric
- ½ teaspoon black pepper
- 3 cups tomato puree
- 20 oz green Jackfruit drained and rinsed
- Salt to taste
- 3 cups water

How to

1. Put the oil, onions, garlic, ginger, bay leaves, salt and red chilli into the instant pot.
2. 'Sauté' for 2 minutes. Stir in the remaining ingredients.
3. Secure the lid and cook on 'manual' for 8 minutes at high pressure.
4. After the beep, 'natural release' the steam and remove the lid.
5. Stir well and serve hot.

Nutrition Values (Per Serving)

- Calories: 319
- Carbohydrate: 70.2g
- Protein: 5.4g
- Fat: 4.8g
- Sugar: 1.8g
- Sodium: 49mg

Potato Cauliflower

(**Serves**: 8 / **Prep Time:** 15 minutes / **Cooking Time**: 8 minutes)

Ingredients

- 1 small onion
- 4 tomatoes
- 4 garlic cloves, chopped
- 2-inch ginger, chopped
- 2 teaspoons oil
- 1 teaspoon turmeric
- 2 teaspoons ground cumin
- Salt to taste
- 1 teaspoon paprika
- 4 medium potatoes, cubed small
- 2 small cauliflowers, diced

How to

1. Blend the tomato, garlic, ginger and onion in a blender.
2. Put the oil and cumin into the instant pot and 'sauté' for 1 minute.
3. Stir in the blended mixture and remaining spices.
4. Add the potatoes and cook for 5 minutes on 'sauté'
5. Add the cauliflower chunks and secure the lid.
6. Cook on 'manual' for 2 minutes at high pressure.
7. 'Quick release' the steam and remove the lid.
8. Stir and serve with the cilantro on top.

Nutrition Values (Per Serving)

- Calories: 113
- Carbohydrate: 23.3g
- Protein: 4g
- Fat: 1.7g
- Sugar: 4.3g
- Sodium: 53mg

Sweet Potato Curry

(**Serves**: 8 / **Prep time:** 5 minutes / **Cooking time**: 8 minutes)

Ingredients

- 2 large brown onions, finely diced
- 4 tablespoons olive oil
- 4 teaspoons salt
- 4 large garlic cloves, diced
- 1 red chili, sliced
- 4 tablespoons cilantro, chopped
- 4 teaspoons ground cumin
- 2 teaspoons ground coriander
- 2 teaspoons paprika
- 2 lbs sweet potato, diced
- 4 cups chopped, tinned tomatoes
- 2 cups water
- 2 cups vegetable stock
- Lemon juice and cilantro (garnish)

How to

1. Put the oil and onions into the instant pot and 'sauté' for 5 minutes.
2. Stir in the remaining ingredients and secure the lid.
3. Cook on 'manual' function for 3 minutes at high pressure.
4. 'Quick release' the steam and remove the lid.
5. Garnish with cilantro and lemon juice.
6. Serve.

Nutrition Values (Per Serving)

- Calories: 203
- Carbohydrate: 32g
- Protein: 4g
- Fat: 7.8g
- Sugar: 11.6g
- Sodium: 1227mg

Potato Scallion Stew

(**Serves**: 8 / **Prep time:** 5 minutes / **Cooking time**: 8 minutes)

Ingredients

- 2 large brown onions, finely diced
- 4 tablespoons olive oil
- ½ teaspoon ground turmeric
- 4 teaspoons salt
- 4 large garlic cloves, diced
- 4 medium length scallions, chopped
- 4 teaspoons ground cumin
- 2 teaspoons paprika
- 2 lbs medium potatoes, diced
- 4 cups chopped, tinned tomatoes
- 3 cups water
- 2 cups vegetable stock
- Cilantro (garnish)

How to

1. Put the oil and onions in the instant pot and 'sauté' for 5 minutes.
2. Stir in the remaining ingredients and secure the lid.
3. Cook on 'manual' function for 3 minutes at high pressure.
4. 'Quick release' the steam and remove the lid.
5. Garnish with cilantro and lemon juice.
6. Serve.

Nutrition Values (Per Serving)

- Calories: 496
- Carbohydrate: 99.9g
- Protein: 9.4g
- Fat: 7.6g
- Sugar: 4.4g
- Sodium: 1289g

Sweet Potato with Cauliflower

(**Serves**: 8 / **Prep Time:** 15 minutes / **Cooking Time**: 8 minutes)

Ingredients

- 1 small onion
- 4 tomatoes
- 4 garlic cloves, chopped
- 2-inch ginger, chopped
- 2 teaspoons oil
- 1 teaspoon turmeric
- 2 teaspoons ground cumin
- Salt to taste
- 1 teaspoon paprika
- 2 medium sweet potatoes, cubed small
- 2 small cauliflowers, diced

How to

1. Blend the tomatoes, garlic, ginger and onion in a blender.
2. Put the oil and cumin in the instant pot and 'sauté' for 1 minute.
3. Stir in the blended mixture and remaining spices.
4. Add the sweet potatoes and cook for 5 minutes on 'sauté'
5. Add the cauliflower chunks and secure the lid.
6. Cook on 'manual' for 2 minutes at high pressure.
7. 'Quick release' the steam and remove the lid.
8. Stir and serve with cilantro on top.

Nutrition Values (Per Serving)

- Calories: 118
- Carbohydrate: 24.3g
- Protein: 4.1g
- Fat: 1.7g
- Sugar: 6.7g
- Sodium: 51mg

Stuffed Eggplants

(**Serves**: 4 / **Prep Time:** 15 minutes / **Cooking Time**: 9 minutes)

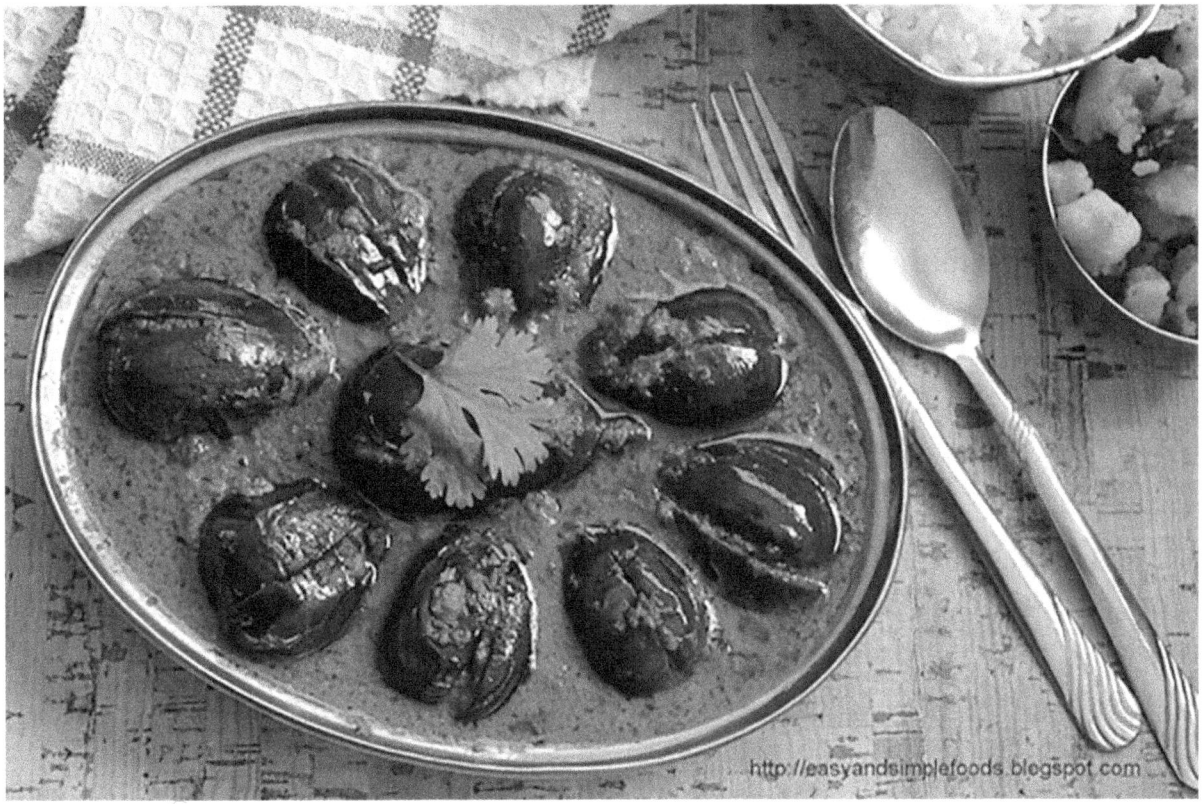

Ingredients

- 1 tablespoon coriander seeds
- ½ teaspoon cumin seeds
- ½ teaspoon mustard seeds
- 2 to 3 tablespoons chickpea flour
- 2 tablespoons chopped peanuts
- 2 tablespoons coconut shreds
- 1-inch ginger, chopped
- 2 cloves garlic, chopped
- 1 hot green chili, chopped
- ½ teaspoon ground cardamom
- a pinch of cinnamon
- ⅓ to ½ teaspoon cayenne
- ½ teaspoon turmeric
- ½ teaspoon raw sugar
- ½ to ¾ teaspoon salt
- 1 teaspoon lemon juice

- Water as needed
- 4 baby eggplants
- Cilantro

How to

1. Put the coriander, mustard seeds and cumin in the instant pot.
2. Roast on 'sauté' function for 2 minutes.
3. Add the chickpea flour, nuts and coconut shred to the pot, and roast for 2 minutes.
4. Blend this mixture in a blender, then transfer to a medium-size bowl.
5. Roughly blend the ginger, garlic, lime, chili, and all the spices in a blender.
6. Add water and the lemon juice to make a paste. Combine it with the dry flour mix.
7. Cut the eggplants from one side and stuff with the spice mixture.
8. Add 1 cup of water to the instant pot and place the stuffed eggplants inside.
9. Sprinkle some salt on top and secure the lid.
10. Cook on 'manual' for 5 minutes at high pressure, then 'quick release' the steam.
11. Remove the lid and serve hot.

Nutrition Values (Per Serving)

- Calories: 316
- Carbohydrate: 64.4g
- Protein: 11.1g
- Fat: 5.7g
- Sugar: 34.4g
- Sodium: 312mg

Sesame Vegetable Teriyaki

(**Serves**: 4 / **Prep time:** 10 minutes / **Cooking time**: 18 minutes)

Ingredients

- ¾ large yellow or white onion, chopped
- 1½ medium carrots, diced
- 1½ ribs celery, chopped
- 1 medium portabella mushroom, diced
- ¾ tablespoon garlic, chopped
- 2 cups water
- 1 lb white potatoes, peeled and diced
- ¼ cup tomato paste
- ½ tablespoon sesame oil
- 2 teaspoons sesame seeds
- ½ tablespoon paprika
- 1 teaspoon fresh rosemary
- ¾ cups peas
- ¼ cup fresh parsley, chopped

How to

1. Put the oil, sesame seeds, and all the vegetables in the instant pot and 'sauté' for 5 minutes.
2. Stir in the remaining ingredients and secure the lid.
3. Cook on 'manual' function for 13 minutes at high pressure.
4. After the beep, 'natural release' the steam and remove the lid.
5. Garnish with fresh parsley and sesame seeds and serve hot.

Nutrition Values (Per Serving)

- Calories: 202
- Carbohydrate: 34.5g
- Protein: 6.2g
- Fat: 5.3g
- Sugar: 9.2g
- Sodium: 49mg

Cauliflower Beans

(**Serves**: 8 / **Prep Time:** 15 minutes / **Cooking Time**: 8 minutes)

Ingredients

- 1 small onion
- 4 tomatoes
- 4 garlic cloves, chopped
- 2-inch ginger, chopped
- 2 teaspoons oil
- 1 teaspoon turmeric
- 2 teaspoons ground cumin
- Salt to taste
- 1 teaspoon paprika
- 4 medium potatoes, cubed small
- 2 small cauliflowers, diced
- ½ cup cooked black beans

How to

1. Blend the tomatoes, garlic, ginger and onion in a blender.
2. Put the oil and cumin into the instant pot and 'sauté' for 1 minute.
3. Stir in the blended mixture and the remaining spices.
4. Add the potatoes and cook for 5 minutes on 'sauté'.
5. Add the cauliflower chunks and secure the lid.
6. Cook on 'manual' for 2 minutes at high pressure.
7. 'Quick release' the steam and remove the lid.
8. Stir in the black beans and serve with the cilantro on top.

Nutrition Values (Per Serving)

- Calories: 153
- Carbohydrate: 30.5g
- Protein: 6.6g
- Fat: 1.8g
- Sugar: 4.5g
- Sodium: 53mg

Potato with Green Beans

(**Serves**: 4 / **Prep time:** 10 minutes / **Cooking time**: 18 minutes)

Ingredients

- ¾ large yellow or white onion, chopped
- 1½ ribs celery, chopped
- ¾ tablespoon garlic, chopped
- 2½ cups water
- 1 lb white potatoes, peeled and diced
- ¼ cup tomato paste
- 1 cup green beans, cut into pieces
- ½ tablespoon paprika
- 1 teaspoon fresh rosemary
- ¾ cups peas
- ¼ cup fresh parsley, chopped

How to

1. Put the oil and all the vegetables in the instant pot and 'sauté' for 5 minutes.
2. Stir in the remaining ingredients and secure the lid.
3. Cook on 'manual' function for 13 minutes at high pressure.
4. After the beep, 'natural release' the steam and remove the lid.
5. Garnish with fresh parsley and serve hot.

Nutrition Values (Per Serving)

- Calories: 167
- Carbohydrate: 32.6g
- Protein: 5.6g
- Fat: 2.5g
- Sugar: 8.1g
- Sodium: 34mg

Corn Potato Chowder

(**Serves**: 4 / **Prep time:** 10 minutes / **Cooking time**: 18 minutes)

Ingredients

- ¾ large yellow or white onion, chopped
- 1½ ribs celery, chopped
- ¼ cup carrots, diced
- ¼ cup corn kernels
- ¾ tablespoon garlic, chopped
- 2½ cups water
- 1 lb white potatoes, peeled and diced
- ¼ cup tomato paste
- ½ tablespoon paprika
- 1 teaspoon fresh rosemary
- ¾ cup peas
- ¼ cup fresh parsley, chopped

How to

1. Put the oil and all the vegetables in the instant pot and 'sauté' for 5 minutes.
2. Stir in the remaining ingredients and secure the lid.
3. Cook on 'manual' function for 13 minutes at high pressure.
4. After the beep, 'natural release' the steam and remove the lid.
5. Garnish with fresh parsley and serve hot.

Nutrition Values (Per Serving)

- Calories: 170
- Carbohydrate: 33.2g
- Protein: 5.4g
- Fat: 2.6g
- Sugar: 8.3g
- Sodium: 39mg

Vegetable Pasta

(**Serves**: 6 / **Prep Time:** 10 minutes / **Cooking Time**: 11 minutes)

Ingredients

- ½ (1lb) pack penne pasta, cooked
- ½ large onion, chopped
- 2 large carrots, diced
- 2 celery sticks, chopped
- ½ small leek, chopped
- 1 tablespoon olive oil
- ½ tablespoon ginger paste
- ½ teaspoon garlic paste
- ½ cup green bell pepper
- ½ tablespoon Worcester sauce
- 1½ tablespoon soy sauce
- ½ teaspoon coriander
- ½ teaspoon parsley
- 1 cup water
- Salt and pepper to taste

How to

1. Put the oil, onion, ginger and garlic paste in the instant pot and 'sauté' for 5 minutes.
2. Stir in the remaining vegetables and stir-fry for 3 minutes.
3. Add the remaining ingredients, except for the pasta, and secure the lid.
4. Cook on 'manual' function for 3 minutes at high pressure.
5. After the beep, 'natural release' the steam and remove the lid.
6. Stir in the cooked pasta and serve warm.

Nutrition Values (Per Serving)

- Calories: 368
- Carbohydrate: 67.4g
- Protein: 13.1g
- Fat: 4.9g
- Sugar: 2.8g
- Sodium: 284mg

Vegetable Bean Rice

(**Serves**: 4 / **Prep Time:** 10 minutes / **Cooking Time**: 13 minutes)

Ingredients

- 1 cup long-grain white rice
- ½ cup chickpeas, soaked
- ½ large onion, chopped
- 2 large carrots, diced
- 2 celery sticks, chopped
- ½ small leek, chopped
- 1 tablespoon olive oil
- ½ tablespoon ginger paste
- ½ teaspoon garlic paste
- ½ tablespoon Worcester Sauce
- ½ teaspoon coriander
- ½ teaspoon parsley
- 2½ cups water
- Salt and pepper, to taste

How to

1. Put the oil, onion, ginger and garlic paste in the instant pot and 'sauté' for 5 minutes.
2. Stir in the remaining vegetables and stir-fry for 3 minutes.
3. Add the remaining ingredients and secure the lid.
4. Cook on 'manual' function for 5 minutes at high pressure.
5. After the beep, 'natural release' the steam and remove the lid.
6. Stir well and serve warm.

Nutrition Values (Per Serving)

- Calories: 341
- Carbohydrate: 64.1g
- Protein: 9.1g
- Fat: 5.5g
- Sugar: 6g
- Sodium: 57mg

Mixed Vegetable Chili

(**Serves**: 3 / **Prep Time:** 15 minutes / **Cooking Time**: 10 minutes)

Ingredients

- ½ tablespoon olive oil
- 1 small yellow onion, chopped
- 4 garlic cloves, minced
- ¾ (15 oz) can diced tomatoes
- 1 oz sugar-free tomato paste
- ½ (4 oz) can green chilies with liquid
- 1 tablespoon Worcestershire sauce
- 2 tablespoons red chili powder
- ½ cup carrots, diced
- ½ cup scallions, chopped
- ½ cup green bell pepper, chopped
- ¼ cup peas
- 1 tablespoon ground cumin
- ½ tablespoon dried oregano, crushed
- Salt and freshly ground black pepper to taste

How to

1. Put the oil, onion, and garlic into the instant pot and 'sauté' for 5 minutes.
2. Stir in the remaining vegetables and stir-fry for 3 minutes.
3. Add the remaining ingredients and secure the lid.
4. Cook on 'manual' function for 2 minutes at high pressure.
5. After the beep, 'natural release' the steam and remove the lid.
6. Stir well and serve warm.

Nutrition Values (Per Serving)

- Calories: 144
- Carbohydrate: 26.2g
- Protein: 4.6g
- Fat: 3.9g
- Sugar: 12g
- Sodium: 219mg

Stuffed Acorn Squash

(**Serves**: 4 / **Prep Time:** 15 minutes / **Cooking Time**: 23 minutes)

Ingredients

- ½ tablespoon olive oil
- 2 medium Acorn squashes
- ¼ small yellow onion, chopped
- 1 jalapeño pepper, chopped
- ½ cup green onions, chopped
- ½ cup carrots, chopped
- ¼ cup cabbage, chopped
- 1 garlic clove, minced
- ½ (6 oz) can sugar-free tomato sauce
- ½ tablespoon chili powder
- ½ tablespoon ground cumin
- Salt and freshly ground black pepper to taste
- 2 cups water
- ¼ cup cheddar cheese, shredded

How to

1. Pour the water into the instant pot and place the trivet inside.
2. Slice the squash into 2 halves and remove the seeds.
3. Place over the trivet, skin side down, and sprinkle some salt and pepper over.
4. Secure the lid and cook on 'manual' for 15 minutes at high pressure.
5. Release the pressure naturally and remove the lid. Empty the pot into a bowl.
6. Now put the oil, onion, and garlic in the instant pot and 'sauté' for 5 minutes.
7. Stir in the remaining vegetables and stir-fry for 3 minutes.
8. Add the remaining ingredients and secure the lid.
9. Cook on 'manual' function for 2 minutes at high pressure.
10. After the beep, 'natural release' the steam and remove the lid.
11. Stuff the squashes with the prepared mixture and serve warm.

Nutrition Values (Per Serving)

- Calories: 154
- Carbohydrate: 27.7g
- Protein: 4.4g
- Fat: 4.7g
- Sugar: 2.1g
- Sodium: 80mg

Spinach Potato Curry

(**Serves**: 4 / **Prep time:** 10 minutes / **Cooking time**: 13 minutes)

Ingredients

- ¾ large yellow or white onion, chopped
- 1½ ribs celery, chopped
- 1 cup baby spinach leaves
- ¾ tablespoon garlic, chopped
- 2½ cups water
- 1 lb white potatoes, peeled and diced
- ¼ cup tomato paste
- ½ tablespoon paprika
- 1 teaspoon fresh rosemary
- ¼ cup fresh parsley, chopped

How to

1. Put the oil and all the vegetables, except the spinach, in the instant pot and 'sauté' for 5 minutes.
2. Stir in the remaining ingredients and secure the lid.
3. Cook on 'manual' function for 8 minutes at high pressure.
4. After the beep, natural release' the steam and remove the lid.
5. Stir in the spinach and cook for 5 minutes on 'sauté'.
6. Garnish with fresh parsley and serve hot.

Nutrition Values (Per Serving)

- Calories: 114
- Carbohydrate: 25.7g
- Protein: 3.6g
- Fat: 0.5g
- Sugar: 4.9g
- Sodium: 49mg

Creamy Vegetable Curry

(**Serves**: 4 / **Prep time**: 10 minutes / **Cooking time**: 18 minutes)

Ingredients

- ¾ large yellow or white onion, chopped
- 1½ ribs celery, chopped
- ¼ cup carrots, diced
- ¼ cup green onions
- ½ cup coconut milk
- ¾ tablespoon garlic, chopped
- 1½ cups water
- 1 lb white potatoes, peeled and diced
- ¼ cup heavy cream
- ¼ teaspoon thyme
- ¼ teaspoon rosemary
- ½ tablespoon black pepper
- ¾ cup peas
- Salt to taste

How to

1. Put the oil and all the vegetables in the instant pot and 'sauté' for 5 minutes.
2. Stir in the remaining ingredients and secure the lid.
3. Cook on 'manual' function for 13 minutes at high pressure.
4. After the beep, 'natural release' the steam and remove the lid.
5. Garnish with herbs and serve hot.

Nutrition Values (Per Serving)

- Calories: 218
- Carbohydrate: 29g
- Protein: 5g
- Fat: 10.3g
- Sugar: 5.8g
- Sodium: 77mg

Enticing Spaghetti Squash

(**Serves**: 2 / **Prep Time:** 15 minutes / **Cooking Time**: 25 minutes)

Ingredients

- ½ tablespoon olive oil
- 1 large spaghetti squash
- ¼ small yellow onion, chopped
- 1 jalapeño pepper, chopped
- ½ cup green onions, chopped
- ½ cup carrots, chopped
- ¼ cup cabbage, chopped
- 1 garlic clove, minced
- ½ (6 oz) can sugar-free tomato sauce
- ½ tablespoon chili powder
- ½ tablespoon ground cumin
- Salt and freshly ground black pepper to taste
- 2 cups water
- ¼ cup cheddar cheese, shredded

How to

1. Pour the water into the instant pot and place the trivet inside.
2. Slice the squash into 2 halves and remove the seeds.
3. Place them over the trivet, skin side down, and sprinkle some salt and pepper over.
4. Secure the lid and cook on 'manual' for 15 minutes at high pressure.
5. Release the pressure naturally and remove the lid. Empty the pot.
6. Shred the squash with a fork and keep the shredded pieces to one side.
7. Now put the oil, onion, and garlic in the instant pot and 'sauté' for 5 minutes.
8. Stir in the remaining vegetables and stir-fry for 3 minutes.
9. Add the remaining ingredients and secure the lid.
10. Cook on 'manual' function for 2 minutes at high pressure.
11. After the beep, 'natural release' the steam and remove the lid.
12. Stir in the spaghetti squash shreds.
13. Garnish with herbs and cheese. Serve warm.

Nutrition Values (Per Serving)

- Calories: 194
- Carbohydrate: 19.4g
- Protein: 5.4g
- Fat: 9g
- Sugar: 4.1g
- Sodium: 147mg

Stuffed Sweet Peppers

(**Serves**: 7 / **Prep Time:** 15 minutes / **Cooking Time**: 8 minutes)

Ingredients

- 7 mini sweet peppers
- 1 cup button mushrooms, minced
- 5 oz organic baby spinach
- ½ teaspoon of fresh garlic
- ½ teaspoon of coarse sea salt
- ¼ teaspoon of cracked mixed pepper
- 2 tablespoons water
- 1 tablespoon olive oil
- Organic mozzarella, diced

How to

1. Put the sweet peppers and water in the instant pot and 'sauté' for 2 minutes.
2. Remove the peppers and put the olive oil into the pot.
3. Stir in the mushrooms, garlic, spices and spinach.
4. Cook on 'sauté' until the mixture is dry.
5. Stuff each sweet pepper with cheese and spinach mixture.
6. Bake the stuffed peppers in an oven for 6 minutes at 400° F.
7. Once done, serve hot.

Nutrition Values (Per Serving)

- Calories: 74
- Carbohydrate: 10.3g
- Protein: 3.2g
- Fat: 3.1g
- Sugar: 6.3g
- Sodium: 93mg

Spinach Lentils

(**Serves**: 2 / **Prep Time:** 5 minutes / **Cooking Time**: 18 minutes)

Ingredients

- 1 teaspoon olive oil
- ½ small yellow onion, diced
- 1 medium carrot, peeled and diced
- ½ medium stalk celery, diced
- 2 medium garlic cloves, minced
- 1 teaspoon ground cumin
- ½ teaspoon ground turmeric
- ½ teaspoon dried thyme
- Salt to taste
- Freshly ground black pepper to taste
- ½ cup dry lentils, rinsed well
- 2 cups vegetable broth
- 4 oz baby spinach

How to

1. Put the oil, onions, celery and carrots into the instant pot and 'sauté' for 5 minutes.
2. Add the thyme, cumin, garlic, pepper and salt, and cook for 1 minute.
3. Stir in the broth, along with the lentils, then secure the lid.
4. Press the 'manual' key and set the cooking time to 12 minutes at medium pressure.
5. After the beep, 'quick release' the steam and remove the lid.
6. Add the spinach and salt and pepper to taste, then serve.

Nutrition Values (Per Serving)

- Calories: 294
- Carbohydrate: 43g
- Protein: 20.5g
- Fat: 4.9g
- Sugar: 4.2g
- Sodium: 1014mg

Vegetable Cheese Macaroni

(**Serves**: 4 / **Prep Time:** 10 minutes / **Cooking Time**: 11 minutes)

Ingredients

- 1 (1 lb) pack macaroni pasta, cooked
- ½ large onion, chopped
- 2 large carrots, diced
- ¼ cup cheddar cheese, shredded
- ¼ cup mozzarella cheese, shredded
- 2 celery sticks, chopped
- ½ small leek, chopped
- 1 tablespoon olive oil
- ½ tablespoon ginger paste
- ½ teaspoon garlic paste
- ½ cup green bell pepper, chopped
- ½ tablespoon Worcestershire sauce
- 1½ tablespoon soy sauce
- ½ teaspoon Parsley
- 1 cup water
- Salt and pepper to taste

How to

1. Put the oil, onion, ginger and garlic paste into the instant pot and 'sauté' for 5 minutes.
2. Stir in the remaining vegetables and stir-fry for 3 minutes.
3. Add the remaining ingredients, except for the pasta, and secure the lid.
4. Cook on 'manual' function for 3 minutes at high pressure.
5. After the beep, 'natural release' the steam and remove the lid.
6. Stir in the cooked macaroni and cheeses. Stir well while the cheese melts in.
7. Serve warm.

Nutrition Values (Per Serving)

- Calories: 331
- Carbohydrate: 54.4g
- Protein: 10.7g
- Fat: 7.3g
- Sugar: 6g
- Sodium: 428mg

Delicious Minestrone Curry

(**Serves**: 6 / **Prep Time:** 10 minutes / **Cooking Time**: 11 minutes)

Ingredients

- 2 tablespoons olive oil
- 2 stalks celery, diced
- 1 large onion, diced
- 1 large carrot, diced
- 3 cloves garlic, minced
- 1 teaspoon dried oregano
- 1 teaspoon dried basil
- Salt and pepper to taste
- 1 cup tomatoes, chopped
- 1 (15 oz) can cannellini beans
- 2 cups vegetable broth
- 1 bay leaf
- ½ cup fresh spinach
- 1 cup gluten-free elbow pasta
- 1/3 cup finely grated parmesan cheese
- 2 tablespoons fresh pesto

How to

1. Put the oil, onion, garlic and celery in the instant pot and 'sauté' for 5 minutes.
2. Drizzle over salt, pepper, oregano and basil to add more flavour.
3. Add the broth, spinach, pasta, tomatoes and bay leaf to the pot.
4. Secure the lid and cook on 'manual' settings for 6 minutes at high pressure.
5. 'Quick release' the steam and remove the lid carefully.
6. Stir in the white kidney beans.
7. Add the parmesan cheese and pesto on top then serve.

Nutrition Values (Per Serving)

- Calories: 447
- Carbohydrate: 73g
- Protein: 13.5g
- Fat: 10.6g
- Sugar: 3.5g
- Sodium: 351mg

Vegetable Tortilla Bowl

(**Serves**: 4 / **Prep Time:** 10 minutes / **Cooking Time**: 8 minutes)

Ingredients

- 1½ cups vegetable broth
- ½ cup tomatoes, undrained diced
- 1 small onion, diced
- 2 garlic cloves, finely minced
- 1 teaspoon chili powder
- 1 teaspoon cumin
- ½ teaspoon paprika
- ½ teaspoon ground coriander
- Salt and pepper to taste
- ½ cup carrots, diced
- 2 small potatoes, cubed
- ½ cup bell pepper, chopped
- ½ can black beans, drained and rinsed
- 1 cup frozen corn kernels
- ½ tablespoon lime juice
- 2 tablespoons cilantro, chopped
- Tortilla chips

How to

1. Put the oil and all the vegetables into the instant pot and 'sauté' for 3 minutes.
2. Add all the spices, corn and broth, along with the beans, to the pot.
3. Seal the lid and cook on 'manual' setting at high pressure for 5 minutes.
4. 'Natural release' the steam when the timer goes off. Remove the lid.
5. To serve, put the prepared mixture into a bowl.
6. Top with tortilla chips and fresh cilantro

Nutrition Values (Per Serving)

- Calories: 234
- Carbohydrate: 46.5g
- Protein: 10.9g
- Fat: 1.7g
- Sugar: 6.2g
- Sodium: 409mg

Vegetable Ramen

(**Serves**: 4 / **Prep Time:** 10 minutes / **Cooking Time**: 10 minutes)

Ingredients

- ½ cup cabbage, roughly chopped
- ½ cup carrot, diced
- 1 tablespoon cooking oil
- 1 large onion, peeled, thick sliced
- 1½ cloves garlic, smashed
- 1 teaspoon ginger, grated
- Soy sauce, or salt, to taste
- 1 cup boiled egg noodles
- 1 cup vegetable broth
- ¼ cup green onion, chopped.
- 1 boiled egg, diced

How to

1. Put the onion and oil in the instant pot and 'sauté' for 5 minutes.
2. Add all the remaining ingredients to the onions in the pot.
4. Secure the lid and cook on 'manual' for 5 minutes at high pressure.
5. After the beep, 'natural release' the steam and remove the lid.
6. Add the boiled noodles, chopped green onions and boiled egg on top.
7. Serve hot.

Nutrition Values (Per Serving)

- Calories: 141
- Carbohydrate: 17.4g
- Protein: 5.4g
- Fat: 5.8g
- Sugar: 3.3g
- Sodium: 233mg

Vegetable Barley

(**Serves**: 6 / **Prep Time:** 10 minutes / **Cooking Time**: 13 minutes)

Ingredients

- 2 tablespoons oil
- 10 baby Bella mushrooms, quartered
- 1 cup onions, chopped
- 1 cup carrots, chopped
- 4 celery stalks, chopped
- 6 cloves garlic, minced
- 6 cups vegetable broth
- 1 cup water
- 2 bay leaves
- ½ teaspoon dried thyme
- 1 large potato, shredded
- 2/3 cup pearl barley, rinsed
- Salt and pepper to taste

How to

1. Put the onions, mushrooms, carrot and celery in the pot and cook for 5 minutes stirring constantly.
2. Add the garlic and cook for another minute.
3. Now add the thyme, bay leaves, water and broth, and secure the lid.
4. Cook the mixture on the "manual' function at high pressure for 3 minutes.
5. 'Natural release' the steam and remove the lid.
6. Stir in the potatoes and barley, then cover the lid.
7. Cook on 'manual' for 5 minutes at high pressure
8. Remove the lid and serve hot.

Nutrition Values (Per Serving)

- Calories: 245
- Carbohydrate: 37.7g
- Protein: 10.7g
- Fat: 6.5g
- Sugar: 4.5g
- Sodium: 797mg

Scrumptious Celery Chowder

(**Serves**: 8 / **Prep Time:** 10 minutes / **Cooking Time**: 8 minutes)

Ingredients

- 2 bunches celery, diced
- 2 sweet yellow onions, diced
- ½ cup leek, chopped
- 1 cup coconut milk
- 1 cup vegetable broth
- 1 teaspoon dill
- 1 teaspoon black pepper
- 1 teaspoon red paprika
- ½ cup shredded cheddar cheese
- Sea salt to taste

How to

1. Put all the ingredients, except the cheese, in the instant pot.
2. Secure the lid and set the cooker to 'manual' for 5 minutes at high pressure.
3. After the beep, 'natural release' the steam, then remove the lid.
4. Stir in the cheese and let it cook on 'sauté' for 3 minutes.
5. Serve hot.

Nutrition Values (Per Serving)

- Calories: 121
- Carbohydrate: 5g
- Protein: 3.8g
- Fat: 9.8g
- Sugar: 3.2g
- Sodium: 216mg

Cauliflower Butternut Gravy

(**Serves**: 3 / **Prep Time:** 5 minutes / **Cooking Time**: 7 minutes)

Ingredients

- ½ medium onion, diced
- 2 teaspoons oil
- 1 garlic clove, minced
- ½ cup tomato paste
- ½ lb frozen cauliflower
- ½ lb frozen, cubed butternut squash
- ½ cup vegetable broth
- ½ teaspoon paprika
- ¼ teaspoon dried thyme
- 2 pinches of sea salt

How to

1. Put the oil, onion and garlic into the instant pot and 'sauté' for 2 minutes.
2. Add the broth, tomato paste, cauliflower, butternut, and all the spices, to the pot.
3. Secure the lid. Cook on the 'manual' setting at high pressure for 5 minutes.
4. After the beep, 'quick release' the steam and remove the lid.
5. Stir well, garnish with cilantro and serve hot.

Nutrition Values (Per Serving)

- Calories: 128
- Carbohydrate: 22.6g
- Protein: 5.2g
- Fat: 3.7g
- Sugar: 9.6g
- Sodium: 353mg

Vegetable Lasagne

(**Serves**: 4 / **Prep Time:** 10 minutes / **Cooking Time**: 12 minutes)

Ingredients

- 2 tablespoons olive oil
- 1 medium onion, chopped
- ½ green pepper, chopped
- 2 carrots, chopped
- 1 medium zucchini, chopped
- 1 cup bell pepper sliced
- 1 large can diced tomatoes
- 3 cups vegetable stock
- ½ box of lasagne noodles (small pieces)
- ½ teaspoon onion powder
- 1 teaspoon black pepper
- 1 teaspoon oregano
- Sea salt to taste

How to

1. Put the oil, green pepper, onion and carrots in the instant pot and "sauté for 5 minutes.
2. Stir in the zucchini and all the spices to cook for 3 minutes
3. Add the broth, tomatoes, and lasagne noodles to the cooker and secure the lid.
4. Cook on the 'manual' setting at high pressure for 4 minutes.
5. After the beep, 'quick release' the steam and remove the lid.
6. Serve hot.

Nutrition Values (Per Serving)

- Calories: 468
- Carbohydrate: 90.6g
- Protein: 10.3g
- Fat: 8.3g
- Sugar: 8.4g
- Sodium: 197mg

Cauliflower with Broccoli Florets

(**Serves**: 3 / **Prep Time:** 5 minutes / **Cooking Time**: 7 minutes)

Ingredients

- ½ medium onion, diced
- 2 teaspoons oil
- 1 garlic clove, minced
- ½ cup tomato paste
- ½ lb frozen cauliflower
- ½ lb broccoli florets
- ½ cup vegetable broth
- ½ teaspoon paprika
- ¼ teaspoon dried thyme
- 2 pinches sea salt

How to

1. Put the oil, onion and garlic into the instant pot and 'sauté' for 2 minutes.
2. Add the broth, tomato paste, cauliflower, broccoli, and all the spices, to the pot.
3. Secure the lid. Cook on the 'manual' setting at with pressure for 5 minutes.
4. After the beep, 'quick release' the steam and remove the lid.
5. Stir well and serve hot.

Nurition Values (Per Serving)

- Calories: 124
- Carbohydrate: 19.7g
- Protein: 6.6g
- Fat: 3.9g
- Sugar: 9.4g
- Sodium: 375mg

Chinese Vegetable Congee

(**Serves**: 3 / **Prep Time:** 5 minutes / **Cooking Time**: 20 minutes)

Ingredients

- 1 cup carrots, diced
- ½ cup radish, diced
- 6 cups vegetable broth
- Salt to taste
- 1½ cups short grain rice, rinsed
- 1 tablespoon grated fresh ginger
- 4 cups cabbage, shredded
- Green onions to garnish

How to

1. Put all the ingredients, except the cabbage and green onions, into the instant pot.
2. Select the 'porridge' function and cook on the default time and settings.
3. After the beep, 'quick release' the steam and remove the lid
4. Stir in the shredded cabbage and cover with the lid.
5. Serve after 10 minutes with chopped green onions on top.

Nutrition Values (Per Serving)

- Calories: 189
- Carbohydrate: 26.6g
- Protein: 12.8g
- Fat: 3.1g
- Sugar: 7g
- Sodium: 1606mg

Spicy Pickled Potatoes

(**Serves**: 4 / **Prep Time:** 10 minutes / **Cooking Time**: 15 minutes)

Ingredients

- 1 tablespoon cumin seeds
- 1 tablespoon coriander seeds, pounded
- 5 cloves
- 1 bay leaf
- 1 teaspoon salt
- ½ teaspoon red chili powder
- ½ teaspoon turmeric powder
- 1 teaspoon dry pomegranate powder
- 2 teaspoons dried fenugreek leaves
- 1 tablespoon mango pickle
- 2 tablespoon oil
- 5 potatoes, boiled and cubed

How to

1. Put the oil and all the spices in the instant pot and 'sauté' for 1 minute.
2. Add the remaining ingredients to the pot and secure the lid.
3. Use the 'manual' function on your cooker to cook for 2 minutes at high pressure.
4. After the beep, 'quick release' the steam and remove the lid.
5. Stir well to coat the potatoes and serve hot.

Nutrition Values (Per Serving)

- Calories: 260
- Carbohydrate: 44.7g
- Protein: 5.3g
- Fat: 7.6g
- Sugar: 3.3g
- Sodium: 635mg

Delectable Carrot Medley

(**Serves**: 3 / **Prep Time:** 10 minutes / **Cooking Time**: 20 minutes)

Ingredients

- 1 tablespoon olive oil
- ½ onion white, diced
- 1½ cloves garlic, finely chopped
- 1 lb potatoes, cut into chunks
- 1lb broccoli florets, diced
- 1 lb baby carrots, cut in half
- ¼ cup vegetable broth
- ½ teaspoon Italian seasoning
- ½ teaspoon Spike original seasoning,
- Fresh parsley for garnish

How to

1. Put the oil and onion into the instant pot and 'sauté' for 5 minutes.
2. Stir in the carrots and stir-fry for 5 minutes.
3. Add the remaining ingredients and secure the lid.
4. Cook on the 'manual' function for 10 minutes at high pressure.
5. After the beep, 'quick release' the steam and remove the lid.
6. Stir gently and serve.

Nutrition Values (Per Serving)

- Calories: 317
- Carbohydrate: 62.4g
- Protein: 6.8g
- Fat: 5.5g
- Sugar: 11.6g
- Sodium: 308mg

Vegetable Quinoa

(**Serves**: 5 / **Prep Time:** 10 minutes / **Cooking Time**: 23 minutes)

Ingredients

- 1 cup onion, diced
- 2 cloves garlic, minced
- ½ teaspoon olive oil
- ½ green bell pepper, diced
- ½ red bell pepper, diced
- ½ cup corn kernels
- ½ can spicy chili beans in sauce
- ½ can black beans, drained and rinsed
- 1¼ tablespoons chili powder
- ¾ tablespoon cumin
- ½ teaspoon dried oregano
- ¼ teaspoon smoked paprika,
- Salt and pepper to taste
- ¼ cup quinoa
- ¼ cup dried red lentils
- 1¼ cups vegetable broth
- 1 cup crushed tomatoes

How to

1. Put the oil and the onions into the instant pot and 'sauté' for 5 minutes.
2. Add the remaining vegetables to the pot and stir-fry for 3 minutes.
3. Stir in the remaining ingredients and secure the lid.
4. Cook on the 'manual' function for 15 minutes at high pressure.
5. After the beep, 'natural release' the steam and remove the lid.
6. Stir well and garnish with cilantro.
7. Serve hot.

Nutrition Values (Per Serving)

- Calories: 232
- Carbohydrate: 38.6g
- Protein: 12.1g
- Fat: 3.9g
- Sugar: 6.1g
- Sodium: 447mg

Spicy Vegetable Salsa

(**Serves**: 4 / **Prep Time:** 10 minutes / **Cooking Time**: 12 minutes)

Ingredients

- 1 tablespoon olive oil
- 1 onion, diced
- 1 cup potatoes, diced
- ½ cup carrots, diced
- ½ cup bell pepper, diced
- 1 cup vegetable broth
- 2 cans diced tomatoes
- ½ teaspoon ground cumin
- ½ teaspoon kosher salt
- ¼ teaspoon chili powder
- 1 cup salsa
- 2 cups shredded cheese
- ½ cup milk

How to

1. Put the oil and the onion into the instant pot and "Sauté" for 3 minutes.
2. Stir in all the vegetables and 'sauté' for a further 5 minutes.
3. Add the remaining ingredients, except the salsa, to the pot and secure the lid.
4. Select 'manual' setting and cook at high pressure for 4 minutes.
5. After the beep, 'quick release' the steam and remove the lid.
6. Stir in the salsa and serve hot.

Nutrition Values (Per Serving)

- Calories: 365
- Carbohydrate: 21.2g
- Protein: 19.3g
- Fat: 23.7g
- Sugar: 9.2g
- Sodium: 1256mg

Cheese Potato

(**Serves**: 4 / **Prep Time:** 10 minutes / **Cooking Time**: 15 minutes)

Ingredients

- 1 tablespoon butter
- ¼ cup chopped onion
- 3 cups potatoes, peeled and cubed
- 1½ cup vegetable broth
- ½ teaspoon salt
- ¼ teaspoon black pepper
- 1 tablespoon dried parsley
- 1½ oz cream cheese, cut into cubes
- ½ cup shredded cheddar cheese
- ½ cup frozen corn
- 3 slices crisp-cooked bacon, crumbled

How to

1. Put the butter and the onion into the instant pot and cook for 5 minutes using the 'sauté' function.
2. Add the broth, pepper, salt and parsley to the onions.
3. Place the steamer trivet in the pot and arrange the diced potatoes on it.
4. Secure the lid and select the 'manual' function. Cook for 4 minutes at high pressure.
5. After the beep, 'quick release' the steam and remove the lid.
6. Remove the steamer trivet along with the potatoes.
7. Add the remaining ingredients, including the potatoes, and cook for 5 minutes.
8. Serve hot.

Nutrition Values (Per Serving)

- Calories: 297
- Carbohydrate: 23.4g
- Protein: 17.4g
- Fat: 15.1g
- Sugar: 2.6g
- Sodium: 1272mg

Cajun Style Vegetable Rice

(**Serves**: 4 / **Prep Time:** 15 minutes / **Cooking Time**: 12 minutes)

Ingredients

- 2 teaspoons olive oil
- 1 onion, diced
- 2 cups white basmati rice
- 1 teaspoon chilli powder
- 2/3 teaspoon dried thyme
- 2/3 teaspoon dried oregano
- 1 teaspoon smoked paprika
- 1 teaspoon ground cumin
- 3 cups frozen vegetables
- 4 tablespoon tomato purée
- Salt and black pepper to taste
- 2 teaspoons lemon juice
- 2 tablespoon chopped fresh coriander

How to

1. Put the oil and the onion into the instant pot and 'sauté' for 5 minutes.
2. Stir in the frozen vegetables and sauté for a further 3 minutes.
3. Add the remaining ingredients and secure the lid.
4. Cook on the 'manual' function for 4 minutes at high pressure.
5. After the beep, 'quick release' the steam and remove the lid
6. Stir gently with a fork and serve hot.

Nutrition Values (Per Serving)

- Calories: 444
- Carbohydrate: 91.3g
- Protein: 11.1g
- Fat: 3.9g
- Sugar: 7.6g
- Sodium: 61mg

Potato Hemp Burgers

(**Serves**: 5 / **Prep Time:** 20 minutes / **Cooking Time**: 21 minutes)

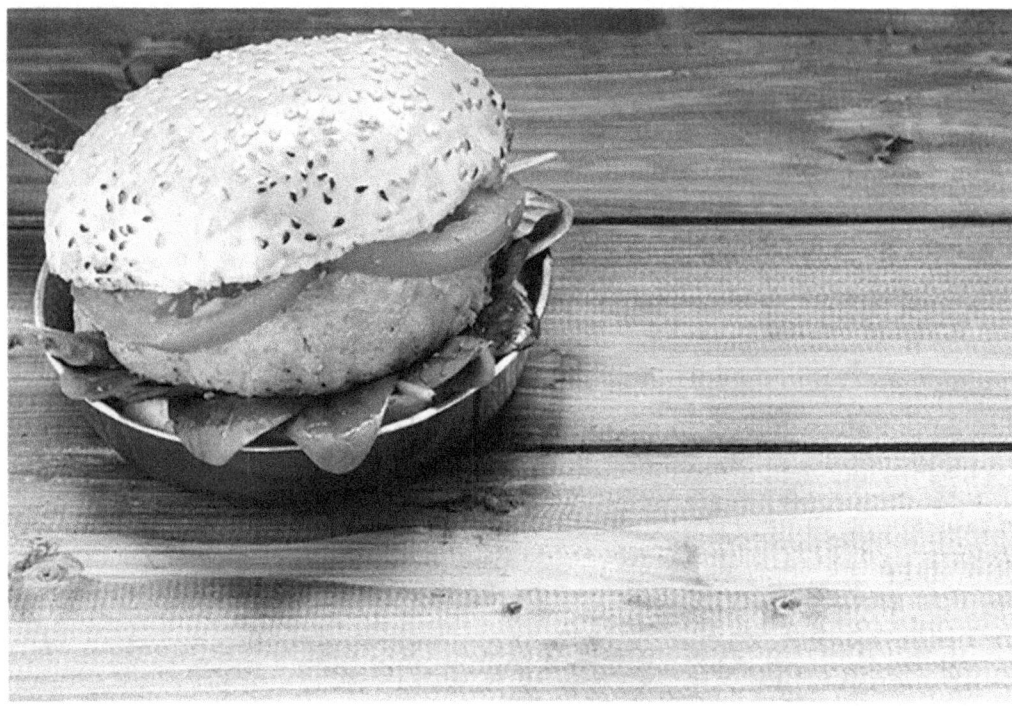

Ingredients

- ½ cup minced onion
- 1 teaspoon grated fresh ginger
- ½ cup minced mushrooms
- ½ cup red lentils, rinsed
- ¾ sweet potato, peeled and diced
- 1 cup vegetable stock
- 2 tablespoons hemp seeds
- 2 tablespoons chopped parsley
- 2 tablespoons chopped cilantro
- 1 tablespoon curry powder
- 1 cup quick oats
- 5 tomato slices
- Lettuce leaves
- 5 wheat buns

How to

1. Put the oil, ginger, mushrooms and onion into the instant pot and 'sauté' for 5 minutes.
2. Stir in the lentils, the stock, and the sweet potato.
3. Secure the lid and cook on the 'manual' function for 6 minutes at high pressure.
4. After the beep, 'natural release' the steam and remove the lid.
5. Meanwhile, heat the oven to 375º F and line a baking tray with parchment paper.
6. Mash the prepared lentil mixture with a potato masher.
7. Add the oats and the remaining spices. Put in some brown rice flour if the mixture is not thick enough.
8. Wet your hands and prepare 5 patties, using the mixture, and place them on the baking tray.
9. Bake the patties for 10 minutes in the preheated oven.
10. Slice the buns in half and stack each with a tomato slice, a vegetable patty and lettuce leaves.
11. Serve and enjoy.

Nutrition Values (Per Serving)

- Calories: 518
- Carbohydrate: 96.5g
- Protein: 21.3g
- Fat: 6g
- Sugar: 2.9g
- Sodium: 892mg

Potato Spinach Corn Mix

(**Serves**: 6 / **Prep Time:** 10 minutes / **Cooking Time**: 10 minutes)

Ingredients

- 1 tablespoon olive oil
- 3 scallions, chopped
- ½ cup onion, chopped
- 2 large white potatoes, peeled and diced
- 1 tablespoon ginger, grated
- 3 cups frozen corn kernels
- 1 cup vegetable stock
- 1 tablespoon fish sauce
- 2 tablespoons light soy sauce
- 2 large cloves of garlic, diced
- ⅓ teaspoon white pepper
- 1 teaspoon salt
- 3-4 handfuls of baby spinach leaves
- Juice of ½ lemon

How to

1. Put the oil ginger, garlic and onions in the instant pot and 'sauté' for 5 minutes.
2. Add all the remaining ingredients - except the spinach.
3. Secure the lid and cook on the 'manual' setting for 5 minutes at high pressure.
4. After the beep, 'quick release' the steam and remove the lid.
5. Add the spinach and cook for 3 minutes on 'sauté'
6. Drizzle the lime juice over the dish and serve hot.

Nutrition Values (Per Serving)

- Calories: 210
- Carbohydrate: 45.4g
- Protein: 7.3g
- Fat: 3.6g
- Sugar: 8.6g
- Sodium: 2275 mg

INSTANT POT STOCKS AND SAUCES

Chicken Stock

(**Serves**: 8 / **Prep time:** 6 minutes / **Cooking time**: 60 minutes)

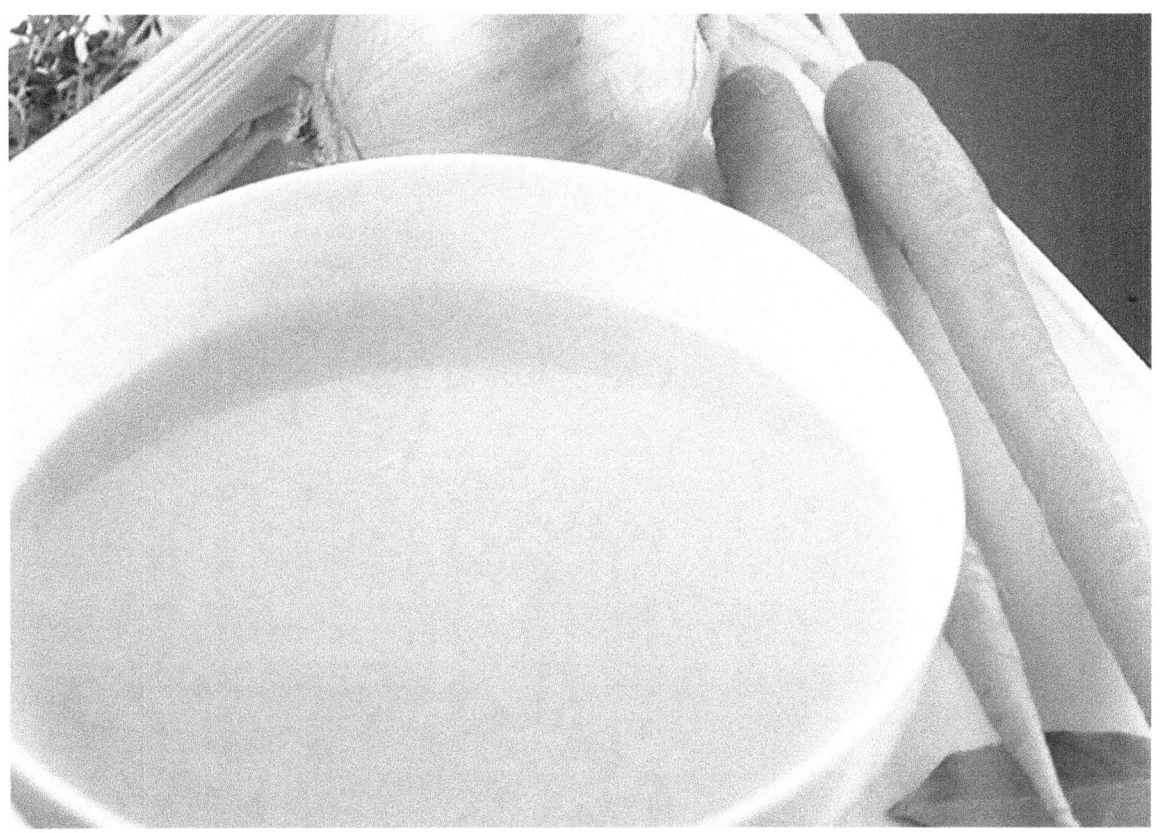

Ingredients

- 2½ lbs chicken carcass
- 1 celery stalk, chopped into thirds
- 1 small onion, unpeeled and halved
- 1 teaspoon dried bay leaf
- 1 sprig fresh parsley
- 1 teaspoon kosher salt
- ½ teaspoon whole black peppercorns
- 10 cups water

How to

1. Pour the water into the instant pot.
2. Add all the ingredients to the water.

3. Secure the lid. Turn the pressure release handle to the 'sealed' position.

4. Select the 'manual' function. Set to high pressure and adjust the time to 60 minutes.

5. After the beep, 'natural release' the steam for 10 minutes and remove the lid.

6. Strain the prepared stock through a mesh strainer and discard all the solids.

7. Skim off all the surface fats and serve hot.

Nutrition Values (Per Serving)

- Calories: 306
- Carbohydrate: 1g
- Protein: 25.2g
- Fat: 21.3g
- Sugar: 0.4g
- Sodium: 408mg

Chicken Vegetable Stock

(**Serves**: 8 / **Prep time:** 6 minutes / **Cooking time**: 60 minutes)

Ingredients

- 2½ lbs chicken (bones only)
- 1 celery stalk, chopped into thirds
- ¼ cup carrots, chopped
- ¼ cup green onions, chopped
- ¼ cup green bell pepper, chopped
- 1 small onion, unpeeled and halved
- 1 sprig fresh parsley
- Salt and black pepper to taste
- 8 cups water

How to

1. Pour the water into the instant pot.
2. Add all the ingredients to the water.
3. Secure the lid and turn the pressure release handle to the 'sealed' position.
4. Select the 'manual' function, set on high pressure and adjust the timer to 60 minutes.
5. After the beep, 'natural release' the steam for 10 minutes and remove the lid.
6. Strain the prepared stock through a mesh strainer and discard all the solids.
7. Skim off all the surface fats and serve hot.

Nutrition Values (Per Serving)

- Calories: 224
- Carbohydrate: 2.2g
- Protein: 41.5g
- Fat: 4.3g
- Sugar: 1g
- Sodium: 101mg

Chicken Mushroom Stock

(**Serves**: 8 / **Prep time**: 6 minutes / **Cooking time**: 60 minutes)

Ingredients

- 2½ lbs chicken (bones only)
- 1 leek, finely chopped
- 1 small onion, unpeeled and halved
- 1 teaspoon dried bay leaf
- 1 teaspoon kosher salt
- ½ teaspoon whole black peppercorns
- 1 cup cremini mushrooms, diced
- ½ teaspoon white pepper
- 8 cups water

How to

1. Pour the water into the instant pot.
2. Put all the ingredients into the water.
3. Secure the lid and turn the pressure release handle to the 'sealed' position.
4. Select the 'manual' function, set on high pressure and adjust the timer to 60 minutes.
5. After the beep, 'natural release' the steam for 10 minutes and remove the lid.
6. Strain the prepared stock through a mesh strainer and discard all the solids.
7. Skim off all the surface fats and serve hot.

Nutrition Values (Per Serving)

- Calories: 228
- Carbohydrate: 3.1g
- Protein: 41.6g
- Fat: 4.4g
- Sugar: 1g
- Sodium: 390g

Chicken with Herbs Stock

(**Serves**: 8 / **Prep time:** 6 minutes / **Cooking time**: 60 minutes)

Ingredients

- 2½ lbs chicken (bones only)
- 1 small onion, unpeeled and halved
- ¼ teaspoon oregano
- ¼ teaspoon dried basil
- 1 teaspoon dried bay leaf
- 1 sprig fresh parsley
- 1 teaspoon sea salt
- ½ teaspoon whole black peppercorns
- 8 cups water

How to

1. Pour the water into the instant pot.
2. Put all the ingredients into the water.
3. Secure the lid and turn the pressure release handle to the 'sealed' position.
4. Select the 'manual' function, set on high pressure and adjust the timer to 60 minutes.
5. After the beep, 'natural release' the steam for 10 minutes and remove the lid.
6. Strain the prepared stock through a mesh strainer and discard all the solids.
7. Skim off all the surface fats and serve hot.

Nutrition Values (Per Serving)

- Calories: 221
- Carbohydrate: 3.3g
- Protein: 41.2g
- Fat: 4.6g
- Sugar: 0.1g
- Sodium: 378mg

Chicken Kale Stock

(**Serves**: 8 / **Prep time:** 6 minutes / **Cooking time**: 60 minutes)

Ingredients

- 2½ lbs chicken (bones only)
- 1 celery stalk, chopped into thirds
- 1 small onion, unpeeled and halved
- 1 teaspoon dried bay leaf
- 1 sprig fresh kale
- Salt and black pepper to taste
- 8 cups water

How to

1. Pour the water into the instant pot.
2. Put all the ingredients into the water.
3. Secure the lid and turn the pressure release handle to the 'sealed' position.
4. Select the 'manual' function, set on high pressure and adjust the timer to 60 minutes.
5. After the beep, 'natural release' the steam for 10 minutes and remove the lid.
6. Strain the prepared stock through a mesh strainer and discard all the solids.
7. Skim off all the surface fats and serve hot.

Nutrition Values (Per Serving)

- Calories: 218
- Carbohydrate: 2.5g
- Protein: 42.1g
- Fat: 3.9g
- Sugar: 1g
- Sodium: 387mg

Chicken Corn Stock

(**Serves**: 8 / **Prep time:** 6 minutes / **Cooking time**: 60 minutes)

Ingredients

- 2½ lbs chicken (bones only)
- 1 cup corn kernels
- ½ cup green onion, chopped
- ½ cup carrots, chopped
- ½ teaspoon white pepper
- 1 teaspoon kosher salt
- ½ teaspoon whole black peppercorns
- 8 cups water

How to

1. Pour the water into the instant pot.
2. Put all the ingredients into the water.
3. Secure the lid and turn the pressure release handle to the 'sealed' position.
4. Select the 'manual' function, set on high pressure and adjust the timer to 60 minutes.
5. After the beep, 'natural release' the steam for 10 minutes and remove the lid.
6. Strain the prepared stock through a mesh strainer and discard all the solids.
7. Skim off all the surface fats and serve hot.

Nutrition Values (Per Serving)

- Calories: 243
- Carbohydrate: 7.8g
- Protein: 45.1g
- Fat: 5.3g
- Sugar: 0.2g
- Sodium: 431mg

Brown Beef Stock

(**Serves**: 10 / **Prep time:** 6 minutes / **Cooking time**: 2 hours 5 minutes)

Ingredients

- 2 tablespoons olive oil
- 4 lbs beef stock bones
- 1 celery stalk, chopped into thirds
- 1 small onion, unpeeled and halved
- 2 garlic cloves, chopped
- 1 tablespoon apple cider vinegar
- 1 teaspoon dried bay leaf
- 1 sprig fresh parsley
- 1 teaspoon kosher salt
- ½ teaspoon whole black peppercorns

How to

1. Grease a baking tray with olive oil and place the beef bones on it.
2. Roast the bones for 30 minutes in an oven at 420º F. Flip the bones over and roast for another 20 minutes
3. Fill the instant pot with water up to one inch below the 'max line'.
4. Add all the ingredients, including the roasted beef bones, to the water.
5. Secure the lid. Turn the pressure release handle to the 'sealed' position.
6. Select the 'manual' function, set to high pressure and adjust the time to 75 minutes.
7. After the beep, 'natural release' the steam for 10 minutes and remove the lid.
8. Strain the prepared stock through a mesh strainer and discard all the solids.
9. Skim off all the surface fats and serve hot.

Nutrition Values (Per Serving)

- Calories: 388
- Carbohydrate: 1g
- Protein: 49.8g
- Fat: 19.1g
- Sugar: 0.3g
- Sodium: 363mg

Beef Vegetable Stock

(**Serves**: 10 / **Prep time:** 6 minutes / **Cooking time**: 2 hours 5 minutes)

Ingredients

- 2 tablespoons olive oil
- 4 lbs beef stock bones
- 1 celery stalk, chopped into thirds
- 1 small onion, unpeeled and halved
- 2 garlic cloves, chopped
- 1 tablespoon apple cider vinegar
- 1 cup carrots, chopped
- ½ cup bell peppers, sliced
- ¼ cabbage, chopped
- 1 sprig fresh parsley
- 1 teaspoon kosher salt
- ½ teaspoon whole black peppercorns

How to

1. Grease the baking tray with olive oil and place the beef bones on it.
2. Roast the bones for 30 minutes in an oven at 420º F. Flip the bones over and roast for another 20 minutes
3. Fill the instant pot with water up to one inch below the 'max line'.
4. Add all the ingredients, including the roasted beef bones to the water.
5. Secure the lid. Turn the pressure release handle to the 'sealed' position.
6. Select the 'manual' function, set to high pressure and adjust the time to 75 minutes.
7. After the beep, 'natural release' the steam for 10 minutes and remove the lid.
8. Strain the prepared stock through a mesh strainer and discard all the solids.
9. Skim off all the surface fats and serve hot.

Nutrition Values (Per Serving)

- Calories: 396
- Carbohydrate: 1.3g
- Protein: 48.4g
- Fat: 18.9g
- Sugar: 0.4g
- Sodium: 365smg

Roasted Beef Mushroom Stock

(**Serves**: 10 / **Prep time:** 6 minutes / **Cooking time**: 2 hours 5 minutes)

Ingredients

- 2 tablespoons olive oil
- 4 lbs beef stock bones
- 1 cup cremini mushrooms, sliced
- 1 celery stalk, chopped into thirds
- 1 small onion, unpeeled and halved
- 2 garlic cloves, chopped
- 1 tablespoon apple cider vinegar
- 1 teaspoon kosher salt
- ½ teaspoon white pepper
- 1 teaspoon black pepper ground

How to

1. Grease the baking tray with olive oil and place the beef bones on it.
2. Roast the bones for 30 minutes in an oven at 420° F. Flip the bones over and roast for another 20 minutes
3. Fill the instant pot with water up to one inch below the 'max line'.
4. Add all the ingredients, including the roasted beef bones to the water.
5. Secure the lid. Turn the pressure release handle to the 'sealed' position.
6. Select the 'manual' function, set to high pressure and adjust the time to 75 minutes.
7. After the beep, 'natural release' the steam for 10 minutes and remove the lid.
8. Strain the prepared stock through a mesh strainer and discard all the solids.
9. Skim off all the surface fats and serve hot.

Nutrition Values (Per Serving)

- Calories: 393
- Carbohydrate: 1.2g
- Protein: 47.4g
- Fat: 20g
- Sugar: 0.4g
- Sodium: 365mg

Beef Pepper Stock

(**Serves**: 10 / **Prep time:** 6 minutes / **Cooking time**: 2 hours 5 minutes)

Ingredients

- 2 tablespoons olive oil
- 4 lbs beef stock bones
- 1 celery stalk, chopped into thirds
- 1 small onion, unpeeled and halved
- 2 garlic cloves, chopped
- 1 cup red bell pepper
- ¼ teaspoon red pepper flakes
- ¼ teaspoon turmeric ground
- 1 teaspoon kosher salt
- ½ teaspoon whole black peppercorns

How to

1. Grease the baking tray with olive oil and place the beef bones on it.
2. Roast the bones for 30 minutes in an oven at 420º F. Flip the bones over and roast for another 20 minutes
3. Fill the instant pot with water up to one inch below the 'max line'.
4. Add all the ingredients, including the roasted beef bones to the water.
5. Secure the lid. Turn the pressure release handle to the 'sealed' position.
6. Select the 'manual' function, set to high pressure and adjust the time to 75 minutes.
7. After the beep, 'natural release' the steam for 10 minutes and remove the lid.
8. Strain the prepared stock through a mesh strainer and discard all the solids.
9. Skim off all the surface fats and serve hot.

Nutrition Values (Per Serving)

- Calories: 378
- Carbohydrate: 2.1g
- Protein: 48.6g
- Fat: 18.3g
- Sugar: 0.4g
- Sodium: 350mg

Beef Bacon Stock

(**Serves**: 10 / **Prep time:** 6 minutes / **Cooking time**: 2 hours 8 minutes)

Ingredients

- 2 tablespoons olive oil
- 4 lbs beef stock bones
- 6 bacon strips
- 1 celery stalk, chopped into thirds
- 1 small onion, unpeeled and halved
- 2 garlic cloves, chopped
- 1 teaspoon kosher salt
- ½ teaspoon whole black peppercorns

How to

1. Grease the baking tray with olive oil and place the beef bones on it.
2. Roast the bones for 30 minutes in an oven at 420º F. Flip the bones over and roast for another 20 minutes
3. Add the bacon and the rest of the oil to the instant pot and 'sauté' for 3 minutes.
4. Now fill the instant pot with water up to one inch below the 'max line'.
5. Put all the ingredients, including the roasted beef bones, into the water.
6. Secure the lid, and turn the pressure release handle to the 'sealed' position.
7. Select the 'manual' function. Set to high pressure and adjust the time to 75 minutes.
8. After the beep, 'natural release' the steam for 10 minutes and remove the lid.
9. Strain the prepared stock through a fine mesh strainer and discard all the solids.
10. Skim off all the surface fats and serve hot.

Nutrition Values (Per Serving)

- Calories: 397
- Carbohydrate: 2g
- Protein: 50.1g
- Fat: 20.7g
- Sugar: 0.2g
- Sodium: 383mg

Mixed Vegetable Stock

(**Serves**: 8 / **Prep time:** 10 minutes / **Cooking time**: 15 minutes)

Ingredients

- 1 celery stalk, chopped into thirds
- 1 small onion, unpeeled and halved
- 1 cup carrots, diced
- 1 cup potatoes, diced
- ½ cup green onions, chopped
- ½ cup bell peppers, chopped
- 1 tablespoon ginger, grated
- 1 teaspoon dried bay leaf
- ½ teaspoon ground turmeric
- 1 sprig fresh parsley
- 1 teaspoon kosher salt
- ½ teaspoon whole black peppercorns
- 8 cups water

How to

1. Pour the water into the instant pot.
2. Add all the ingredients to the water.
3. Secure the lid and turn the pressure release handle to the 'sealed' position.
4. Select the 'manual' function and set to high pressure. Adjust the time to 15 minutes.
5. After the beep, 'natural release' the steam for 10 minutes and remove the lid.
6. Strain the prepared stock through a mesh strainer and discard all the solids.
7. Serve hot.

Nutrition Values (Per Serving)

- Calories: 30
- Carbohydrate: 6.9g
- Protein: 0.8g
- Fat: 0.1g
- Sugar: 1.9g
- Sodium: 312mg

Corn and Mushroom Stock

(**Serves**: 8 / **Prep time:** 5 minutes / **Cooking time**: 15 minutes)

Ingredients

- 2 cobs of corns
- 4 large mushrooms, diced
- 1 celery stalk, chopped into thirds
- 1 small onion, unpeeled and halved
- 1 teaspoon dried bay leaf
- ½ teaspoon turmeric ground
- 1 teaspoon ginger, grated
- 1 sprig fresh parsley
- 1 teaspoon kosher salt
- ½ teaspoon whole black peppercorns
- 8 cups water

How to

1. Pour the water into the instant pot.
2. Add all the ingredients to the water.
3. Secure the lid and turn the pressure release handle to the 'sealed' position.
4. Select the 'manual' function and set to high pressure. Adjust the time to 15 minutes.
5. After the beep, 'natural release' the steam for 10 minutes and remove the lid.
6. Strain the prepared stock through a mesh strainer and discard all the solids.
7. Serve hot.

Nutrition Values (Per Serving)

- Calories: 47
- Carbohydrate: 9.6g
- Protein: 1.6g
- Fat: 0.9g
- Sugar: 0.6g
- Sodium: 308mg

Fish Anchovy Stock

(**Serves**: 8 / **Prep time:** 5 minutes / **Cooking time**: 20 minutes)

Ingredients

- 2 oz dried anchovies
- 1 celery stalk, chopped into thirds
- 6 small pieces kombu*
- 1 teaspoon kosher salt
- ½ teaspoon whole black peppercorns
- 8 cups water

How to

1. Pour the water into the instant pot.
2. Put all the ingredients into the water.
3. Secure the lid and turn the pressure release handle to the 'sealed' position.
4. Select the 'manual' function. Set to high pressure and adjust the timer to 20 minutes.
5. After the beep, 'natural release' the steam for 10 minutes and remove the lid.
6. Strain the prepared stock through a mesh strainer and discard all the solids.
7. Skim off all the surface fats and serve hot.

Nutrition Values (Per Serving)

- Calories: 20
- Carbohydrate: 0.9g
- Protein: 2.3g
- Fat: 0.7g
- Sugar: 0g
- Sodium: 638mg

(**Note: Kombu*** - a brown seaweed used in Japanese cooking, especially as a base for stock.)

Tunisian Chickpea Stock

(**Serves**: 8 / **Prep time:** 10 minutes / **Cooking time**: 20 minutes)

Ingredients

- 2 cups chickpeas, rinsed and drained
- 1 cup carrots, diced
- ½ cup green onions, chopped
- 1 teaspoon dried bay leaf
- ½ teaspoon apple cider vinegar
- 1 teaspoon kosher salt
- 1 tablespoon thyme leaves
- ½ teaspoon red pepper flakes
- 8 cups water

How to

1. Pour the water into the instant pot.
2. Put all the ingredients into the water.
3. Secure the lid and turn the pressure release handle to the 'sealed' position.
4. Select the 'manual' function. Set to high pressure and adjust the timer to 20 minutes.
5. After the beep, 'natural release' the steam for 10 minutes and remove the lid.
6. Strain the prepared stock through a mesh strainer and discard all the solids.
7. Serve hot.

Nutrition Values (Per Serving)

- Calories: 191
- Carbohydrate: 32.4g
- Protein: 9.9g
- Fat: 3.1g
- Sugar: 6.2g
- Sodium: 321mg

Crab and Tomato Stock

(**Serves**: 8 / **Prep time:** 10 minutes / **Cooking time**: 1 hour 20 minutes)

Ingredients

- 2 lbs crab shells
- 1 onion, rough chop – skin on
- 1 cup carrots, rough chop
- 2 stalks of celery, rough chop
- 4 cloves of garlic
- 1 teaspoon black peppercorns
- 1 teaspoon parsley flakes
- 2 bay leaves
- 4 sprigs fresh thyme
- 2 tablespoons tomato paste
- 10 cups water

How to

1. Put the oil, the crab shells and vegetables in the instant pot and 'sauté' for 5 minutes.
2. Pour the water into the instant pot.
3. Add all the remaining ingredients to the water.
4. Secure the lid and turn the pressure release handle to the 'sealed' position.
5. Select the 'manual' function, set to high pressure and adjust the timer to 80 minutes.
6. After the beep, 'natural release' the steam for 10 minutes and remove the lid.
7. Strain the prepared stock through a mesh strainer and discard all the solids.
8. Serve.

Nutrition Values (Per Serving)

- Calories: 156
- Carbohydrate: 5.2g
- Protein: 27.4g
- Fat: 1.5g
- Sugar: 1.9g
- Sodium: 468mg

Salmon Fish Stock

(**Serves**: 6 / **Prep time:** 6 minutes / **Cooking time**: 53 minutes)

Ingredients

- 2 salmon heads (2 to 2½ lbs)
- 1 small onion, quartered
- 2 cloves garlic
- 1 carrot, diced
- 1 bay leaf
- 3 sprigs fresh thyme
- 5 peppercorns
- 6 cups cold water
- 1 cup dry white wine

How to

1. Put the oil and the salmon heads in the instant pot and 'sauté' for 5 minutes.
2. Pour the water into the pot.
3. Add all the remaining ingredients to the water.
4. Secure the lid and turn the pressure release handle to the 'sealed' position.
5. Select the 'manual' function, set to high pressure and adjust the timer to 48 minutes.
6. After the beep, 'natural release' the steam for 10 minutes and remove the lid.
7. Strain the prepared stock through a mesh strainer and discard all the solids.
8. Skim off all the surface fats and serve hot.

Nutrition Values (Per Serving)

- Calories: 123
- Carbohydrate: 3.9g
- Protein: 11.9g
- Fat: 3.7g
- Sugar: 1.3g
- Sodium: 43mg

Seafood Gumbo Stock

(**Serves**: 8 / **Prep time:** 6 minutes / **Cooking time**: 60 minutes)

Ingredients

- 1 salmon head
- ½ lb crab shells
- ½ lb shrimp shells
- 1 small onion, quartered
- 2 cloves garlic
- 1 carrot, diced
- 1 bay leaf
- 3 sprigs fresh thyme
- 5 peppercorns
- 6 cups cold water
- 1 cup dry white wine

How to

1. Put the oil, the salmon head, crab shells and shrimp shells in the instant pot and 'sauté' for 5 minutes.
2. Pour the water into the instant pot.
3. Add all the remaining ingredients to the water.
4. Secure the lid and turn the pressure release handle to the 'sealed' position.
5. Select the 'manual' function, set to high pressure and adjust the timer to 48 minutes.
6. After the beep, 'natural release' the steam for 10 minutes and remove the lid.
7. Strain the prepared stock through a mesh strainer and discard all the solids.
8. Skim off all the surface fats and serve hot.

Nutrition Values (Per Serving)

- Calories: 126
- Carbohydrate: 3.4g
- Protein: 16.8g
- Fat: 2.4g
- Sugar: 1g
- Sodium: 171mg

Turkey Bone Stock

(**Serves**: 8 / **Prep time:** 6 minutes / **Cooking time**: 60 minutes)

Ingredients

- 1 turkey carcass
- 1 celery stalk, chopped into thirds
- 1 small onion, unpeeled and halved
- 1 teaspoon dried bay leaf
- 1 sprig fresh parsley
- 1 teaspoon kosher salt
- ½ teaspoon whole black peppercorns
- 10 cups water

How to

1. Pour the water into the instant pot.
2. Add all the ingredients to the water.
3. Secure the lid and turn the pressure release handle to the 'sealed' position.
4. Select the 'manual' function. Set to high pressure and adjust the timer to 60 minutes.
5. After the beep, 'natural release' the steam for 10 minutes and remove the lid.
6. Strain the prepared stock through a mesh strainer and discard all the solids.
7. Skim off all the surface fats and serve hot.

Nutrition Values (Per Serving)

- Calories: 39
- Carbohydrate: 1g
- Protein: 5g
- Fat: 1.4g
- Sugar: 0.4g
- Sodium: 312mg

Pork Bone Stock

(**Serves**: 8 / **Prep time:** 6 minutes / **Cooking time**: 20 minutes)

Ingredients

- 3 lbs pastured pork bones
- 1 celery stalk, chopped into thirds
- 1 small onion, unpeeled and halved
- 1 teaspoon dried bay leaf
- 1 sprig fresh parsley
- 1 teaspoon kosher salt
- ½ teaspoon whole black peppercorns
- 8 cups water

How to

1. Pour the water into the instant pot.
2. Add all the ingredients to the water.
3. Secure the lid and turn the pressure release handle to the 'sealed' position.
4. Select the 'manual' function, set to high pressure and adjust the timer to 20 minutes.
5. After the beep, 'natural release' the steam for 10 minutes and remove the lid.
6. Strain the prepared stock through a mesh strainer and discard all the solids.
7. Skim off all the surface fats and serve hot.

Nutrition Values (Per Serving)

- Calories: 445
- Carbohydrate: 7g
- Protein: 22.1g
- Fat: 36g
- Sugar: 0.4g
- Sodium: 1601mg

Pork Beef Stock

(**Serves**: 8 / **Prep time:** 6 minutes / **Cooking time**: 60 minutes)

Ingredients

- 2 lbs pastured pork bones
- 1 lb beef stew meat
- 1 celery stalk, chopped into thirds
- 1 small onion, unpeeled and halved
- 1 teaspoon dried bay leaf
- 1 sprig fresh parsley
- 1 teaspoon kosher salt
- ½ teaspoon whole black peppercorns
- 8 cups water

How to

1. Pour the water into the instant pot.
2. Add all the ingredients to the water.
3. Secure the lid and turn the pressure release handle to the 'sealed' position.
4. Select the 'manual' function, set to high pressure and adjust the timer to 60 minutes.
5. After the beep, 'natural release' the steam for 10 minutes and remove the lid.
6. Strain the prepared stock through a mesh strainer and discard all the solids.
7. Skim off all the surface fats and serve hot.

Nutrition Values (Per Serving)

- Calories: 464
- Carbohydrate: 6.7g
- Protein: 32.1g
- Fat: 37g
- Sugar: 0.4g
- Sodium: 1578mg

Pork and Vegetable Stock

(**Serves**: 8 / **Prep time:** 6 minutes / **Cooking time**: 60 minutes)

Ingredients

- 2 lbs pastured pork bones
- ½ cup carrots, chopped
- ½ cup bell peppers
- ½ cup green onions, chopped
- 1 celery stalk, chopped into thirds
- 1 small onion, unpeeled and halved
- 1 teaspoon dried bay leaf
- 1 sprig fresh parsley
- 1 teaspoon kosher salt
- ½ teaspoon whole black peppercorns
- 8 cups water

How to

1. Pour the water into the instant pot.
2. Add all the ingredients to the water.
3. Secure the lid and turn the pressure release handle to the 'sealed' position.
4. Select the 'manual' function, set to high pressure and adjust the timer to 20 minutes.
5. After the beep, 'natural release' the steam for 10 minutes and remove the lid.
6. Strain the prepared stock through a mesh strainer and discard all the solids.
7. Skim off all the surface fats and serve hot.

Nutrition Values (Per Serving)

- Calories: 443
- Carbohydrate: 7.1g
- Protein: 25.1g
- Fat: 32g
- Sugar: 0.4g
- Sodium: 1611mg

Chicken Green Beans Stock

(**Serves**: 8 / **Prep time:** 6 minutes / **Cooking time**: 60 minutes)

Ingredients

- 2½ lbs chicken (bones only)
- 1 cup green beans, sliced
- 1 celery stalk, chopped into thirds
- 1 small onion, unpeeled and halved
- 1 teaspoon dried bay leaf
- 1 sprig fresh parsley
- 1 teaspoon kosher salt
- ½ teaspoon whole black peppercorns
- 8 cups water

How to

1. Pour the water into the instant pot.
2. Add all the ingredients to the water.
3. Secure the lid and turn the pressure release handle to the 'sealed' position.
4. Select the 'manual' function, set to high pressure and adjust the timer to 20 minutes.
5. After the beep, 'natural release' the steam for 10 minutes and remove the lid.
6. Strain the prepared stock through a mesh strainer and discard all the solids.
7. Skim off all the surface fats and serve hot.

Nutrition Values (Per Serving)

- Calories: 480
- Carbohydrate: 2g
- Protein: 30.8g
- Fat: 9.5g
- Sugar: 0.6g
- Sodium: 495mg

Red Hot Sauce

(**Serves**: 4 / **Prep Time:** 5 minutes / **Cooking Time**: 2 minutes)

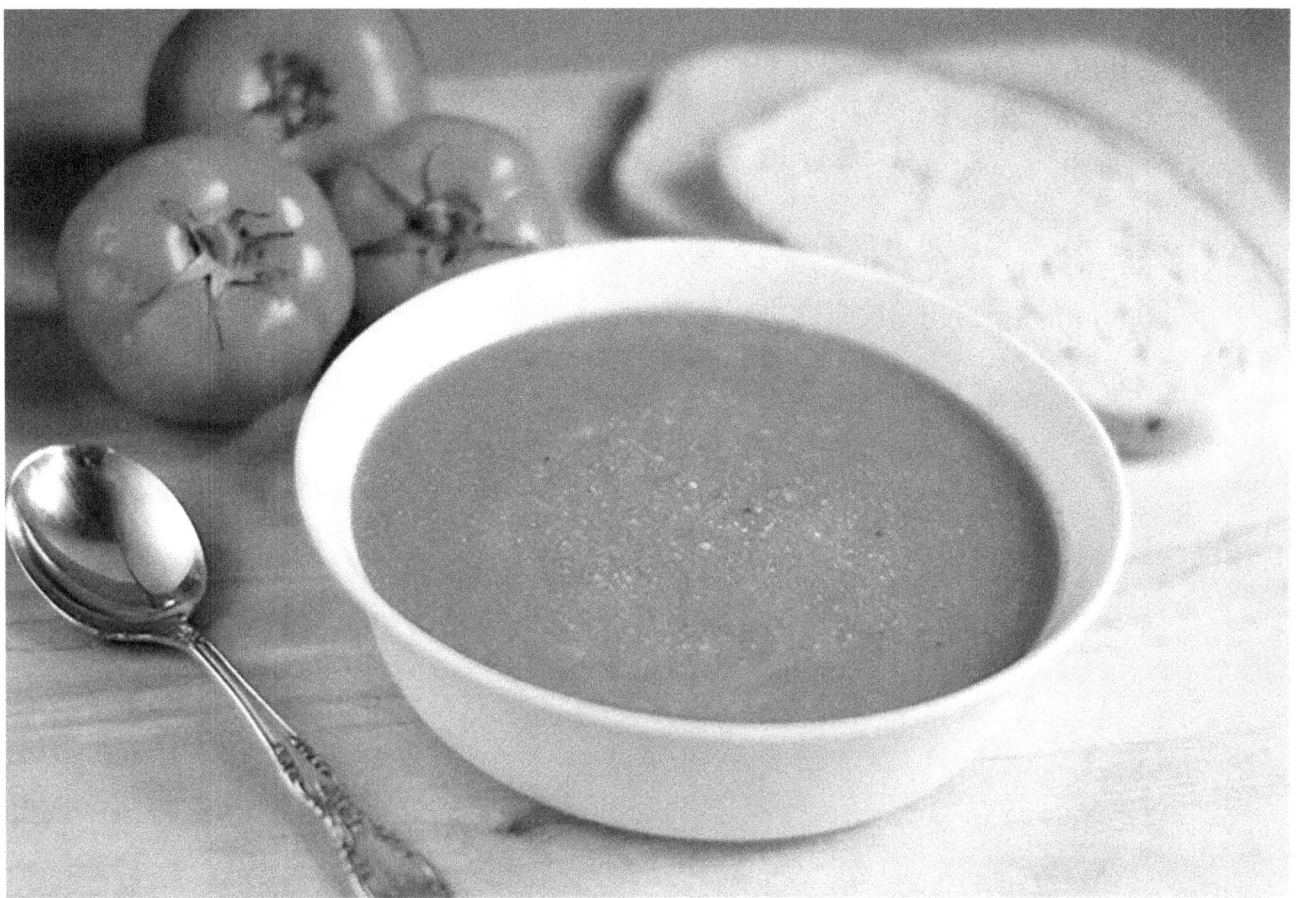

Ingredients

- 1 lb Fresno peppers
- ¼ cup carrot, shredded
- 6 garlic cloves, peeled and smashed
- 1 roasted red pepper, chopped
- 1 cup white vinegar
- ¼ cup apple cider vinegar
- ½ cup water
- 1 tablespoon sea salt

How to

1. Put all the ingredients into the instant pot.
2. Secure the lid and turn the pressure release handle to the 'sealed' position.
3. Select the 'manual' function. Set to high pressure and adjust the timer to 2 minutes.
4. After the beep, 'quick release' the steam and remove the lid.

5. Transfer the sauce to a blender and blend well to form a smooth mixture.
6. Use immediately or save in a bottle for later use.

Nutrition Values (Per Serving)

- Calories: 43
- Carbohydrate: 9.5g
- Protein: 0.5g
- Fat: 0.1g
- Sugar: 1.4g
- Sodium: 457mg

Green Hot Sauce

(**Serves**: 8 / **Prep Time:** 5 minutes / **Cooking Time**: 2 minutes)

Ingredients

- 16 oz green chilies
- 8 garlic cloves, peeled and smashed
- 1 green bell pepper, chopped
- 1 cup white vinegar
- ¼ cup apple cider vinegar
- ½ cup water
- 1 tablespoon sea salt

How to

1. Put all the ingredients into the instant pot.
2. Secure the lid and turn the pressure release handle to the 'sealed' position.
3. Select the 'manual' function. Set to high pressure and adjust the timer to 2 minutes.
4. After the beep, 'quick release' the steam and remove the lid.
5. Transfer the sauce to a blender and blend well to form a smooth mixture.
6. Use immediately or save in a bottle for later use.

Nutrition Values (Per Serving)

- Calories: 34
- Carbohydrate: 6.2g
- Protein: 0.3g
- Fat: 0.1g
- Sugar: 2.8g
- Sodium: 932mg

Mushroom Sauce

(**Serves**: 3 / **Prep Time:** 5 minutes / **Cooking Time**: 5 minutes)

Ingredients

- ½ tablespoon butter
- 1 tablespoon oil
- 2½ cups portabella mushrooms, sliced
- 1 sprig fresh thyme
- 1 garlic clove, crushed
- ½ cup cream
- ½ cup milk
- 3 teaspoons corn starch
- 1 tablespoon lemon juice
- Salt and pepper to taste
- ½ cup water
- 1 tablespoon chopped parsley

How to

1. Select the 'sauté' function on the instant pot and heat the oil and butter.
2. Add the garlic, mushrooms and thyme to the oil. Stir-fry for 5 minutes.
3. Add the salt, pepper, cream and water to the mushrooms.
4. Secure the lid and turn the pressure release handle to the 'sealed' position.
5. Select the 'manual' function, set to high pressure and adjust the timer to 3 minutes.
6. After the beep, 'quick release' the steam and remove the lid.
7. Prepare a slurry by mixing the cornstarch with half a cup of milk. Add this slurry to the mushroom sauce.
8. Stir in the parsley and lemon juice, then serve.

Nutrition Values (Per Serving)

- Calories: 69
- Carbohydrate: 5.3g
- Protein: 1.8g
- Fat: 4.9g
- Sugar: 2g
- Sodium: 27mg

Super Quick Garlic Sauce

(**Serves**: 2 / **Prep Time:** 5 minutes / **Cooking Time**: 3 minutes)

Ingredients

- 1 cup water, (divided as explained in **How to** below)
- 4 tablespoons chopped garlic
- 2 teaspoon garlic powder
- 4 cups heavy cream
- 2 tablespoon chopped fresh parsley
- Salt and pepper to taste
- 4 tablespoons cornstarch

How to

1. Put half the water, garlic, garlic powder, cream, salt and pepper in the instant pot.
2. Secure the lid and turn the pressure release handle to the 'sealed' position.
3. Select the 'manual' function, set to high pressure and adjust the timer to 3 minutes.
4. After the beep, 'quick release' the steam and remove the lid.
5. Mix the cornstarch with the remaining water. Add this slurry to the garlic sauce.
6. Stir in the parsley and serve.

Nutrition Values (Per Serving)

- Calories: 231
- Carbohydrate: 7.3g
- Protein: 1.7g
- Fat: 22.2g
- Sugar: 0.3g
- Sodium: 25mg

Special BBQ Sauce

(**Serves**: 6 / **Prep Time:** 10 minutes / **Cooking Time**: 5 minutes)

Ingredients

- 8 oz Heinz ketchup
- 4 oz water
- 2½ tablespoons brown sugar
- 2½ tablespoons white sugar
- ¼ tablespoon black pepper, freshly ground
- ¼ tablespoon onion powder
- ¼ tablespoon dry mustard powder
- ½ oz lemon juice
- ½ oz Worcestershire sauce
- 2 oz apple cider vinegar
- ½ oz light corn syrup
- ½ tablespoon jerk rub

How to

1. Put all the ingredients in the instant pot.
2. Secure the lid and turn the pressure release handle to the 'sealed' position.
3. Select the 'manual' function, set to high pressure and adjust the time to 5 minutes.
4. After the beep, 'natural release' the steam for 10 minutes and remove the lid.
5. Use immediately or save in a bottle for later use.

Nutrition Values (Per Serving)

- Calories: 85
- Carbohydrate: 21.1g
- Protein: 0.5g
- Fat: 0.2g
- Sugar: 18.6g
- Sodium: 475mg

Watermelon BBQ Sauce

(**Serves**: 8 / **Prep Time:** 15 minutes / **Cooking Time**: 20 minutes)

Ingredients

- 2 cups watermelon pulp
- 2 cups dark corn syrup
- ½ cup watermelon juice
- ½ cup Heinz ketchup
- ½ cup distilled vinegar
- ½ teaspoon crushed red pepper flakes
- 1 teaspoon liquid smoke
- ½ teaspoon freshly ground black pepper

How to

1. Put the diced, red part of the watermelon into a food processor and blend.
2. Strain the watermelon pulp from its water. Keep it aside for later use.
3. Put all the ingredients, including 1 cup watermelon pulp, in the instant pot.
4. Secure the lid and turn the pressure release handle to the 'sealed' position.
5. Select the 'manual' function, set to high pressure and adjust the timer to 20 minutes.
6. After the beep, 'natural release' the steam for 10 minutes and remove the lid.
7. Let it simmer for 5 minutes.
8. Use immediately or save in a jar for later use.

Nutrition Values (Per Serving)

- Calories: 244
- Carbohydrate: 64.9g
- Protein: 0.3g
- Fat: 0.1g
- Sugar: 25.6g
- Sodium: 170mg

Instant Pot Barbeque Sauce

(**Serves**: 5 / **Prep Time:** 10 minutes / **Cooking Time**: 13 minutes)

Ingredients

- 2 tablespoons sesame seed oil
- 2 medium onions, roughly chopped
- 1 cup tomato puree
- 1 cup water
- ½ cup honey
- ½ cup white vinegar
- 2 teaspoons sea salt
- 1 teaspoon granulated garlic
- 2 teaspoons hot sauce
- 2 teaspoons liquid smoke
- ¼ teaspoon clove ground
- ¼ teaspoon cumin powder
- 1½ cups seedless dried plums

How to

1. Put the oil, onion and garlic into the instant pot and 'sauté' for 3 minutes.
2. Stir in all the ingredients and mix them well.
3. Secure the lid and turn the pressure release handle to the 'sealed' position.
4. Select the 'manual' function, set to high pressure and adjust the timer to 10 minutes.
5. After the beep, 'quick release' the steam and remove the lid.
6. Transfer the sauce to a blender and blend well to form a smooth mixture
7. Use immediately or save in a bottle for later use.

Nutrition Values (Per Serving)

- Calories: 229
- Carbohydrate: 44.8g
- Protein: 1.8g
- Fat: 5.6g
- Sugar: 37.8g
- Sodium: 820mg

Bolognese Bacon Sauce

(**Serves**: 6 / **Prep Time**: 5 minutes / **Cooking Time**: 45 minutes)

Ingredients

- ½ large onion, finely chopped
- 1 carrot, finely chopped
- 1½ celery stalks, finely chopped
- 1½ garlic cloves, minced or pressed
- ½ tablespoon olive oil
- ½ (6 oz) can tomato paste
- 1 lb ground beef
- ½ cup bacon, diced
- ½ tablespoon salt
- ½ teaspoon black pepper
- ¾ teaspoon dried thyme
- 1 teaspoon dried oregano
- 1 (28 oz) can crushed tomatoes
- 1 cup whole milk
- 1 cup dry red wine

How to

1. Pour the oil into the instant pot and select the 'sauté' function.
2. Add all the vegetables to the oil and stir-fry for 10 minutes.
3. Stir in the tomato paste and all the spices. Use an immerse blender to blend the sauce.
4. Now put all the remaining ingredients into the instant pot.
5. Secure the lid and turn the pressure release handle to the 'sealed' position.
6. Select the 'meat stew' function and adjust the timer to 35 minutes.
7. After the beep, 'quick release' the steam and remove the lid.
8. Stir well and serve with pasta.

Nutrition Values (Per Serving)

- Calories: 322
- Carbohydrate: 25.8g
- Protein: 29.7g
- Fat: 7.9g
- Sugar: 16.3g
- Sodium: 978mg

Cashew Cheese Sauce

(**Serves**: 5 / **Prep Time:** 10 minutes / **Cooking Time**: 5 minutes)

Ingredients

- 1 cup water
- ¼ white onion, peeled and quartered
- 1 garlic clove, peeled
- ½ cup carrots, peeled and sliced
- ¾ cup Yukon Gold potatoes, peeled and chopped
- ¼ cup raw cashews
- ¼ cup nutritional yeast
- 1 tablespoon mellow white miso
- ½ teaspoon smoked or sweet paprika
- 1 tablespoon lemon juice
- 1 tablespoon apple cider vinegar
- 1 teaspoon sea salt

How to

1. Put all the ingredients into the instant pot.
2. Secure the lid and turn the pressure release handle to the 'sealed' position.
3. Select the 'manual' function, set to high pressure and adjust the timer to 5 minutes.
4. After the beep, 'quick release' the steam and remove the lid.
5. Transfer the sauce to a blender and blend well to form a smooth mixture.
6. Use immediately or save in a bottle for later use.

Nutrition Values (Per Serving)

- Calories: 103
- Carbohydrate: 13.4g
- Protein: 5.5g
- Fat: 3.7g
- Sugar: 1.4g
- Sodium: 501mg

Strawberry Sauce

(**Serves**: 5 / **Prep Time:** 02 minutes / **Cooking Time**: 8 minutes)

Ingredients

- 8 oz fresh strawberries
- 2 tablespoons raw honey
- ½ cup pure squeezed orange juice
- ½ teaspoon cinnamon or 2 cinnamon sticks
- 1 tablespoon stevia

How to

1. Put all the ingredients in the instant pot.
2. Secure the lid and turn the pressure release handle to the 'sealed' position.
3. Select the 'manual' function, set to high pressure and adjust the timer to 8 minutes.
4. After the beep, 'quick release' the steam and remove the lid.
5. Use an immerse blender to puree the sauce.
6. Serve when cool, or save in a bottle for later use.

Nutrition Values (Per Serving)

- Calories: 63
- Carbohydrate: 15.6g
- Protein: 0.5g
- Fat: 0.1g
- Sugar: 13.9g
- Sodium: 4mg

Cranberry Sauce

(**Serves**: 5 / **Prep Time:** 2 minutes / **Cooking Time**: 8 minutes)

Ingredients

- 8 oz fresh cranberries
- 2 tablespoons raw honey
- ½ cup pure squeezed orange juice
- ½ teaspoon cinnamon or 2 cinnamon sticks
- 1 tablespoon stevia

How to

1. Put all the ingredients in the instant pot.
2. Secure the lid and turn the pressure release handle to the 'sealed position.
3. Select the 'manual' function, set to high pressure and adjust the timer to 8 minutes.
4. After the beep, 'quick release' the steam and remove the lid.
5. Serve when cool, or save in a bottle for later use.

Nutrition Values (Per Serving)

- Calories: 62
- Carbohydrate: 13.7g
- Protein: 0.1g
- Fat: 0g
- Sugar: 11g
- Sodium: 2mg

Sweet Caramel Dipping Sauce

(**Serves**: 4 / **Prep Time:** 10 minutes / **Cooking Time**: 50 minutes)

Ingredients

- 2 (14 oz.) cans sweetened condensed milk
- 6 (3 oz) canning jars
- 1 cup water

How to

1. Pour the cup of water into the instant pot and place the trivet inside.
2. Pour the condensed milk into the canning jars. Place the jars on the trivet.
3. Secure the lid and turn the pressure release handle to the 'sealed' position.
4. Select the 'manual' function, set to high pressure and adjust the timer to 50 minutes.
5. After the beep, 'quick release' the steam and remove the lid.
6. Stir each jar and store in the refrigerator for later use.

Nutrition Values (Per Serving)

- Calories: 11
- Carbohydrate: 1.9g
- Protein: 0.3g
- Fat: 0.3g
- Sugar: 1.9g
- Sodium: 5mg

Roasted Tomato Sauce

(**Serves**: 4 / **Prep Time:** 10 minutes / **Cooking Time**: 10 minutes)

Ingredients

- 1 red onion, chopped
- 1 green bell pepper, chopped
- 1 jalapeño pepper, sliced
- 8 garlic cloves
- 4 chipotle chilies in adobo sauce
- 2 teaspoon powdered cumin
- 4 teaspoons Mexican red chili powder
- 4 teaspoons salt
- 1 cup water
- 28 oz canned, fire-roasted, diced tomatoes

How to

1. Put all the ingredients in the instant pot.
2. Secure the lid and turn the pressure release handle to the 'sealed' position.
3. Select the 'manual' function, set to high pressure and adjust the timer to 10 minutes.
4. After the beep, 'quick release' the steam and remove the lid.
5. Transfer the sauce to a blender and blend well to form a smooth mixture
6. Use immediately or save in a bottle for later use.

Nutrition Values (Per Serving)

- Calories: 96
- Carbohydrate: 18.4g
- Protein: 3.9g
- Fat: 1.4g
- Sugar: 7.9g
- Sodium: 3109mg

Tomato Basil Sauce

(**Serves**: 8 / **Prep Time:** 5 minutes / **Cooking Time**: 15 minutes)

Ingredients

- 4 tablespoons olive oil
- ½ garlic cloves, minced
- 2 onions, diced
- 8 lbs Romas tomatoes, diced
- 2 tablespoons salt
- 1 tablespoon pepper
- 1 tablespoon garlic powder
- 3 tablespoons Italian seasoning
- ½ teaspoon crushed peppers
- 2 bay leaves
- 1 cup chopped fresh basil

How to

1. Pour the oil into the instant pot and select the 'sauté' function.
2. Add the garlic and onions to the oil and stir-fry for 5 minutes.
3. Now add all the remaining ingredients, except the basil to the instant pot.
4. Secure the lid and turn the pressure release handle to the 'sealed' position.
5. Select the 'manual' function, set to high pressure and adjust the timer to 10 minutes.
6. After the beep, 'quick release' the steam and remove the lid.
7. Stir well, remove the bay leaves and add the basil to the sauce.
8. Serve.

Nutrition Values (Per Serving)

- Calories: 197
- Carbohydrate: 25.2g
- Protein: 0.7g
- Fat: 8.7g
- Sugar: 15.5g
- Sodium: 2433 mg

Bolognese Eggplant Sauce

(**Serves**: 6 / **Prep Time:** 10 minutes / **Cooking Time**: 35 minutes)

Ingredients

- ½ large onion, finely chopped
- 1 carrot, finely chopped
- 1½ celery stalk, finely chopped
- 1½ garlic clove, minced or pressed
- ½ tablespoon olive oil
- ½ (6 oz) can tomato paste
- 1 lb ground beef
- 1 eggplant, diced
- ½ tablespoon salt
- ½ teaspoon black pepper
- ¾ teaspoon dried thyme
- 1 teaspoon dried oregano
- 1 (28 oz) can crushed tomatoes
- 1 cup whole milk
- 1 cup dry red wine

How to

1. Pour the oil into the instant pot. Select the 'sauté' function.
2. Put all the vegetables into the oil and stir-fry for 10 minutes.
3. Stir in the tomato paste and all the spices. Use an immerse blender to blend the sauce.
4. Now put all the remaining ingredients in the instant pot.
5. Secure the lid and turn the pressure release handle to the 'sealed' position.
6. Select the 'manual' function, set to high pressure and adjust the timer to 35 minutes.
7. After the beep, 'quick release' the steam and remove the lid.
8. Stir well and serve with pasta.

Nutrition Values (Per Serving)

- Calories: 259
- Carbohydrate: 14.7g
- Protein: 26.5g
- Fat: 7.5g
- Sugar: 8.8g
- Sodium: 716mg

Beets Nomato Sauce

(**Serves**: 4 / **Prep Time:** 10 minutes / **Cooking Time**: 10 minutes)

Ingredients

- 1 tablespoon olive oil
- ½ large onion, diced
- 2½ ribs of celery, diced
- 4 carrots, diced
- 4 garlic cloves, diced
- ½ cup butternut squash, peeled and cubed
- 2 beets, peeled and diced
- 2 tablespoons fresh lemon juice
- ½ cup broth
- 1 bay leaf
- ½ small bunch fresh basil, roughly chopped
- ¼ teaspoon sea salt

How to

1. Pour the oil into the instant pot. Select the 'sauté' function.
2. Put all the vegetables into the oil and stir-fry for 5 minutes.
3. Stir in all the remaining ingredients.
4. Secure the lid and turn the pressure release handle to the 'sealed' position.
5. Select the 'manual' function, set to high pressure and adjust the timer to 10 minutes.
6. After the beep, 'quick release' the steam and remove the lid.
7. Remove the bay leaf then transfer the sauce to a blender and blend well to form a smooth mixture
8. Use immediately or save in a bottle for later use.

Nutrition Values (Per Serving)

- Calories: 108
- Carbohydrate: 16.9g
- Protein: 2.8g
- Fat: 3.9g
- Sugar: 8.8g
- Sodium: 316mg

Bolognese Lentil Sauce

(**Serves**: 6 / **Prep Time:** 15 minutes / **Cooking Time**: 20 minutes)

Ingredients

- ½ large onion, finely chopped
- 1 carrot, finely chopped
- 1½ celery stalks, finely chopped
- 1½ garlic cloves, minced or pressed
- ½ tablespoon olive oil
- ½ can tomato paste (6 oz)
- ½ cup lentils, soaked, rinsed and drained
- ½ tablespoon salt
- ½ teaspoon black pepper
- ¾ teaspoon dried thyme
- 1 teaspoon dried oregano
- 1 can crushed tomatoes (28 oz)
- 1 cup whole milk
- 1 cup dry red wine

How to

1. Pour the oil into the instant pot and select the 'sauté' function.
2. Put all the vegetables into the oil and stir-fry for 10 minutes.
3. Stir in the tomato paste and all the spices. Use an immerse blender to blend the sauce.
4. Now put all the remaining ingredients into the instant pot.
5. Secure the lid and turn the pressure release handle to the 'sealed' position.
6. Select the 'manual' function, set to high pressure and adjust the timer to 20 minutes.
7. After the beep, 'quick release' the steam and remove the lid.
8. Stir well and serve with pasta.

Nutrition Values (Per Serving)

- Calories: 156
- Carbohydrate: 19.8g
- Protein: 6.9g
- Fat: 2.8g
- Sugar: 6.8g
- Sodium: 666mg

Apple Cinnamon Sauce

(**Serves**: 6 / **Prep Time**: 10 minutes / **Cooking Time**: 7 minutes)

Ingredients

- 1 lb Fuji apples, unpeeled, quartered
- 1 lb Golden Delicious apples, unpeeled, quartered
- ½ lb Granny Smith apples, unpeeled, quartered
- ½ cup cold water
- 1 teaspoon pure vanilla extract or vanilla bean paste
- ½ tablespoon ground cinnamon
- ⅛ teaspoon ground cardamom
- 1 large pinch kosher salt

How to

1. Put all the ingredients into the instant pot.
2. Secure the lid and turn the pressure release handle to the 'sealed' position.
3. Select the 'manual' function, set to high pressure and adjust the timer to 7 minutes.
4. After the beep, 'natural release' the steam and remove the lid.
5. Transfer the sauce to a blender and blend well to form a smooth mixture.
6. Use immediately or save in a bottle for later use.

Nutrition Values (Per Serving)

- Calories: 98
- Carbohydrate: 26.2g
- Protein: 0.3g
- Fat: 0.2g
- Sugar: 20g
- Sodium: 99mg

Spicy Indian Sauce

(**Serves**: 4 / **Prep Time:** 10 minutes / **Cooking Time**: 25 minutes)

Ingredients

- 1 tablespoon olive oil
- 1½ large onions, finely diced
- 1½ garlic cloves, finely chopped
- ½ inch knob fresh ginger, peeled and grated
- Sea salt to taste
- ½ tablespoon ground coriander
- ½ tablespoon ground cumin
- ¼ teaspoon cayenne pepper
- ½ teaspoon ground turmeric
- ½ tablespoon sweet paprika
- ½ (28 oz) can whole tomatoes
- ½ cup water

How to

1. Pour the oil into the instant pot and select the 'sauté' function.
2. Put all the vegetables into the oil and stir-fry for 10 minutes.
3. Stir in the tomato paste and all the spices.
4. Now add all the remaining ingredients to the instant pot.
5. Secure the lid and turn the pressure release handle to the 'sealed' position.
6. Select the 'manual' function, set to high pressure and adjust the timer to 15 minutes.
7. After the beep, 'quick release' the steam and remove the lid.
8. Stir well and serve with pasta.

Nutrition Values (Per Serving)

- Calories: 83
- Carbohydrate: 9.8g
- Protein: 1.6g
- Fat: 3.9g
- Sugar: 2.5g
- Sodium: 181mg

Instant Marinara Sauce

(**Serves**: 6 / **Prep Time:** 10 minutes / **Cooking Time**: 16 minutes)

Ingredients

- 4 tablespoons olive oil
- 2 small onions, chopped
- 2 cloves garlic, minced
- 2 carrots, diced
- 4 cans tomatoes, diced
- 3 teaspoons dried basil
- 3 teaspoons dried oregano
- 1½ teaspoons sea salt
- freshly ground black pepper to taste
- 2 tablespoons butter, unsalted
- Parsley, fresh

How to

1. Pour the oil into the instant pot and 'select the 'sauté' function.
2. Put all the vegetables into the oil and stir-fry for 5 minutes.
3. Now put all the remaining ingredients, except the butter and black pepper, into the instant pot.
4. Secure the lid and turn the pressure release handle to the 'sealed' position.
5. Select the 'manual' function, set to high pressure and adjust the timer to 10 minutes.
6. After the beep, 'quick release' the steam and remove the lid.
7. Use an immerse blender to blend the sauce into a smooth paste.
8. Add the butter and black pepper, and cook for 1 minute on the 'sauté' function.
9. Stir well and serve with pasta.

Nutrition Values (Per Serving)

- Calories: 148
- Carbohydrate: 6.1g
- Protein: 0.9g
- Fat: 13.3g
- Sugar: 3.1g
- Sodium: 649mg

Bolognese Pasta Sauce

(**Serves**: 6 / **Prep Time:** 5 minutes / **Cooking Time**: 45 minutes)

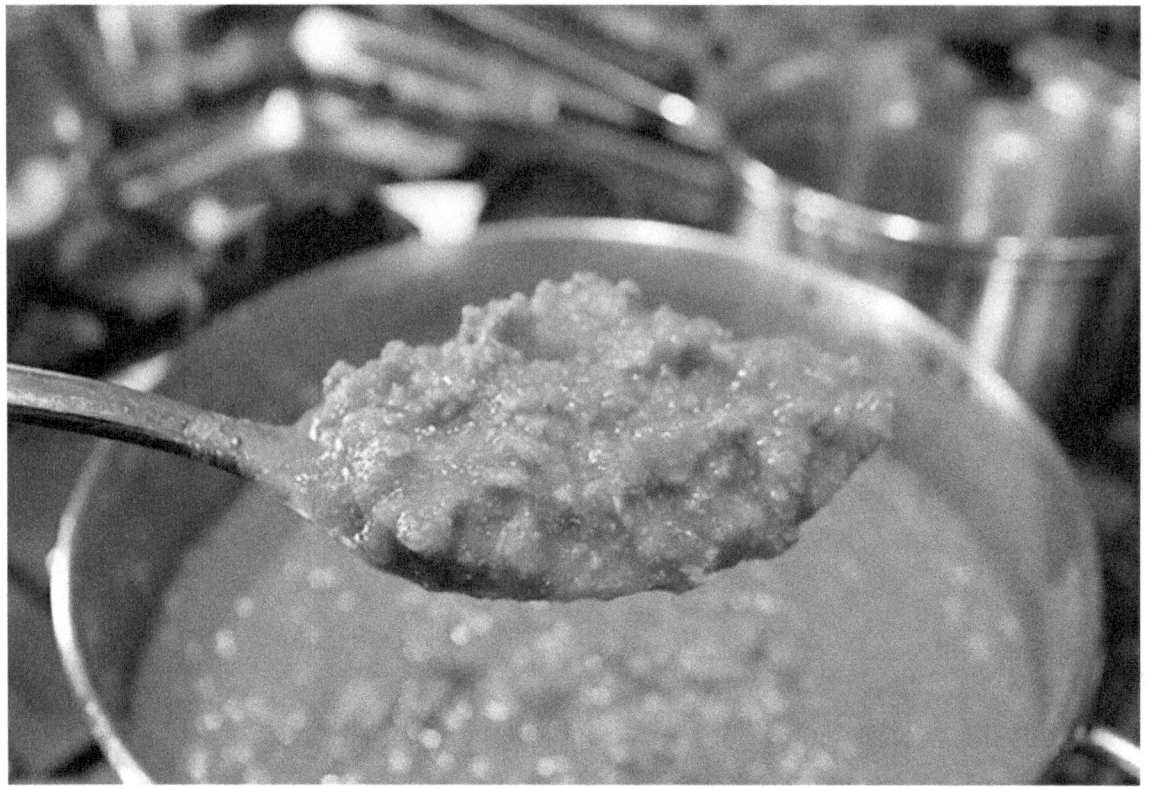

Ingredients

- ½ large onion, finely chopped
- 1 carrot, finely chopped
- 1½ celery stalks, finely chopped
- 1½ garlic cloves, minced or pressed
- ½ tablespoon olive oil
- ½ (6 oz) can tomato paste
- 1 lb ground beef
- ½ tablespoon salt
- ½ teaspoon black pepper
- ¾ teaspoon dried thyme
- 1 teaspoon dried oregano
- 1 (28 oz) can crushed tomatoes
- 1 cup whole milk
- 1 cup dry red wine

How to

1. Pour the oil into the instant pot and select the 'sauté' function.
2. Put all the vegetables into the oil and stir-fry for 10 minutes.
3. Stir in the tomato paste and all the spices. Use an immerse blender to blend the sauce.
4. Now put all the remaining ingredients into the instant pot.
5. Secure the lid and turn the pressure release handle to the 'sealed' position.
6. Select the 'meat/stew' function and adjust the timer to 35 minutes.
7. After the beep, 'quick release' the steam and remove the lid.
8. Stir well and serve with pasta.

Nutrition Values (Per Serving)

- Calories: 148
- Carbohydrate: 6.1g
- Protein: 0.9g
- Fat: 13.3g
- Sugar: 3.1g
- Sodium: 649mg

Ancho Chilies

(**Serves**: 4 / **Prep Time:** 10 minutes / **Cooking Time**: 8 minutes)

Ingredients

- 4 oz dried ancho chilies (without stems)
- 4 garlic cloves, lightly smashed
- 3 cups water
- 4 teaspoons kosher salt
- 3 teaspoons sugar
- 1 teaspoon dried oregano
- 1 teaspoon ground cumin
- 2 tablespoons apple cider vinegar

How to

1. Put all the ingredients into the instant pot.
2. Secure the lid and turn the pressure release handle to the 'sealed' position.
3. Select the 'manual' function, set to high pressure and adjust the timer to 8 minutes.
4. After the beep, 'quick release' the steam and remove the lid.
5. Transfer the sauce to a blender and blend well to form a smooth mixture.
6. Use immediately or save in a bottle for later use.

Nutrition Values (Per Serving)

- Calories: 122
- Carbohydrate: 20.7g
- Protein: 4.4g
- Fat: 0.2g
- Sugar: 17.3g
- Sodium: 2343mg

DESSERTS

Wine-Glazed Apples

(**Serves**: 4 / **Prep time:** 5 minutes / **Cooking time**: 10 minutes)

Ingredients

- 4 apples, cored
- ¾ cup red wine
- 1/3 cup demerara sugar
- ¼ cup raisins
- ¾ teaspoon ground cinnamon

How to

1. Add all the ingredients to the Instant Pot.
2. Secure the lid. Cook on manual function for 10 minutes at high pressure.
3. After the beep, do a quick release and remove the lid.
4. Top the apples with some cooking oil and serve.

Nutrition Values (Per Serving)

- Calories: 227
- Carbohydrate: 51.4g
- Protein: 0.9g
- Fat: 0.5g
- Sugar: 40.6gg
- Sodium: 9mg

Brown Fudge Cake

(**Serves**: 4 / **Prep time:** 6 minutes / **Cooking time**: 6 minutes)

Ingredients

- ¼ cup milk
- 2 tablespoons extra-virgin olive oil
- 1 egg
- ¼ cup all-purpose flour
- ¼ cup sugar
- 1 tablespoon cocoa powder
- ½ teaspoon baking powder
- 2 teaspoons fresh orange zest, grated finely
- Powdered sugar, as required
- 3 ramekins

How to

1. Add all the ingredients to a large bowl except powdered sugar.
2. Whisk all the ingredients well to prepare a smooth mixture.
3. Grease the three ramekins and pour the prepared mixture into the ramekins.
4. Pour a cup of water into the Instant Pot. Place the steamer trivet inside.
5. Arrange the ramekins over the trivet.
6. Secure the lid and cook on manual for 6 minutes at high pressure.
7. After the beep, do a quick release and remove the lid.
8. Let the ramekins cool. Sprinkle powdered sugar on top of each cake.
9. Serve.

Nutrition Values (Per Serving)

- Calories: 166
- Carbohydrate: 21.2g
- Protein: 3g
- Fat: 8.7g
- Sugar: 13.9g
- Sodium: 24mg

Instant Chocolate Cheesecake

(**Serves**: 4 / **Prep time:** 10 minutes / **Cooking time**: 18 minutes)

Ingredients

- ¼ cup Swerve sugar (Sweetener)
- 3/4 tablespoon cocoa powder
- 1 egg
- 8 oz. cream cheese softened
- 1 tablespoon powdered peanut butter
- ½ teaspoon pure vanilla extract

How to

1. Blend the eggs and cream cheese in a blender to form a smooth mixture.
2. Add the brown sugar, peanut butter and vanilla extract to the egg mixture and blend.
3. Transfer the mixture to a greased ramekin.
4. Pour water into the Instant Pot and place the trivet inside.
5. Arrange the ramekin over the trivet.
6. Secure the lid and cook on manual function for 18 minutes at high pressure.
7. After the beep, do a quick release and remove the lid.
8. Let the ramekin cool and refrigerate the cake for 8 hours.
9. Serve.

Nutrition Values (Per Serving)

- Calories: 223
- Carbohydrate: 17.8g
- Protein: 6.5g
- Fat: 21.2g
- Sugar: 15.4g
- Sodium: 195g

Maple-Glazed Flan

(**Serves**: 4 / **Prep Time**: 10 minutes / **Cooking Time**: 9 minutes)

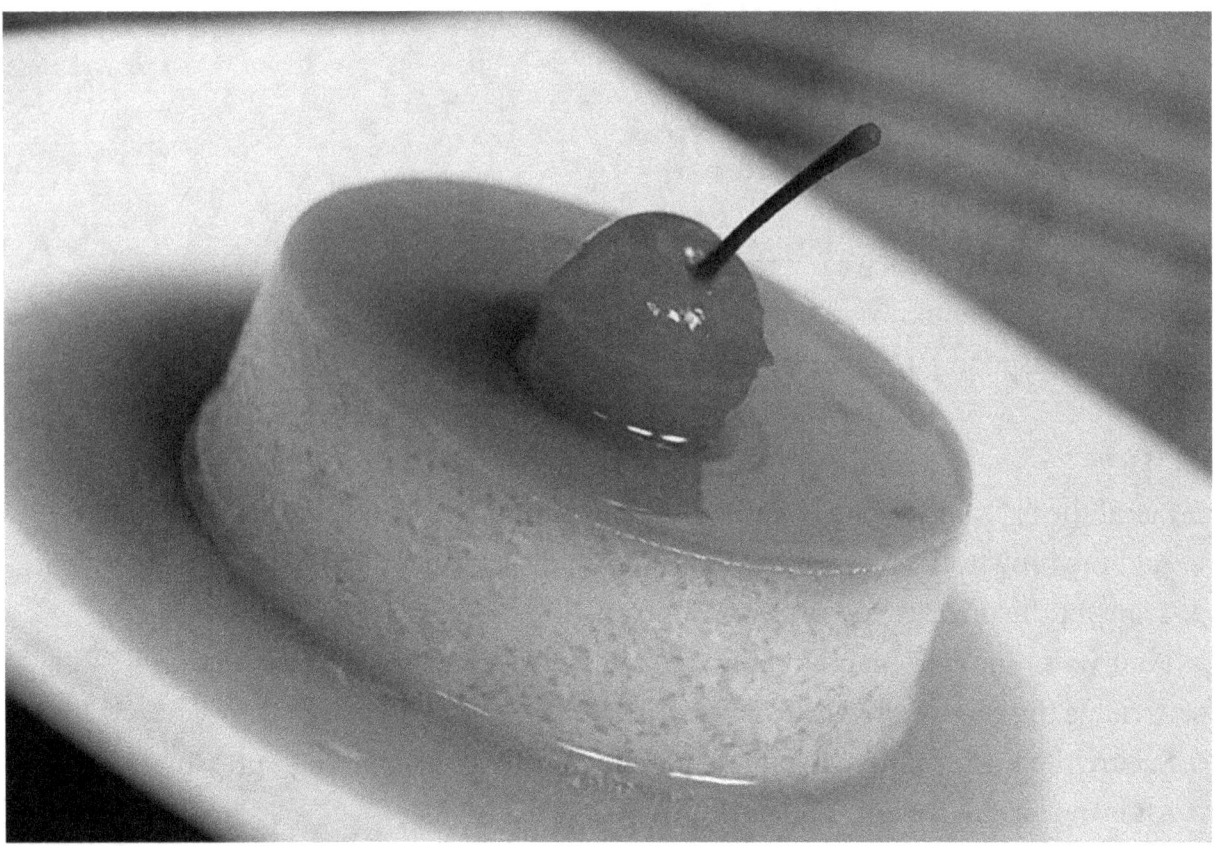

Ingredients

- 2 large eggs
- ½ cup milk
- ½ can sweeten condensed milk
- ¼ cup water
- ½ teaspoon vanilla extract
- Pinch of salt
- ¼ cup maple syrup

How to

1. Beat the eggs in a large bowl and stir in the remaining ingredients except for maple syrup.
2. Glaze a ramekin with maple syrup and transfer the vanilla mixture in it.
3. Pour a cup of water into the Instant Pot and place the trivet inside.
4. Arrange the ramekin over the trivet.
5. Secure the lid and cook on manual function for 9 minutes at high pressure.

6. After the beep, do a quick release and remove the lid.
7. Let the ramekin cool and refrigerate the flan for 3 hours.
8. Top with additional maple glaze and cherry then serve.

Nutrition Values (Per Serving)

- Calories: 227
- Carbohydrate: 35.8g
- Protein: 7.2g
- Fat: 6.5g
- Sugar: 34.2g
- Sodium: 139mg

Almond Cheesecake

(**Serves**: 4 / **Prep time:** 10 minutes / **Cooking time**: 18 minutes)

Ingredients

- ¼ cup powdered sugar
- ¼ cup almonds, thinly sliced
- 1 egg
- 8 oz. cream cheese softened
- 1 tablespoon powdered peanut butter
- ½ teaspoon pure vanilla extract

How to

1. Blend the eggs and cream cheese in a blender to form a smooth mixture.
2. Add the brown sugar, peanut butter and vanilla extract to the egg mixture and blend.
3. Transfer the mixture to a greased ramekin.
4. Pour water into the Instant Pot and place the trivet inside.
5. Arrange the ramekin over the trivet.
6. Secure the lid and cook on manual function for 18 minutes at high pressure.
7. After the beep, do a quick release and remove the lid.
8. Let the ramekin cool and top it with almonds. Refrigerate the cake for 8 hours.
9. Serve.

Nutrition Values (Per Serving)

- Calories: 248
- Carbohydrate: 11g
- Protein: 7.6g
- Fat: 24g
- Sugar: 8g
- Sodium: 195mg

Delightful Crème Brûlée

(**Serves**: 4 / **Prep Time:** 10 minutes / **Cooking Time**: 13 minutes)

Ingredients

- 4 ramekins
- 5 egg yolks
- 2 cups heavy cream
- 1 tablespoon vanilla extract
- ½ cup sugar
- ¼ cup superfine sugar

How to

1. Beat the egg yolks, cream, vanilla extract and sugar in a large bowl.
2. Divide the mixture into 4 ramekins.
3. Pour a cup of water into the Instant Pot and place the trivet inside.
4. Arrange the ramekins over the trivet.
5. Secure the lid and cook on manual function for 13 minutes at high pressure.
6. After the beep, do a quick release and remove the lid.
7. Let the ramekin cool and refrigerate for 4 hours.
8. Sprinkle superfine sugar on top and serve.

Nutrition Values (Per Serving)

- Calories: 377
- Carbohydrate: 27.8g
- Protein: 4.6g
- Fat: 27.8g
- Sugar: 25.6g
- Sodium: 33mg

Nutmeg Apple Crisp

(**Serves**: 4 / **Prep Time:** 10 minutes / **Cooking Time**: 8 minutes)

Ingredients

- 5 medium apples, peeled, cored and diced
- 2 teaspoons cinnamon ground
- ¼ teaspoon ginger ground
- ¼ teaspoon nutmeg ground
- 1 tablespoon pure maple syrup
- ½ cup water
- ¾ cup old-fashioned rolled oats
- ¼ cup flour
- ¼ cup brown sugar
- ¼ cup unsalted butter, melted
- Pinch of salt

How to

1. Combine oats, butter, salt, sugar, and flour in a bowl.
2. Transfer this mixture to the Instant Pot. Place apples on top.
3. Top the apples with maple syrup and water.
4. Secure the lid and cook on manual function for 8 minutes at high pressure.
5. After the beep, do a quick release and remove the lid.
6. Serve and enjoy.

Nutrition Values (Per Serving)

- Calories: 383
- Carbohydrate: 67.8g
- Protein: 3.7g
- Fat: 13.2g
- Sugar: 41g
- Sodium: 128mg

Chocolate Crème Brûlée

(**Serves**: 4 / **Prep Time:** 10 minutes / **Cooking Time**: 13 minutes)

Ingredients

- 4 ramekins
- 5 egg yolks
- 2 cups heavy cream
- 1 tablespoon vanilla extract
- ½ tablespoon cocoa powder
- ½ cup sugar
- ¼ cup superfine sugar
- ½ tablespoon grated chocolate

How to

1. Beat the egg yolks, cream, cocoa powder, vanilla extract and sugar in a large bowl.
2. Divide the mixture into 4 ramekins.
3. Pour a cup of water into the Instant Pot and place the trivet inside.
4. Arrange the ramekins over the trivet.
5. Secure the lid and cook on manual function for 13 minutes at high pressure.
6. After the beep, do a quick release and remove the lid.
7. Let the ramekin cool and refrigerate for 4 hours.
8. Sprinkle superfine sugar and grated chocolate on top and serve.

Nutrition Values (Per Serving)

- Calories: 386
- Carbohydrate: 29g
- Protein: 4.8g
- Fat: 28.3g
- Sugar: 26.3g
- Sodium: 34mg

Blueberry Cheesecake

(**Serves**: 4 / **Prep Time**: 10 minutes / **Cooking Time**: 40 minutes)

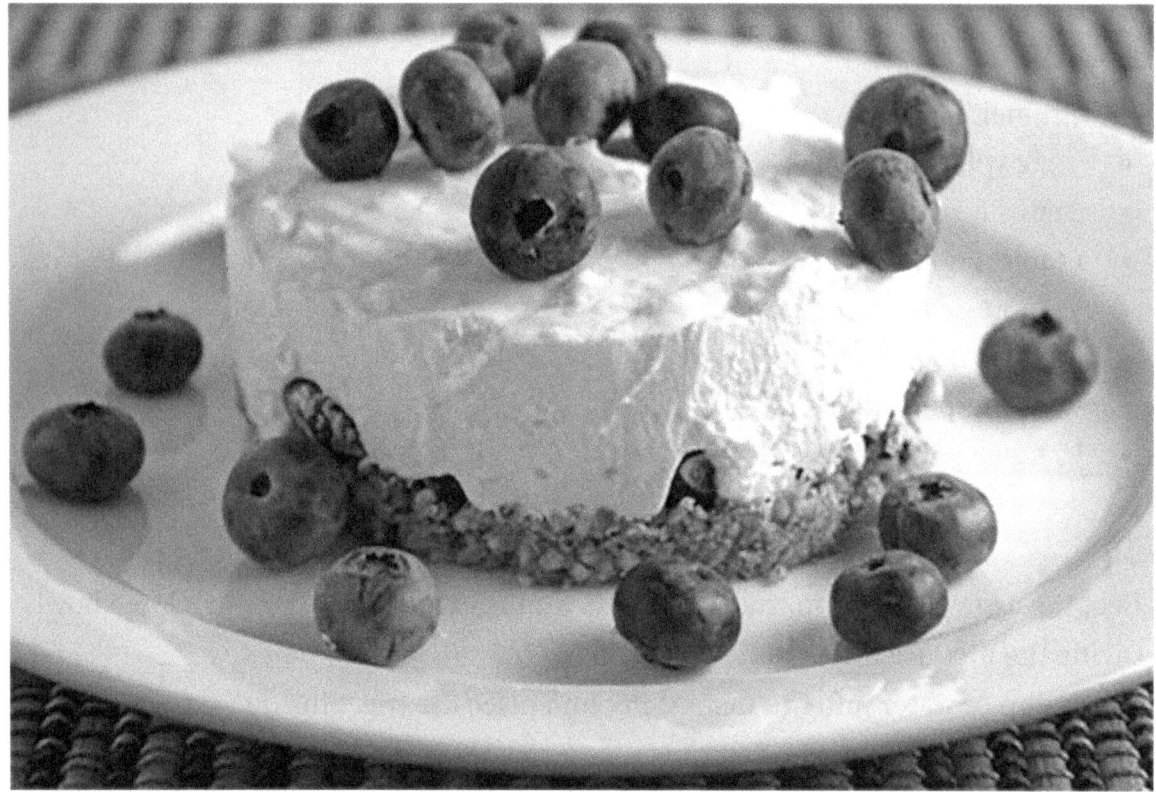

Ingredients

- 8 oz. cream cheese
- ½ cup powdered sugar
- 2 eggs
- ¼ cup sour cream
- 1 tablespoon vanilla extract
- 10 butter cookies, crushed
- 2 tablespoons unsalted butter, melted
- 2 tablespoons powdered sugar
- ¼ cup fresh blueberries, pitted

How to

1. Blend eggs, ricotta, sugar and cream cheese in a blender.
2. Stir in vanilla extract and sour cream.
3. Mix crushed cookies with butter.
4. Layer a 7-inch springform pan with the cookies and cream cheese mixture.
5. Pour water into the Instant Pot and place the trivet inside.

6. Arrange the pan over the trivet.
7. Secure the lid and cook on manual function for 40 minutes at high pressure.
8. After the beep, do a quick release and remove the lid.
9. Let the ramekin cool and top it with powdered sugar and blueberries. Refrigerate the cake for 12 hours.
10. Serve.

Nutrition Values (Per Serving)

- Calories: 471
- Carbohydrate: 29.4g
- Protein: 9g
- Fat: 35.5g
- Sugar: 19.1g
- Sodium: 368mg

Tapioca Pudding

(**Serves**: 4 / **Prep Time:** 05 minutes / **Cooking Time**: 9 minutes)

Ingredients

- 1½ cups water
- ½ cup small pearl tapioca
- ½ cup sugar
- Pinch of salt
- ½ cup milk
- 2 egg yolks
- ½ teaspoon vanilla extract
- ¼ cup fresh raspberries

How to

1. Add water and tapioca to the Instant Pot and mix well.
2. Secure the lid and cook on manual for 6 minutes at high pressure.
3. Do a quick release and remove the lid.
4. Whisk egg and milk in a bowl using a beater then add this mix to the pot.
5. Cook on sauté for 3 minutes and stir in vanilla extract.
6. Let it chill in the refrigerator for 30 minutes.
7. Top with raspberries and then serve.

Nutrition Values (Per Serving)

- Calories: 295
- Carbohydrate: 63.7g
- Protein: 3.3g
- Fat: 3.9g
- Sugar: 35.8g
- Sodium: 88mg

Cherry Cheesecake

(**Serves**: 6 / **Prep Time:** 10 minutes / **Cooking Time**: 40 minutes)

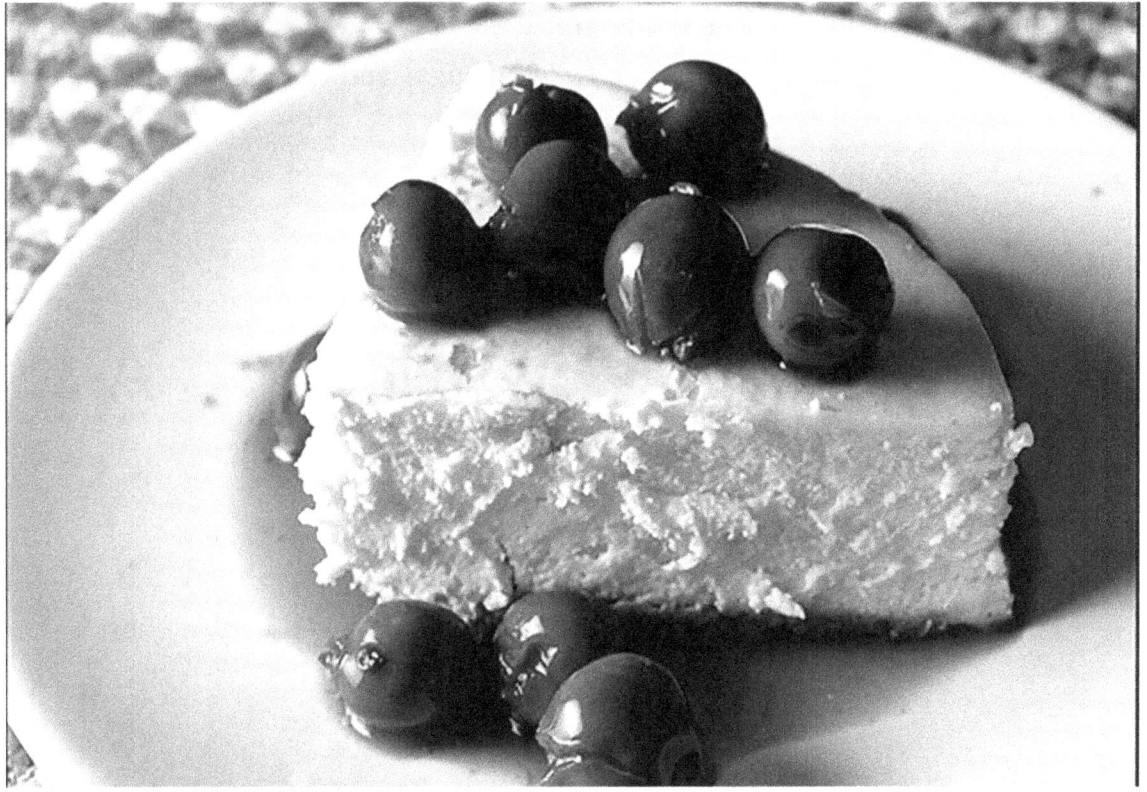

Ingredients

- 8 oz. cream cheese
- 8oz. ricotta cheese
- ¼ cup powdered sugar
- 2 eggs
- ¼ cup sour cream
- 1 tablespoon vanilla extract
- 10 Oreo cookies, crushed
- 2 tablespoons unsalted butter, melted
- 2 tablespoons powdered sugar
- ¼ cup fresh cherries, pitted

How to

1. Blend the eggs, ricotta, sugar and cream cheese in a blender.
2. Stir in vanilla extract and sour cream.
3. Mix crushed Oreos with butter.
4. Layer a 7-inch springform pan with the cookies and cream cheese mixture.

5. Pour water into the Instant Pot and place the trivet inside.
6. Arrange the pan over the trivet.
7. Secure the lid and cook on manual function for 40 minutes at high pressure.
8. After the beep, do a quick release and remove the lid.
9. Let the ramekin cool and top it with powdered sugar and cherries. Refrigerate the cake for ½ hours.
10. Serve.

Nutrition Values (Per Serving)

- Calories: 366
- Carbohydrate: 21.5g
- Protein: 10.3g
- Fat: 26.7g
- Sugar: 12.3g
- Sodium: 293mg

Lavender Crème Brûlée

(**Serves**: 4 / **Prep Time:** 10 minutes / **Cooking Time**: 13 minutes)

Ingredients

- 4 ramekins
- 5 egg yolks
- 2 cups heavy cream
- 1 tablespoon vanilla extract
- ½ cup sugar
- ¼ cup superfine sugar
- ½ tablespoon lavender buds

How to

1. Beat the egg yolks, cream, vanilla extract and sugar in a large bowl.
2. Divide the mixture into 4 ramekins.
3. Pour a cup of water into the Instant Pot and place the trivet inside.
4. Arrange the ramekins over the trivet.
5. Secure the lid and cook on manual function for 13 minutes at high pressure.
6. After the beep, do a quick release and remove the lid.
7. Let the ramekin cool and refrigerate for 4 hours.
8. Sprinkle superfine sugar and lavender buds on top and serve.

Nutrition Values (Per Serving)

- Calories: 377
- Carbohydrate: 27.8g
- Protein: 4.6g
- Fat: 27.8g
- Sugar: 25.6g
- Sodium: 33mg

Pumpkin Bundt Cake

(**Serves**: 3 / **Prep Time:** 15 minutes / **Cooking Time**: 35 minutes)

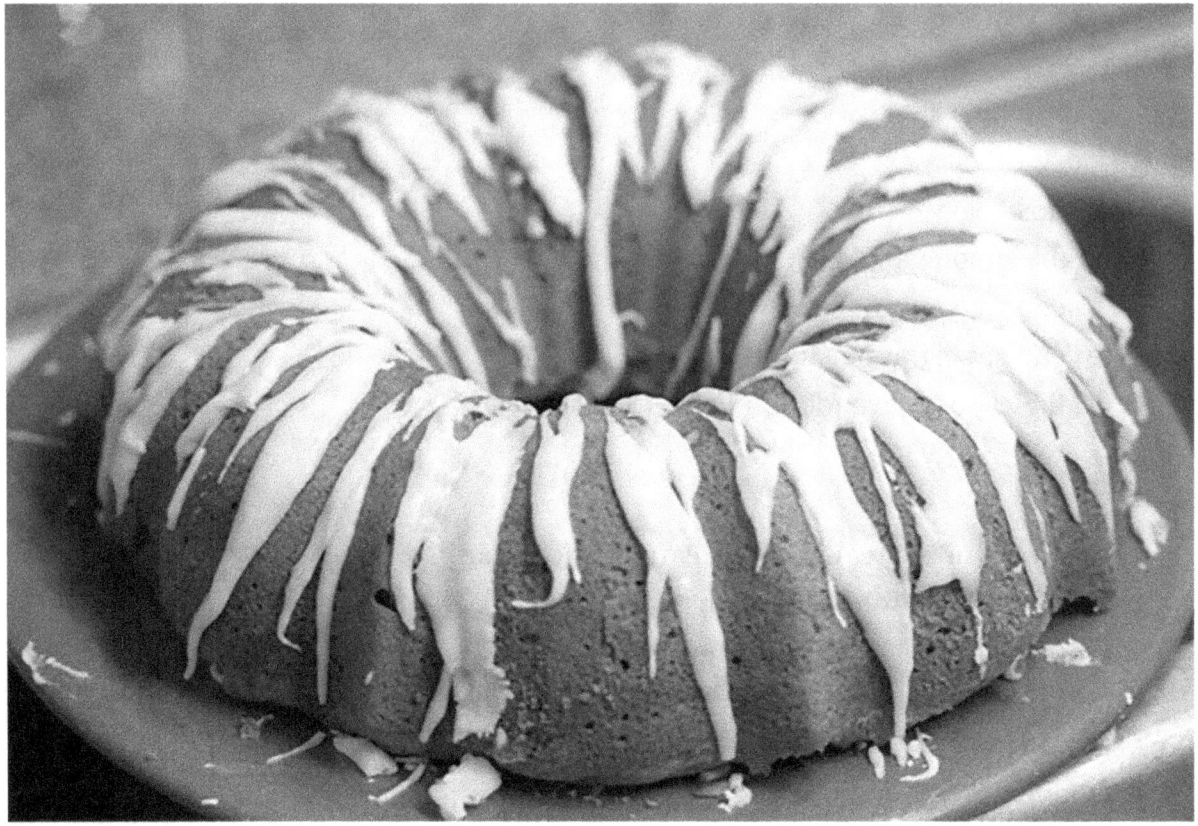

Ingredients

- 6 tablespoons whole wheat flour
- 6 tablespoons unbleached all-purpose flour
- ¼ teaspoon salt
- ½ teaspoon baking soda
- ¼ teaspoon baking powder
- ¼ teaspoon pumpkin pie spice
- 6 tablespoons sugar
- ½ medium banana mashed
- 1 tablespoon canola oil
- ¼ cup Greek yoghurt
- ¼ (15 oz.) can pumpkin puree
- ½ egg
- ¼ teaspoon pure vanilla extract
- ¼ cup chocolate chips

How to

1. Combine all the dry ingredients in a bowl and keep them aside.
2. Mix banana, sugar, oil, yoghurt, egg, vanilla and pureed pumpkin with the electric mixer.
3. Add all the dry ingredients to the egg mixture and beat until smooth.
4. Fold in chocolate chips and divide the mixture into 3 mini Bundt pans.
5. Pour a cup of water into the Instant Pot and place the trivet inside.
6. Arrange the Bundt pans over the trivet.
7. Secure the lid and cook on manual function for 35 minutes at high pressure.
8. After the beep, do a natural release and remove the lid.
9. Let the Bundt cool then remove the cake.
10. Garnish with fresh cream and serve.

Nutrition Values (Per Serving)

- Calories: 356
- Carbohydrate: 59.7g
- Protein: 6.7g
- Fat: 10.5g
- Sugar: 36.1g
- Sodium: 453mg

Triple Layer Cheesecake

(**Serves**: 6 / **Prep Time:** 10 minutes / **Cooking Time**: 40 minutes)

Ingredients

- 8 oz. cream cheese
- ¼ cup powdered sugar
- 2 eggs
- ¼ cup sour cream
- 1 tablespoon vanilla extract
- 10 Oreo cookies, crushed
- 2 tablespoons unsalted butter, melted
- 2 tablespoons powdered sugar
- ¼ cup fresh blueberries, pitted
- ¼ cup melted chocolate

How to

1. Blend the eggs, ricotta, sugar and half of cream cheese in a blender.
2. Stir in vanilla extract and sour cream in half of this mix. Add melted chocolate to the other half.
3. Mix crushed Oreos with butter.
4. Layer a 7-inch springform pan with the cookies then cream cheese mix and top with the chocolate layer.
5. Pour water into the Instant Pot and place the trivet inside.
6. Arrange the pan over the trivet.
7. Secure the lid and cook on manual function for 40 minutes at high pressure.
8. After the beep, do a quick release and remove the lid.
9. Let the ramekin cool and top it with powdered sugar and blueberries. Refrigerate the cake for ½ hours.
10. Serve.

Nutrition Values (Per Serving)

- Calories: 317
- Carbohydrate: 20g
- Protein: 6g
- Fat: 23.9g
- Sugar: 13.1g
- Sodium: 246mg

Cinnamon Applesauce

(**Serves**: 3 / **Prep Time**: 10 minutes / **Cooking Time**: 8 minutes)

Ingredients

- 6 large apples
- 1 cup water
- 1-2 drops cinnamon essential oil
- 1 teaspoon organic cinnamon

How to

1. Add all the ingredients to the Instant Pot.
2. Secure the lid and cook on manual for 8 minutes at high pressure.
3. After the beep, do a quick release and remove the lid.
4. Let it cool then blend the mixture using an immerse blender.
5. Garnish with cinnamon ground and serve.

Nutrition Values (Per Serving)

- Calories: 321
- Carbohydrate: 62.2g
- Protein: 1.2g
- Fat: 10.1g
- Sugar: 46.4g
- Sodium: 6mg

Apple Bread Pudding

(**Serves**: 8 / **Prep Time:** 15 minutes / **Cooking Time**: 70 minutes)

Ingredients

- 3 cups apples peeled, cored, and cubed
- 1 cup sugar
- 2 eggs
- 1 tablespoon vanilla
- 1 tablespoon apple pie spice
- 2 cups flour
- 1 tablespoon baking powder

Topping:

- 1 stick butter
- 2 cups brown sugar
- 1 cup heavy cream

How to

1. Combine flour and baking powder in a bowl and set aside.
2. Mix butter, eggs sugar and apple pie spice with the electric mixer.
3. Add all the dry ingredients to the egg mixture and beat until smooth.
4. Fold in apples and pour the mixture into a 7-inch springform pan.
5. Pour a cup of water into the Instant Pot and place the trivet inside.
6. Arrange the pan over the trivet. Secure the lid.
7. Cook on manual function for 70 minutes at high pressure.
8. After the beep, do a natural release and remove the lid.
9. Boil the butter with brown sugar in a skillet over medium heat for 3 minutes.
10. Stir in cream. Mix well on low heat.
11. Pour this mixture over the pudding and serve.

Nutrition Values (Per Serving)

- Calories: 554
- Carbohydrate: 95.4g
- Protein: 5.1g
- Fat: 18.5g
- Sugar: 67g
- Sodium: 234mg

Orange Cheesecake

(**Serves**: 3 / **Prep Time:** 10 minutes / **Cooking Time**: 8 minutes)

Ingredients

- 3 half pint mason jars
- 8 oz. cream cheese
- ¼ cup sugar
- ½ teaspoon flour
- ¼ teaspoon vanilla
- 2 tablespoons sour cream
- ½ tablespoon orange Juice
- zest of ¼ orange
- 1 ½ eggs
- ½ jar Greek yoghurt
- 3 raspberries
- 1 cup water

How to

1. Beat the cream cheese, flour and sugar in a large bowl.
2. Add sour cream, orange juice, zest, vanilla and eggs. Beat again.
3. Layer each Mason jar with the cheese batter and drop of yoghurt on top.
4. Pour a cup of water into the Instant Pot and place the trivet inside.
5. Cover the jars with aluminium foil and arrange them over the trivet.
6. Secure the lid and cook on manual for 8 minutes at high pressure.
7. After the beep, do a quick release and remove the lid.
8. Let the cakes cool then garnish with yoghurt and raspberries.
9. Serve.

Nutrition Values (Per Serving)

- Calories: 382
- Carbohydrate: 23.3g
- Protein: 9.6g
- Fat: 28.8g
- Sugar: 19.3g
- Sodium: 241mg

Banana Chocolate Chip Cake

(**Serves**: 3 / **Prep Time:** 10 minutes / **Cooking Time**: 35 minutes)

Ingredients

- 6 tablespoons whole wheat flour
- 6 tablespoons unbleached all-purpose flour
- ¼ teaspoon salt
- ½ teaspoon baking soda
- ¼ teaspoon baking powder
- 6 tablespoons sugar
- 2 medium bananas mashed
- 1 tablespoon canola oil
- 1/2 cup Greek yoghurt
- ½ egg
- ¼ teaspoon pure vanilla extract

How to

1. Combine all the dry ingredients in a bowl and set aside.
2. Mix banana, sugar, oil, yoghurt, egg and vanilla with electric mixer.
3. Add all the dry ingredients to the egg mixture and beat until smooth.
4. Fold in chocolate chips and divide the mixture into 3 mini Bundt pans.
5. Pour a cup of water into the Instant Pot and place the trivet inside.
6. Arrange the Bundt pans over the trivet.
7. Secure the lid and cook on manual function for 35 minutes at high pressure.
8. After the beep, do a natural release and remove the lid.
9. Let the Bundt cool then remove the pan.
10. Serve and enjoy.

Nutrition Values (Per Serving)

- Calories: 332
- Carbohydrate: 63.2g
- Protein: 7.7g
- Fat: 6.5g
- Sugar: 35.4g
- Sodium: 427mg

Lemon Cheesecake

(**Serves**: 3 / **Prep Time:** 5 minutes / **Cooking Time**: 8 minutes)

Ingredients

- 3 half pint mason jars
- 8 oz. cream cheese
- ¼ cup sugar
- ½ teaspoon flour
- ¼ teaspoon vanilla
- 2 tablespoons sour cream
- ½ tablespoon lemon juice
- zest of half lemon
- 1 ½ eggs
- ½ jar lemon curd
- 3 raspberries
- 1 cup water

How to

1. Beat the cream cheese, flour and sugar in a large bowl.
2. Add the sour cream, lemon juice, zest, vanilla and eggs. Beat again.
3. Layer each Mason jar with the cheese batter and lemon curd on top.
4. Pour a cup of water into the Instant Pot and place the trivet inside.
5. Cover the jars with aluminium foil and arrange them over the trivet.
6. Secure the lid and cook on manual for 8 minutes at high pressure.
7. After the beep, do a quick release and remove the lid.
8. Let the cakes cool then garnish with lemon curd and raspberries.
9. Serve.

Nutrition Values (Per Serving)

- Calories: 385
- Carbohydrate: 23.6g
- Protein: 8.9g
- Fat: 28.5g
- Sugar: 19.3g
- Sodium: 237mg

Delicious Breakfast Cake

(**Serves**: 3 / **Prep Time:** 15 minutes / **Cooking Time**: 35 minutes)

Ingredients

- 6 tablespoons whole wheat flour
- 6 tablespoons all-purpose flour
- ¼ teaspoon salt
- ½ teaspoon baking soda
- ¼ teaspoon baking powder
- 6 tablespoons sugar
- ¼ cup berry compote
- 1 tablespoon canola oil
- 1/2 cup 2% vanilla yogurt
- 2 ½ eggs
- ¼ teaspoon pure vanilla extract

How to

1. Combine all the dry ingredients in a bowl and set aside.
2. Mix sugar, oil, yoghurt, egg and vanilla with electric mixer.
3. Add all the dry ingredients to the egg mixture and beat until smooth.
4. Fold in berry compote and divide the mixture into 3 mini Bundt pans.
5. Pour a cup of water into the Instant Pot and place the trivet inside.
6. Arrange the Bundt pans over the trivet.
7. Secure the lid and cook on manual function for 35 minutes at high pressure.
8. After the beep, do a natural release and remove the lid.
9. Let the Bundt cool then remove the pan.
10. Serve and enjoy.

Nutrition Values (Per Serving)

- Calories: 299
- Carbohydrate: 43.2g
- Protein: 10g
- Fat: 9.9g
- Sugar: 29g
- Sodium: 519mg

Sweet Honey Yogurt

(**Serves**: 6 / **Prep Time:** 15 minutes / **Cooking Time**: 9 hours)

Ingredients

- 1-gallon milk
- 1 tablespoon vanilla extract
- 1/3 cup Greek yoghurt
- ¼ cup honey
- Cheesecloth
- Wire sieve

How to

1. Add the milk to the Instant Pot and lock the lid.
2. Boil on the "yogurt function" for 1 hour. Remove the lid after the beep.
3. Stir in Greek yoghurt, honey and vanilla extract then secure the lid.
4. Press the yogurt key and adjust the time to 8 hours.
5. After the beep, do a natural release then remove the lid.
6. Place the wire sieve in a bowl layer it with cheesecloth.
7. Pour the prepared curd into the bowl and strain the excess liquid.
8. Let it strain for 45 minutes then remove the thick yoghurt.
9. Serve or store for later use.

Nutrition Values (Per Serving)

- Calories: 383
- Carbohydrate: 44.4g
- Protein: 22.5g
- Fat: 13.6g
- Sugar: 41.6g
- Sodium: 311mg

Chocolate Bundt Cake

(**Serves**: 3 / **Prep Time:** 15 minutes / **Cooking Time**: 35 minutes)

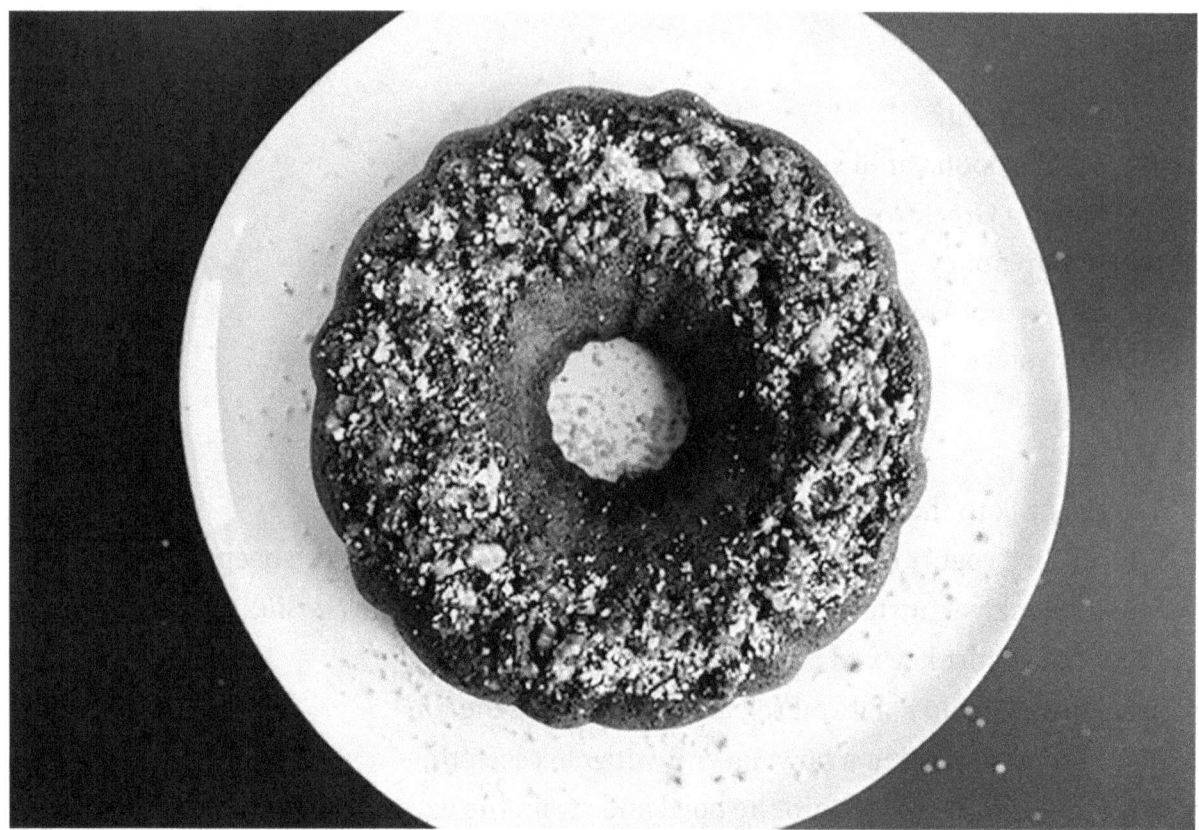

Ingredients

- 6 tablespoons whole wheat flour
- 6 tablespoons all-purpose flour
- ¼ teaspoon salt
- ½ teaspoon baking soda
- ¼ teaspoon baking powder
- 6 tablespoons sugar
- 2 teaspoons cocoa powder
- 1 tablespoon canola oil
- ¼ cup chocolate chips
- 1/2 cup Greek yoghurt
- ½ egg
- ¼ teaspoon pure vanilla extract

How to

1. Combine all the dry ingredients in a bowl and set aside.
2. Mix banana, sugar, oil, yoghurt, egg and vanilla with electric mixer.
3. Add all the dry ingredients to the egg mixture and beat until smooth.
4. Fold in chocolate chips and divide the mixture into 3 mini Bundt pans.
5. Pour a cup of water into the Instant Pot and place the trivet inside.
6. Arrange the Bundt pans over the trivet.
7. Secure the lid and cook on manual function for 35 minutes at high pressure.
8. After the beep, do a natural release and remove the lid.
9. Let the Bundt cool then remove the pan.
10. Serve and enjoy.

Nutrition Values (Per Serving)

- Calories: 312
- Carbohydrate: 48.5g
- Protein: 7.4g
- Fat: 10.5g
- Sugar: 32.8g
- Sodium: 438mg

Fruity Yogurt Bowls

(**Serves**: 6 / **Prep Time:** 20 minutes / **Cooking Time**: 9 hours)

Ingredients

- 1-gallon milk
- 1 tablespoon vanilla extract
- ¼ cup honey
- ¼ cup raspberries, sliced
- ¼ cup kiwi, sliced
- ¼ cup blueberries sliced
- ¼ cup pomegranate seeds
- 1/3 cup Greek yoghurt
- Cheesecloth
- Wire sieve

How to

1. Add the milk to the Instant Pot and lock the lid.
2. Boil on the yogurt function for 1 hour. Remove the lid after the beep.
3. Stir in Greek yoghurt, honey and vanilla extract then secure the lid.
4. Press yogurt key and adjust the time to 8 hours.
5. After the beep, do a natural release then remove the lid.
6. Place the wire sieve in a bowl layer it with cheesecloth.
7. Pour the prepared curd into the bowl and strain the excess liquid.
8. Let it strain for 45 minutes then remove the thick yoghurt.
9. Divide the yoghurt in the serving bowls.
10. Top it with all the fruits and few drops of honey then serve

Nutrition Values (Per Serving)

- Calories: 392
  - Carbohydrate: 44.3g
  - Protein: 23.1g
  - Fat: 14.2g
  - Sugar: 42.3g
  - Sodium: 301mg

Traditional Egg Custard

(**Serves**: 4 / **Prep Time:** 15 minutes / **Cooking Time**: 7 minutes)

Ingredients

- 4 cups milk
- 6 eggs
- 3/4 cup sugar
- 1 teaspoon vanilla extract
- 1 pinch sea salt
- ¼ teaspoon ground cinnamon
- Round stainless-steel pan
- Nutmeg, grated
- Fresh fruits, diced

How to

1. Beat the milk, eggs, sugar, cinnamon, vanilla extract and salt in the bowl until they become smooth.
2. Transfer the mixture to the steel pan.
3. Pour a cup of water into the Instant Pot and place the trivet inside.
4. Cover the bowl with tin foil, poke some holes in it, then place it over the trivet.
5. Secure the lid and cook on manual for 7 minutes at high pressure.
6. After the beep, do a quick release and remove the lid.
7. Top the custard with fruits and nutmeg then serve.

Nutrition Values (Per Serving)

- Calories: 360
- Carbohydrate: 50.3g
- Protein: 16.3g
- Fat: 11.6g
- Sugar: 49.1g
- Sodium: 266mg

Pineapple Cheesecake

(**Serves**: 6 / **Prep Time:** 10 minutes / **Cooking Time**: 40 minutes)

Ingredients

- 8 oz. cream cheese
- 8 oz. ricotta cheese
- 2 tablespoons pineapple juice
- ¼ cup powdered sugar
- 2 eggs
- ¼ cup sour cream
- 1 tablespoon vanilla extract
- 10 Oreo cookies, crushed
- 2 tablespoons unsalted butter, melted
- 1 cup pineapple, slices
- ¼ cup raspberries

How to

1. Blend the eggs, ricotta, sugar and cream cheese in a blender.
2. Stir in vanilla extract and sour cream.
3. Mix crushed Oreos with butter.
4. Layer a 7-inch springform pan with the cookies and cream cheese mixture.
5. Pour water into the Instant Pot and place the trivet inside.
6. Arrange the pan over the trivet.
7. Secure the lid and cook on manual function for 40 minutes at high pressure.
8. After the beep, do a quick release and remove the lid.
9. Allow the ramekin to cool and top it with pineapple slices and raspberries
10. Refrigerate the cake for 12 hours then serve.

Nutrition Values (Per Serving)

- Calories: 393
- Carbohydrate: 31.2g
- Protein: 6.4g
- Fat: 27.2g
- Sugar: 22.5g
- Sodium: 239mg

Apple Custard Trifle

(**Serves**: 4 / **Prep Time:** 15 minutes / **Cooking Time**: 12 minutes)

Ingredients

- 4 cups milk
- 6 eggs
- 3/4 cup sugar
- 1 teaspoon vanilla extract
- 1 pinch sea salt
- ¼ teaspoon ground cinnamon
- Round stainless-steel pan
- 4 tablespoons sugar
- 2 tablespoons water
- 1 medium apple thinly sliced

How to

1. Beat the milk, eggs, sugar, cinnamon, vanilla extract and salt in the bowl until they become smooth.
2. Transfer the mixture to the steel pan.
3. Pour a cup of water into the Instant Pot and place the trivet inside.
4. Cover the bowl with tin foil, poke some holes in it, then place it over the trivet.
5. Secure the lid and cook on manual for 7 minutes at high pressure.
6. After the beep, do a quick release and remove the lid.
7. Transfer the custard to the serving bowl and cover the top with apple slices.
8. Boil the sugar with 2 tablespoons of water in the skillet and let it caramelize.
9. Glaze the top of custard apples with this mixture and serve when cool.

Nutrition Values (Per Serving)

- Calories: 375
- Carbohydrate: 54.1g
- Protein: 16.4g
- Fat: 11.6g
- Sugar: 52g
- Sodium: 266mg

Refreshing Apple Cider

(**Serves**: 4 / **Prep Time:** 5 minutes / **Cooking Time**: 20minutes)

Ingredients

- 3 green apples, sliced
  - 4 red apples, sliced
  - 3 golden apples, sliced
  - 1 orange, quartered
  - 2 cinnamon sticks
  - 1 cup brown sugar
  - 2 teaspoon cloves
  - 1 teaspoon cardamom
  - 4 cups water

How to

1. Add all the ingredients to the Instant Pot.
2. Secure the lid and cook on manual for 10 minutes at high pressure.
3. After the beep, do a natural release and remove the lid.
4. Stir and mash the fruits using a spatula. Lock the lid again.
5. Cook for another 5 minutes on manual and high pressure.
6. Release the pressure and strain the prepared mixture.
7. Discard all the solids and serve with fresh apple slices.

Nutrition Values (Per Serving)

- Calories: 232
- Carbohydrate: 13.2g
- Protein: 2.1g
- Fat: 7.1g
- Sugar: 23.2g
- Sodium: 181mg

Fruity Custard Delight

(**Serves**: 6 / **Prep Time:** 15 minutes / **Cooking Time**: 7 minutes)

Ingredients

- 4 cups milk
- 6 eggs
- 3/4 cup sugar
- 1 teaspoon vanilla extract
- 1 pinch sea salt
- ¼ teaspoon ground cinnamon
- Round stainless-steel pan
- 1 cup whipped cream
- 1 lb. sponge cake, sliced
- Fresh fruits, sliced
- 1 cup homemade fruit jelly

How to

1. Beat milk, eggs, sugar, cinnamon, vanilla extract and salt in the bowl until they become smooth.
2. Transfer the mixture to the steel pan.
3. Pour a cup of water into the Instant Pot and place the trivet inside.
4. Cover the bowl with tin foil, poke some holes in it, then place it over the trivet.
5. Secure the lid and cook on manual for 7 minutes at high pressure.
6. After the beep, do a quick release and remove the lid.
7. In a serving bowl add a thin layer of sponge cake then the custard, fruits and cream on top.
8. Garnish with jelly cubes and refrigerate overnight.
9. Serve and enjoy.

Nutrition Values (Per Serving)

- Calories: 517
- Carbohydrate: 80.3g
- Protein: 15.4g
- Fat: 15.9g
- Sugar: 60.5g
- Sodium: 369mg

Chocolate Cream Custard

(**Serves**: 4 / **Prep Time:** 15 minutes / **Cooking Time**: 7 minutes)

Ingredients

- 4 cups milk
- 6 eggs
- 3/4 cup sugar
- 1 teaspoon vanilla extract
- 1 teaspoon cocoa powder
- ¼ teaspoon ground cinnamon
- Round stainless-steel pan
- Milk chocolate, grated
- Whipped cream

How to

1. Beat milk, eggs, sugar, cocoa powder, cinnamon, vanilla extract and salt in the bowl until they become smooth.
2. Transfer the mixture to the steel pan.
3. Pour a cup to water into the Instant Pot and place the trivet inside.
4. Cover the bowl with tin foil, poke some holes in it, then place it over the trivet.
5. Secure the lid and cook on manual for 7 minutes at high pressure.
6. After the beep, do a quick release and remove the lid.
7. Top with grated chocolate and whipped cream then serve.

Nutrition Values (Per Serving)

- Calories: 458
- Carbohydrate: 54.1g
- Protein: 14.3g
- Fat: 22.1g
- Sugar: 48.4g
- Sodium: 252mg

Instant Lemon Custard

(**Serves**: 4 / **Prep Time:** 15 minutes / **Cooking Time**: 7 minutes)

Ingredients

- 4 cups milk
- 6 egg yolks
- 3/4 cup sugar
- 1 teaspoon vanilla extract
- Zest of 1 lemon
- ¼ cup fresh cream
- Round stainless-steel pan
- ½ cup fresh blackberries

How to

1. Boil cream, milk and lemon zest in a pot over medium heat.
2. Strain this mixture and keep it aside
3. Beat eggs yolks, sugar, vanilla extract and salt in the bowl until they become smooth.
5. Stir in boiled milk and cheese. Transfer the mixture to the steel pan.
6. Pour a cup of water into the Instant Pot and place the trivet inside.
7. Cover the bowl with tin foil, poke some holes in it, then place it over the trivet.
8. Secure the lid and cook on manual for 7 minutes at high pressure.
9. After the beep, do a quick release and remove the lid.
10. Top with blackberries then serve.

Nutrition Values (Per Serving)

- Calories: 364
- Carbohydrate: 52.8g
- Protein: 12.4g
- Fat: 12.7g
- Sugar: 50g
- Sodium: 132mg

Caramel Cheesecake

(**Serves**: 6 / **Prep Time:** 10 minutes / **Cooking Time**: 40 minutes)

Ingredients

- 8 oz. cream cheese
- ¼ cup powdered sugar
- 2 eggs
- ¼ cup sour cream
- 1 tablespoon vanilla extract
- 10 Oreo cookies, crushed
- 2 tablespoons unsalted butter, melted
- 10 caramels, unwrapped
- 2 tablespoons heavy cream
- ¼ cup melted chocolate

How to

1. Blend the eggs, ricotta, sugar and cream cheese in a blender.
2. Stir in vanilla extract and sour cream.
3. Mix crushed Oreos with butter.
4. Layer a 7-inch springform pan with the cookies and cream cheese mixture.
5. Pour water into the Instant Pot and place the trivet inside.
6. Arrange the pan over the trivet.
7. Secure the lid and cook on manual function for 40 minutes at high pressure.
8. After the beep, do a quick release and remove the lid.
9. Let the ramekin cool and top it with powdered sugar and blueberries. Refrigerate the cake for 4 hours.
10. Microwave cream with caramels for 3 minutes and pour the mixture over the cake.
11. Top with melted chocolate and serve.

Nutrition Values (Per Serving)

- Calories: 395
- Carbohydrate: 32.2g
- Protein: 6.8g
- Fat: 27.1g
- Sugar: 23.5g
- Sodium: 289mg

Caramel Egg Custard

(**Serves**: 4 / **Prep Time:** 15 minutes / **Cooking Time**: 12 minutes)

Ingredients

- 4 cups milk
- 6 eggs
- 3/4 cup sugar
- 1 teaspoon vanilla extract
- 1 pinch sea salt
- ¼ teaspoon ground cinnamon
- Round stainless-steel pan
- 4 tablespoons sugar
- 2 tablespoons water

How to

1. Beat the milk, eggs, sugar, cinnamon, vanilla extract and salt in the bowl until they become smooth.
2. Transfer the mixture to the steel pan.
3. Pour a cup of water into the Instant Pot and place the trivet inside.
4. Cover the bowl with tin foil, poke some holes in it, then place it over the trivet.
5. Secure the lid and cook on manual for 7 minutes at high pressure.
6. After the beep, do a quick release and remove the lid.
7. Boil the sugar with 2 tablespoons of water in the skillet and let it caramelize.
8. Pour this mixture on top of custard then serve when cool.

Nutrition Values (Per Serving)

- Calories: 360
- Carbohydrate: 50.3g
- Protein: 16.3g
- Fat: 11.6g
- Sugar: 49.1g
- Sodium: 266mg

Inviting Toffee Pudding

(**Serves**: 4 / **Prep Time:** 10 minutes / **Cooking Time**: 20 minutes)

Ingredients

- 3/4 cup finely chopped dates
- ¼ cup boiling water
- 2 tablespoons blackstrap molasses
- 3/4 cup all-purpose flour
- ½ teaspoon baking powder
- 1 pinch salt
- 6 tablespoons brown sugar
- 1/6 cup unsalted butter
- ½ egg
- ½ teaspoon vanilla extract

How to

1. Mix the dates, molasses and boiling water in a bowl and keep it aside.
2. Combine flour with salt and baking powder in another bowl.
3. Beat brown sugar with butter and cream until fluffy. Beat in vanilla and egg.
4. In a large bowl, combine all the three prepared mixtures and beat well.
5. Divide the batter into 4 greased ramekins and cover with tin foil.
6. Pour a cup of water into the Instant Pot and place the trivet inside.
7. Arrange the ramekins over the trivet and secure the lid.
8. Cook on manual for 20 minutes at high pressure.
9. After the beep, do a natural release and remove the lid.
10. Let the ramekins cool then serve.

Nutrition Values (Per Serving)

- Calories: 338
- Carbohydrate: 64.1g
- Protein: 4g
- Fat: 8.6g
- Sugar: 40g
- Sodium: 111mg

Pumpkin Puree

(**Serves**: 6 / **Prep Time:** 05 minutes / **Cooking Time**: 13 minutes)

Ingredients

- 4 lbs. pie pumpkin
- 1 cup water

How to

1. Pour water into the Instant pot and place the steamer trivet over it.
2. Remove the stem of the pumpkin and arrange it over the trivet.
3. Secure the lid and cook for 13 minutes at high pressure.
4. Do a natural release after the beep, and remove the lid.
5. Slice the pumpkin in half, remove the seeds and peel the skin.
6. Add the pumpkin chunks to a blender and pulse to form the puree.
7. Serve or store for later use.

Nutrition Values (Per Serving)

- Calories: 343
- Carbohydrate: 15.4g
- Protein: 4.7g
- Fat: 6g
- Sugar: 24.4g
- Sodium: 145mg

Pineapple Custard

(**Serves**: 4 / **Prep Time:** 15 minutes / **Cooking Time**: 7 minutes)

Ingredients

- 4 cups milk
- 6 eggs
- 3/4 cup sugar
- 1 teaspoon vanilla extract
- 2 tablespoons pineapple juice
- 1 pinch sea salt
- Round stainless-steel pan
- 3 pineapple slices
- Whipped cream

How to

1. Beat the milk, eggs, sugar, pineapple juice, vanilla extract and salt in the bowl until they become smooth.
2. Transfer the mixture to the steel pan.
3. Pour a cup of water into the Instant Pot and place the trivet inside.
4. Cover the bowl with tin foil, poke some holes in it, then place it over the trivet.
5. Secure the lid and cook on manual for 7 minutes at high pressure.
6. After the beep, do a quick release and remove the lid.
7. Transfer the custard to the serving bowl and cover the top with pineapple slices.
8. Add whipped cream and serve.

Nutrition Values (Per Serving)

- Calories: 375
- Carbohydrate: 54.1g
- Protein: 16.4g
- Fat: 11.6g
- Sugar: 52g
- Sodium:266mg

Peach Parfait

(**Serves**: 4 / **Prep Time:** 15 minutes / **Cooking Time**: 9 hours)

Ingredients

- 1-gallon milk
- 1 tablespoon vanilla extract
- 1/3 cup Greek yoghurt
- ¼ cup honey
- ½ cup blackberries
- ½ cup peaches, peeled and diced
- Cheesecloth
- Wire sieve

How to

1. Add the milk to the Instant Pot and lock the lid.
2. Boil on yogurt function for 1 hour. Remove the lid after the beep.
3. Stir in Greek yoghurt, honey and vanilla extract then secure the lid.
4. Press yogurt key and adjust the time to 8 hours.
5. After the beep, do a natural release then remove the lid.
6. Place the wire sieve in a bowl layer it with cheesecloth.
7. Pour the prepared curd into the bowl and strain the excess liquid.
8. Let it strain for 45 minutes then remove the thick yoghurt.
9. In a serving glass, repeat the layer of yoghurt, blackberries and peaches.
10. Chill well and serve.

Nutrition Values (Per Serving)

- Calories: 391
- Carbohydrate: 41.3g
- Protein: 21.1g
- Fat: 11.2g
- Sugar: 46.3g
- Sodium: 311mg

Carrot Walnut Cake

(**Serves**: 4 / **Prep Time:** 15 minutes / **Cooking Time**: 40 minutes)

Ingredients

- 1 ½ eggs
- ½ cup almond flour
- 1/3 cup Swerve
- ½ teaspoon baking powder
- 3/4 teaspoons apple pie spice
- 2 tablespoons coconut oil
- ¼ cup heavy whipping cream
- ½ cup carrots shredded
- ¼ cup walnuts chopped

How to

1. Beat the eggs, oil, cream, swerve, four and apple spice in a bowl
2. Stir in carrots and walnuts.
3. Transfer the mixture to a greased 6-inch springform pan. Cover with tin foil.
4. Pour a cup of water into the Instant Pot and place the trivet inside.
5. Set the pan on the trivet and secure the lid.
6. Cook on manual for 40 minutes at high pressure.
7. After the beep, do a natural release and remove the lid.
8. Allow it to cool and serve.

Nutrition Values (Per Serving)

- Calories: 365
- Carbohydrate: 31.2g
- Protein: 6.8g
- Fat: 28.1g
- Sugar: 21.5g
- Sodium: 285mg

Coconut Egg Custard

(**Serves**: 4 / **Prep Time:** 15 minutes / **Cooking Time**: 7 minutes)

Ingredients

- 3 cups milk
- 1 cup coconut milk
- 6 eggs
- 3/4 cup sugar
- 1 teaspoon pandan* extract
- 1 pinch sea salt
- ¼ teaspoon crushed coconut flakes
- Round stainless-steel pan

How to

1. Beat the milk, coconut milk, eggs, sugar, pandan extract and salt in the bowl until they become smooth.
2. Transfer the mixture to the steel pan.
3. Pour a cup of water into the Instant Pot and place the trivet inside.
4. Cover the bowl with tin foil, poke some holes in it, then place it over the trivet.
5. Secure the lid and cook on manual for 7 minutes at high pressure.
6. After the beep, do a quick release and remove the lid.
7. Top with coconut flakes and serve.

Nutrition Values (Per Serving)

- Calories: 468
- Carbohydrate: 50.5g
- Protein: 16.7g
- Fat: 24.7g
- Sugar: 48.4g
- Sodium: 247mg

(**Note: Pandan*** - Pandan (Scientific Name: Pandanus, also known as screw pine or palm pine) is a herbaceous tropical plant that grows in Southeast-Asia. In Chinese, it is known as 'fragrant plant' because of its unique, sweet aroma.)

Enticing Dark Chocolate Cake

(**Serves**: 6 / **Prep Time:** 15 minutes / **Cooking Time**: 20 minutes)

Ingredients

- ½ cup almond flour
- 1/3 cup Swerve
- ½ teaspoon baking powder
- 2 tablespoons walnut, chopped
- 2 tablespoons cocoa powder
- 1 ½ eggs
- 2 tablespoons heavy cream
- 2 tablespoons coconut oil

How to

1. Combine all the dry ingredients in a bowl and set aside.
2. Beat the eggs, oil and cream in a large bowl.
3. Add all the dry ingredients to the egg mixture and beat until smooth.
4. Pour the mixture into a Bundt pan.
5. Pour a cup of water into the Instant Pot and place the trivet inside.
6. Arrange the pan over the trivet.
7. Secure the lid and cook on manual function for 20 minutes at high pressure.
8. After the beep, do a natural release and remove the lid.
9. Let the Bundt cool then remove the pan.
10. Serve and enjoy.

Nutrition Values (Per Serving)

- Calories: 346
- Carbohydrate: 31.2g
- Protein: 5.6g
- Fat: 24.1g
- Sugar: 22.5g
- Sodium: 189mg

Quick Pumpkin Custard

(**Serves**: 4 / **Prep Time:** 15 minutes / **Cooking Time**: 7 minutes)

- Ingredients
- 3 cups milk
- 1 cup pumpkin puree
- 6 eggs
- 3/4 cup sugar
- 1 teaspoon pumpkin spice
- 1 pinch sea salt
- ¼ teaspoon cinnamon ground
- Round stainless-steel pan
- 1 cup heavy cream
- Walnuts, to serve

How to

1. Beat the milk, pumpkin puree, eggs, sugar, pumpkin spice and salt in the bowl until they become smooth.
2. Transfer the mixture to the steel pan.
3. Pour a cup of water into the Instant Pot and place the trivet inside.
4. Cover the bowl with tin foil, poke some holes, then place it over the trivet.
5. Secure the lid and cook on manual for 7 minutes at high pressure.
6. After the beep, do a quick release and remove the lid.
7. Top with heavy cream and crushed walnuts.
8. Serve.

Nutrition Values (Per Serving)

- Calories: 453
- Carbohydrate: 53.2g
- Protein: 15.6g
- Fat: 21.6g
- Sugar: 48.3g
- Sodium: 252mg

Wine-Glazed Peaches

(**Serves**: 4 / **Prep time:** 5 minutes / **Cooking time**: 10 minutes)

Ingredients

- 4 peaches, cored
- 3/4 cup red wine
- 1/3 cup demerara sugar
- ¼ cup raisins
- 3/4 teaspoon ground cinnamon

How to

1. Add all the ingredients to the Instant Pot.
2. Secure the lid. Cook on manual function for 10 minutes at high pressure.
3. After the beep, do a quick release and remove the lid.
4. Top the peaches with some cooking oil and serve.

Nutrition Values (Per Serving)

- Calories: 223
- Carbohydrate: 52.4g
- Protein: 0.8g
- Fat: 0.6g
- Sugar: 41.6gg
- Sodium: 9mg

Molten Lave cake

(**Serves**: 3 / **Prep Time:** 15 minutes / **Cooking Time**: 20 minutes)

Ingredients

- ½ cup almond flour
- 1/3 cup Swerve
- ½ teaspoon baking powder
- 2 tablespoons walnut, chopped
- 2 tablespoons cocoa powder
- 1 ½ eggs
- 2 tablespoons heavy cream
- 2 tablespoons coconut oil
- 3 dark chocolate chunks

How to

1. Combine all the dry ingredients in a bowl and set aside.
2. Beat eggs, oil and cream in a large bowl.
3. Add all the dry ingredients to the egg mixture and beat until smooth.
4. Divide the mixture into 3 greased ramekins.
5. Add and dip the chocolate chunks at the centre of the batter.
6. Pour a cup of water into the Instant Pot and place the trivet inside.
7. Cover the ramekins with tin foil and arrange them over the trivet.
8. Secure the lid and cook on manual function for 20 minutes at high pressure.
9. After the beep, do a natural release and remove the lid.
10. Serve and enjoy.

Nutrition Values (Per Serving)

- Calories: 370
- Carbohydrate: 23.4g
- Protein: 7.1g
- Fat: 14.2g
- Sugar: 10.6g
- Sodium: 176mg

Pineapple Yogurt Parfait

(**Serves**: 4 / **Prep Time:** 25 minutes / **Cooking Time**: 9 hours)

Ingredients

- 1-gallon milk
- 1 tablespoon vanilla extract
- 1/3 cup Greek yoghurt
- ¼ cup honey
- ½ cup pineapples, diced
- ½ cup blueberries, halved
- Cheesecloth
- Wire sieve

How to

1. Add milk to the Instant Pot and lock the lid.
2. Boil on yogurt function for 1 hour. Remove the lid after the beep.
3. Stir in Greek yoghurt, honey and vanilla extract then secure the lid.
4. Press yogurt key and adjust the time to 8 hours.
5. After the beep, do a natural release then remove the lid.
6. Place the wire sieve in a bowl layer it with cheesecloth.
7. Pour the prepared curd into the bowl and strain the excess liquid.
8. Let it strain for 45 minutes then remove the thick yoghurt.
9. Add yoghurt, pineapples and blueberries in three layers to the serving cups.
10. Enjoy.

Nutrition Values (Per Serving)

- Calories: 372
- Carbohydrate: 45.3g
- Protein: 25.1g
- Fat: 13.2g
- Sugar: 44.3g
- Sodium: 321mg

Peanut Butter Cake

(**Serves**: 3 / **Prep Time:** 15 minutes / **Cooking Time**: 20 minutes)

Ingredients

- ½ cup almond flour
- 1/3 cup Swerve
- 1/2 teaspoon baking powder
- 2 tablespoons walnut, chopped
- 2 tablespoons cocoa powder
- 1 ½ eggs
- 2 tablespoons heavy cream
- 2 tablespoons coconut oil
- ¼ cup peanut butter

How to

1. Combine all the dry ingredients in a bowl and set aside.
2. Beat eggs, oil and cream in a large bowl.
3. Add all the dry ingredients to the egg mixture and beat until smooth.
4. Pour the mixture into a greased baking pan. Pour peanut butter at the centre of this batter.
5. Pour a cup of water into the Instant Pot and place the trivet inside.
6. Cover the pan with tin foil and arrange it over the trivet.
7. Secure the lid and cook on manual function for 20 minutes at high pressure.
8. After the beep, do a natural release and remove the lid.
9. Allow the pan to cool down and refrigerate for 30 minutes.
10. Serve.

Nutrition Values (Per Serving)

- Calories: 376
- Carbohydrate: 34.2g
- Protein: 7.2g
- Fat: 25.4g
- Sugar: 21.5g
- Sodium: 291mg

Strawberry Yogurt

(**Serves**: 4 / **Prep Time:** 25 minutes / **Cooking Time**: 9 hours)

Ingredients

- 1-gallon milk
- 1 tablespoon strawberry compote
- 1/3 cup Greek yoghurt
- ¼ cup honey
- ¼ cup strawberries, sliced
- Cheesecloth
- Wire sieve

How to

1. Add milk to the Instant Pot and lock the lid.
2. Boil on yogurt function for 1 hour. Remove the lid after the beep.
3. Stir in Greek yoghurt, honey and strawberry compote then secure the lid.
4. Press yogurt key and adjust the time to 8 hours.
5. After the beep, do a natural release then remove the lid.
6. Place the wire sieve in a bowl layer it with cheesecloth.
7. Pour the prepared curd into the bowl and strain the excess liquid.
8. Let it strain for 45 minutes then remove the thick yoghurt.
9. Top with berries and then serve.

Nutrition Values (Per Serving)

- Calories: 381
- Carbohydrate: 41.3g
- Protein: 21.1g
- Fat: 14.2g
- Sugar: 43.3g
- Sodium: 301mg

Cooking Time Charts

Your pressure cooker may have its own cooking times and temperature, always follow the instructions that came with your appliance.

The following charts provide approximate times for a variety of foods. Because cookers and stoves vary, actual cooking times may be different.

To begin, you may want to cook for a minute or two less than the times listed.

Most times are expressed as a range because natural ingredients can vary in cooking time depending on whether they are frozen, chilled, or room temperature, how large or small the pieces are, and other factors.

When in doubt, start with the suggested time at the lower end of the range, test for doneness, and then cook your food for a few minutes if needed.

COOKING CHARTS

	Cooking Time High Pressure (minutes)	Liquid Needed	Release Method		Cooking Time High Pressure (minutes)	Liquid Needed	Release Method
Poultry							
Chicken Bones for stock	40	6 cups	NATURAL	Chicken Thigh (boneless)	4	1 cup	QUICK
Chicken Breast (bone in)	6	1 cup	QUICK	Chicken, Whole	20	1 ½ cups	NATURAL
Chicken Breast (boneless)	4	1 cup	QUICK	Cornish Game Hen (1 to ½)	8	1 cup	NATURAL
Chicken Thigh (bone in)	7	1 cup	QUICK	Turkey Breast (boneless 2 to 3 pounds)	20 to 25	1 ½ cup	NATURAL
Beef							
Beef Bones for stock	40	6 cups	NATURAL	Meatloaf	35	1 ½ cups	NATURAL
Brisket (3 ½ to 4 pounds)	55 to 65	1 ½ cups	NATURAL	Pot Roast (3 ½ to 4 pounds)	55 to 65	2 cups	NATURAL
Corned Beef Brisket	55	covered	NATURAL	Short Ribs	55	1 ½ cups	NATURAL
Flank Steak (1 pound)	25	1 cup	NATURAL	Stew Meat (1-inch cubes)	15 to 20	1 cup	NATURAL
Ground Beef	5	1 cup	QUICK	Veal Shanks	20 to 25	1 ½ cups	NATURAL
Meatballs	5	1 cup	NATURAL	Veal Stew Meat (1-inch cubes)	20 to 25	1 ½ cups	NATURAL

Pork

Item	Time	Liquid	Release	Item	Time	Liquid	Release
Baby Back Ribs	30	1 cup	NATURAL	Pork Chops (boneless, 1-inch)	4 to 5	1 ½ cups	NATURAL
Country Style Ribs	20 to 25	1 ½ cups	NATURAL	Pork Loin (2 to 2 ½ pounds)	25	1 ½ cups	NATURAL
Ground Pork	5	1 cup	QUICK	Pork Shoulder (3 pounds)	55	1 ½ cups	NATURAL
Ham (bone in, 5 pounds, pre cooked)	25 to 30	1 ½ cups	NATURAL	Sausages	10 to 15	1 ½ cups	QUICK
Meatballs	5	1 cup	NATURAL	Spare Ribs	45	1 cup	NATURAL
Pork Chops (bone in, 1-inch)	6	1/2 cups	NATURAL	Stew Meat (1-inch cubes)	15 to 20	1 cup	NATURAL

Lamb

Item	Time	Liquid	Release	Item	Time	Liquid	Release
Ground Lamb	5	1 cup	QUICK	Leg of Lamb (boneless, 3 ½ to 4 pounds)	35 to 45	1 ½ cups	NATURAL
Lamb Shanks	30	1 ½ cups	NATURAL	Stew Meat (1-inch cubes)	15 to 20	1 cup	NATURAL
Meatballs	5	1 cup	NATURAL				

Fish and Seafood

Item	Time	Liquid	Release	Item	Time	Liquid	Release
Calamari	20	5 cups	QUICK	Mussels	4	2 cups	QUICK
Clams	4	1 cup	QUICK	Salmon	5	4 cups	QUICK
Crabs Legs	4	1 cup	QUICK	Shrimp	2	3 cups	QUICK
Fish Fillet (1-inch thick)	5	6 cups	QUICK				

ELECTRIC PRESSURE COOKING DIRECTIONS
RICE, GRAIN AND BEANS

	Amount	Cooking Time	Temperature
White, long grain rice	1 cup rice-1 ½ cup water	6 minutes	High
White, short grain rice	1 cup rice-1 ½ cup water	6 minutes	High
Brown, long grain rice	1 cup rice-1 ½ cup water	12 minutes	High
Brown short grain rice	1 cup rice-1 ¾ cup water	12 minutes	High
Quinoa	1 cup quinoa-2 cups water	6 minutes	High
Kamut	1 cup kamut- 2 cups water	30 minutes	High
Couscous	1 cup cuscous-2 cups water	3 minutes	High
Amaranth	1 cup grain-3 cups water	4 minutes	High
Millet	1 cup grain-2 cups water	6 minutes	High
Spelt	1 cup grain-3 cups water	30 minutes	High
Steel cut oats	1 cup oats-2 cups water	4 minutes	High
Wheat berries	1 cup wheat-3 cups water	30 minutes	High
Barley, pearl	1 cup barley- 4 cups water	20 minutes	High
Bulgur	1 cup bulgur-3 cups water	10 minutes	High
Pinto Beans	1 cup beans-3 cups water	50 minutes	High
Black Beans	1 cup beans-3 cups water	50 minutes	High
Great Northern/Red Beans	1 cup beans-3 cups water	50 minutes	High
Kidney Beans/Red Beans	1 cup beans-3 cups water	50 minutes	High
Lentils	1 cup beans-3 cups water	30 minutes	High
Black-Eyed Peas	1 cup beans-3 cups water	30 minutes	High
Chick Peas/Garbanzo	1 cup beans-3 cups water	30 minutes	High
Cannellini Beans/White Kidney	1 cup beans-3 cups water	30 minutes	High
Lima Beans	1 cup beans-3 cups water	25 minutes	High

Additional Resources

www.instantpot.com/faq/instant-pot-help-video

www.kitchenstewardship.com/10-basic-instant-pot-techniques

www.hippressurecooking.com/which-instant-pot-model-is-right-for-you

www.aboutthechef.com/instant-pot-pressure-cooker

www.kellythekitchenkop.com/best-ways-to-use-a-pressure-cooker

www.hippressurecooking.com/how-to-pressure-cook-frozen-meat

www.hippressurecooking.com/frozen-veggie-stew-pcs

www.traditionalcookingschool.com/food-preparation/how-to-reheat-frozen-food-in-the-instant-pot-freezer-meals-aw079

www.pressurecookingtoday.com/instant-pot-duo-and-smartcooker

About the Author

Michelle Dorrance is the founder and culinary director of the Brooklyn Springs Cooking Academy. She is a lifestyle coach & educator, Food for Life instructor, chef instructor in the culinary program at the University of New Mexico-Taos, personal chef, career coach, and a corporate consultant offering wellness training, brand representation, and strategic planning services.

Diagnosed with celiac disease, a dairy allergy, and Hashimoto's thyroiditis, Michelle used her knowledge of nutrition, flavor, and fitness to find the best ways to eat and move for her body. She learned how to overcome her autoimmune disease and concurrent conditions by eating a minimally processed, customized, anti-inflammatory diet. It is Michelle's philosophy that no single diet works for every person, but that by understanding how food affects the body, it is possible to customize a way of eating that meets individual needs. She also believes that no matter how restrictive a diet is, it is still possible to prepare delicious foods.

Now, she shares that information--along with her lifelong passion for cooking and her understanding of building flavors--with others in her cookbooks, which help people with special nutritional needs or on restrictive diets find delicious ways to eat. You can find many of Michelle's recipes on her food blog.

Along with being a long-time food blogger and passionate cook, Michelle loves writing about wine and cocktails. She also enjoys bartending and creating signature cocktails for non-profit fundraisers. Additionally, Michelle writes wine, gourmet, cooking, and cocktails articles.

Born and raised in Brooklyn, Michelle lives there with her husband and daughter. She loves anchovies, radishes, chicken feet, and lox but not in that order.

During her spare time, Michelle loves to visit different places around the world, taking pictures, and spending time in the kitchen creating new recipes.

Finally, before you go, I'd like to say "thank you" for purchasing my book and I hope that you had as much fun reading it as I had writing it.

I know you could have picked from dozens of books on Instant Pot Pressure Cooker Recipes, but you took a chance with my guide. So, big thanks for downloading this book and reading all the way to the end.

Now, I'd like to ask for a *small* favor. Could you please take a minute or two and leave a review for this book on Amazon? This feedback will help me continue to write the kind of books that will help you get results.

I bid you farewell and encourage you to move forward and find your true pressure cooking spirit!

Thank you and good luck!

—Michelle Dorrance

Recipe Index

A

Almond Quinoa Meal 59

Almond Risotto 74

Avocado Quinoa Salad 147

Asparagus Sticks 149

All Spice Pork Ribs 260

Alfredo Tuscan Shrimp 359

Appetizing Shrimp Corn Chowder 361

American Clam Chowder 363

Apple Cinnamon Sauce 467

Ancho Chilies 472

Almond Cheesecake 478

Apple Bread Pudding 492

Apple Custard Trifle 503

B

Breakfast Bacon Hash 30

Blueberries Oatmeal 42

Black Bean and Egg Casserole 43

Beans Rice Mix 48

Brown Rice Pudding 69

Black Bean Gravy 71

Bean Barley Stew 85

Bean Mustard Curry 91

Black Beans with Chorizo 100

Brown Chicken Rice	103
Beef Rice	108
Black Beans with Chorizo	128
Boiled Bok Choy	158
Beef with Beans Chili	181
Bacon Tomato Chili	197
Barley Soup	205
Borscht Beet Soup	216
Beef Mushroom Stroganoff	219
Bacon Lamb Chili	229
Beef & Bacon Casserole	238
Beef Potato Tots	240
Beef Broccoli Stew	244
Beef and Pork Gumbo	246
Beef Pot Roast	249
Beef Carne Asada	251
Butter-Dipped Lobsters	342
Butter Shrimp Risotto	360
Brazilian Potato Curry	378
Barbeque Mushroom Tacos	384
Brown Beef Stock	432
Beef Vegetable Stock	433
Beef Pepper Stock	435
Beef Bacon Stock	436
Bolognese Bacon Sauce	457
Bolognese Eggplant Sauce	464
Beets Nomato Sauce	465
Bolognese Lentil Sauce	466
Bolognese Pasta Sauce	470

Brown Fudge Cake 474

Blueberry Cheesecake 482

Banana Chocolate Chip Cake 494

C

Creamy Peach Oatmeal 23

Coconut Cornmeal Porridge 24

Coconut Rice Pudding 26

Cranberry Apricot Steel-Cut Oats 27

Creamy Latte Cut Oats 29

Cashew Mango Oatmeal 45

Cinnamon Quinoa Bowl 66

Coco Quinoa Bowl 68

Chorizo Pinto Beans 72

Comforting Mexican Black Beans 81

Cilantro Rice 82

Coconut Risotto 86

Chipotle Lentil Curry 89

Coconut Rice 99

Cumin Rice 102

Cauliflower Risotto 109

Chickpea Tacos 116

Chickpea Rice 118

Corn Lentil Stew 119

Cucumber Quinoa Salad 121

Cheesy Jacket Potato 151

Chickpea Hummus 152

Cabbage with Bacon 161

Creamy Rich Sweet Potatoes	165
Cheese-filled Sweet Potatoes	167
Comforting Broccoli Soup	188
Coconut Chicken Stew	192
Coconut Celery Soup	206
Cauliflower Butternut Soup	207
Chinese Congee	210
Cheesy Leek Soup	212
Cheese Potato Soup	215
Creamy Buffalo Chicken Soup	217
Chicken Spinach Corn Soup	218
Cheesy Beef Meatballs	234
Coconut Lamb Curry	235
Cauliflower Tourtiere	259
Cheese Pork Schnitzel	262
Curry Chicken with Honey	270
Chicken Bowl with Smoked Paprika	272
Chicken with Lettuce Wrap	275
Chicken with Black Beans	277
Chicken with Cashew Butter	280
Chicken with Grape Tomatoes	284
Chicken Bourbon with Honey	304
Chicken Thighs with Potatoes	306
Chicken Marsala	308
Chicken Salsa	310
Crack Chicken	311
Chicken Garlic Delight	312
Chicken Cacciatore	317
Chicken Noodle Pho	318

Citrus Enriched Salmon	345
Creamy Shrimp Grits	358
Coconut Cod curry	364
Creamy Chipotle Soup	365
Crowd-Pleasing Carrot Stew	381
Cauliflower Beans	394
Corn Potato Chowder	396
Creamy Vegetable Curry	402
Cauliflower Butternut Gravy	412
Cauliflower with Broccoli Florets	414
Chinese Vegetable Congee	415
Cheese Potato	420
Cajun Style Vegetable Rice	421
Chicken Stock	425
Chicken Vegetable Stock	427
Chicken Mushroom Stock	428
Chicken with Herbs Stock	429
Chicken Kale Stock	430
Chicken Corn Stock	431
Corn and Mushroom Stock	438
Crab and Tomato Stock	441
Chicken Green Beans Stock	448
Cashew Cheese Sauce	458
Cranberry Sauce	460
Chocolate Crème Brûlée	481
Cherry Cheesecake	485
Cinnamon Applesauce	491
Chocolate Bundt Cake	498
Chocolate Cream Custard	506

Caramel Cheesecake 508

Caramel Egg Custard 509

Coconut Egg Custard 515

Carrot Walnut Cake 514

D

Delicious Strawberry Compote 37

Delicious Spinach Hash 61

Delicious Lentil Risotto 90

Delectable Rice Pilaf 94

Delicious Potato and Corn Soup 171

Delectable Chicken Soup 180

Delightful Zuppa Toscana 201

Delicious Pork Bo Kho 261

Delicious Cod Wrap 339

Delicious Seafood Jambalaya 324

Delectable Shrimp Curry 350

Delicious Minestrone Curry 407

Delectable Carrot Medley 417

Delightful Crème Brûlée 479

Delicious Breakfast Cake 496

E

Egg Stuffed Bell Pepper 28

Enriched Walnut Oatmeal 36

Eggs with Herbs de Provence 56

Eggs Mushroom Casserole 58

Eggs & Red Beans Casserole 65

Egg Broccoli Casserole	67
Enticing Three-Bean Stew	117
Enticing Chicken and Kale Soup	172
Earthy Bacon and Veggie Soup	187
Eastern Lamb Stew	221
Egg Plant Curry	385
Enticing Spaghetti Squash	403
Enticing Dark Chocolate Cake	516

F

Fresh Fruity Oatmeal	33
Fried Beans Mix	79
Fennel Risotto	80
Flavorsome Bacon Rice	114
Flavorsome Brussels Sprout Salad	136
Fresh Kale Salad	142
Fresh Red Beets	163
Full Meal Turkey Soup	184
Flavorsome Carrot Soup	189
Full Meal Lamb Shanks	233
Flavorsome Tuna Chowder	328
Filling Salmon Teriyaki	356
Flavorsome Vegetable Chow Mein	379
Fish Curry Delight	348
Fish Anchovy Stock	439
Fruity Yogurt Bowls	500
Fruity Custard Delight	505

G

Garlic Eggs 51

Green Beans with Tomatoes 146

Green Beans Salad 155

Garlic with White Beets 159

Green Bean Soup 174

Gourmet Mexican Beef Soup 185

Ground Turkey Chili 195

Garlic Beef Sirloin 222

Greek Style Lamb 243

Green Chilli Adobo Chicken 269

Greek Style Turkey Breast 299

Green Hot Sauce 451

H

Honey-glazed Carrots 139

Ham and White Bean Soup 211

Healthy Prime Rib 227

Healthy Clam Meal 362

I

Inviting Butternut Squash Risotto 77

Instant Black Bean Burrito 87

Instant Sweet Potato 132

Instant Pot Mac & Cheese 134

Instant Mashed Potato 150

Italian Potato Salad 160

Inviting Chicken and Mushroom Stew 176

Instant Lasagne Soup 208

Italian Chicken Soup 209

Instant Pork Thai Curry 256

Instant Dumplings 273

Instant BBQ Chicken Wings 315

Instant Thai Chicken 320

Instant Scampi Chicken 323

Instant Tso's Chicken 282

Irresistible Seafood Gumbo 352

Instant Ratatouille 380

Inviting Cod Platter 340

Italian Vegetable Stew 376

Instant Pot Barbeque Sauce 456

Instant Marinara Sauce 469

Instant Chocolate Cheesecake 475

Instant Lemon Custard 507

Inviting Toffee Pudding 510

J

Juicy Quinoa Olives 166

Japanese Ramen Soup 204

Japanese Beef Bowl 236

Juicy Lamb Leg 241

Jamaican Pork Roast 257

Juicy Mojo Chicken Tacos 313

Jack Fruit Stew 386

K

Kung Pao Turkey 296

Korean Steamed Eggs 54

L

Lime Rich Rice 92

Lime Potatoes 137

Lamb Pepper Stew 193

Lamb Meat Balls 223

Lamb and Zucchini Curry 239

Lamb Chop Irish Stew 252

Lime Chicken with chillies 281

Luscious Shrimp Creole 325

Lime-filled Salmon Fillet 334

Lavender Crème Brûlée 487

Lemon Cheesecake 495

M

Morning Frittatas 46

Minty Pineapple Oatmeal 60

Mung Bean Risotto 84

Mushroom Risotto 104

Mexican-Style Rice 105

Mung Bean Curry 112

Mushrooms with Butternut Squash 124

Maple-glazed Brussel Sprouts 126

Mayo Potato Salad 127

Milk-Soaked Fennels 162

Mayo Mushroom Salad 168

Mouth Watering Lamb Stew 237

Mexican Butter Beef 242

Mustard Chicken with Lime Juice..283

Maple Mustard Turkey Thighs 288

Mouth-Watering Casserole 326

Mahi-Mahi with Tomatoes 338

Mayo-Lobster Rolls 368

Mixed Vegetable Chili..399

Mixed Vegetable Stock 437

Mushroom Sauce 452

Maple-Glazed Flan..476

Molten Lave cake 519

N

Nourishing Banana Oatmeal 57

Nutritious Instant Porridge 64

Nutritious Chickpea Bowl 141

Nutritious Tomato Soup.. 169

Nourishing Chicken Soup 183

Nutrient Rich Beef Soup 186

Nutritious Salmon Soup 329

Nourishing Salmon Curry 330

Nourishing Creamy Lobster 343

Nutritious Vegetable Mix 382

Nutmeg Apple Crisp 480

O

Orange Marmalade Oatmeal	49
Oatmeal with Pistachios	52
Oeufs Cocotte	63
Orange Spice Chicken	271
Omega Rich Seafood Soup	353
Orange Cheesecake	493

P

3 Peppers Morning Hash	32
Peanut Butter Oatmeal	55
Potato Cornmeal Porridge	70
Pea & Corn Rice	95
3 Pepper Salad	148
Potato & Cauliflower Mash	154
Pork and Cabbage Soup	175
3-Pepper Chicken Chili	194
Pork and Beef Chili	196
3 Peppers Lamb	226
Potato Lamb Roast	250
Pork Lettuce Wraps	253
Picante Lamb Chops	254
Pork with Calabacita Squash	255
Pork Sausages with Mushrooms	264
Peppercorns Beef	266
Pork Taco bowl	267
Pork Roast Tacos	268
Potatoes with BBQ Chicken	316

Potato Cauliflower 387

Potato Scallion Stew 389

Potato with Green Beans 395

Potato Hemp Burgers 422

Potato Spinach Corn Mix 424

Pork Bone Stock 445

Pork Beef Stock 446

Pork and Vegetable Stock 447

Pumpkin Bundt Cake 488

Pineapple Cheesecake 502

Pumpkin Puree 511

Pineapple Custard 512

Peach Parfait 513

Pineapple Yogurt Parfait 520

Peanut Butter Cake 521

Q

Quinoa with Bananas 53

Quinoa Brussels Sprout Salad 123

Quinoa Mushroom Salad 129

Quinoa Tomato Salad 135

Quinoa Lime Salad 164

Quick Pumpkin Custard 517

R

Rice Pudding 38

Rich Cheese Salmon 336

Ready-to-Eat Dinner Mussels 341

Rice-Mixed Shrimp 351

Roasted Beef Mushroom Stock 434

Red Hot Sauce 449

Roasted Tomato Sauce 462

Refreshing Apple Cider 504

S

Strawberry Cream Oatmeal 25

Silver Almonds Oatmeal 31

Super Healthy Oatmeal 40

Scrumptious Bread Pudding 41

Spice Filled Oatmeal 47

Spinach Chickpea Curry 73

Spinach Lentils Stew 75

Spicy Red Bean Curry 76

Split Pea Curry 78

Spanish Chorizo Red Beans 96

Shrimp & Rice Paella 98

Sausage Mushroom Rice 106

Saucy Red Beans 107

Scrumptious Black-Eyed Peas 115

Spaghetti Squash 120

Saucy Baked Beans 122

Seasoned Potatoes 125

Sauce Dipped Spinach 138

Steamed Garlic Broccoli 143

Steamed Artichoke 145

Spice Rich Beef Chili	198
Spinach Lentil Soup	199
Scrumptious Veggie Soup	191
Special Minestrone Soup	202
Super Easy Chicken Tortilla Soup	203
Spicy Pork Vindaloo	213
Salsa Chicken Soup	214
Super Easy Hot Dogs	230
Sauce Glazed Lamb Chops	231
Spicy Minced Meat	248
Smokey BBQ Pork Ribs	258
Saucy Pork Brisket	263
Sesame Chicken Teriyaki	274
Steamed Garlic Chicken Breasts	278
Scrumptious Spicy Chicken	279
Stuffed Pepper with Turkey	293
Scrumptious Salmon Casserole	327
Super-Easy Salmon Fillets	332
Spicy Salmon Meal	335
Special Crab Legs Delight	344
Shrimp and Beans Mix	349
Salmon Zucchini Stew	354
Sardines Curry	355
Shrimps with Broccoli Florets	369
Shrimp with Spaghetti Squash	371
Seafood Platter	374
Sweet Potato Curry	388
Sweet Potato with Cauliflower	390
Stuffed Eggplants	391

Sesame Vegetable Teriyaki 393

Stuffed Acorn Squash 400

Spinach Potato Curry 401

Stuffed Sweet Peppers 404

Spinach Lentils 405

Scrumptious Celery Chowder 411

Spicy Pickled Potatoes 416

Spicy Vegetable Salsa 419

Salmon Fish Stock 442

Seafood Gumbo Stock 443

Super Quick Garlic Sauce 453

Special BBQ Sauce 454

Strawberry Sauce 459

Sweet Caramel Dipping Sauce 461

Spicy Indian Sauce 468

Sweet Honey Yogurt 497

Strawberry Yogurt 522

T

Tasty Cornmeal Porridge 35

Tasty Cauliflower Rice 131

Tasty Corn Cobs 156

Traditional Beef and Veggie Stew 177

Tempting Mixed Veggie Stew 178

Three Beans Mix Chili 182

Traditional Country Steak 225

Turmeric Beef Steaks 232

Turkey with Gravy 286

Turkey Breasts 287

Turkey with Cranberry Sauce 289

Turkey Breasts with Tomato and Basil Sauce 290

Turkey Lettuce Stacks 291

Turkey with Garlic Herb Sauce..292

Turkey Meatballs with Marinara Sauce 295

Turkey Stuffed Tacos..298

Turkey Noodle Soup 300

Turkey with Smoked Paprika..302

Turkey Cheese Gnocchi 303

Tasty Taco Bowls 314

Traditional Country Chicken 321

Tangy Mahi-Mahi 337

Tuna with Noodles...367

Teriyaki Scallops.. 372

Tomato Clam & Shrimps 373

Tunisian Chickpea Stock 440

Turkey Bone Stock 444

Tomato Basil Sauce 463

Triple Layer Cheesecake..490

Tapioca Pudding 484

Traditional Egg Custard 501

V

Vanilla Rice Pudding..62

Vegetable Rice... 97

Vegetable & Corn Rice...110

Vegetable Chickpea Salad 157

Vegetable Pasta 397

Vegetable Bean Rice 398

Vegetable Cheese Macaroni 406

Vegetable Tortilla Bowl 408

Vegetable Ramen 409

Vegetable Barley 410

Vegetable Lasagne 413

Vegetable Quinoa 418

W

White Bean Curry 93

Wine-glazed Mushrooms 144

Wine Glazed Short Ribs 247

Wine-Sauce Glazed Cod 347

Watermelon BBQ Sauce 455

Wine-Glazed Apples 473

Wine-Glazed Peaches 518

Y

Yellow Potato Rice 111

www.ingramcontent.com/pod-product-compliance
Lightning Source LLC
Chambersburg PA
CBHW080036100526
44584CB00023BA/3196